Nutritional Ophthalmology

NUTRITION: BASIC AND APPLIED SCIENCE
A SERIES OF MONOGRAPHS

WILLIAM J. DARBY, Editor
Professor of Biochemistry (Nutrition)
Vanderbilt University School of Medicine
Nashville, Tennessee
and
President, The Nutrition Foundation
New York, New York

Anthony W. Norman. *Vitamin D: The Calcium Homeostatic Steroid Hormone*, 1979.

Donald S. McLaren: *Nutritional Ophthalmology (2nd edition of Malnutrition and the Eye)*

Nutritional Ophthalmology

Second Edition of
Malnutrition and the Eye

Donald S. McLaren
Department of Medicine, University Medical School
Edinburgh, Scotland

1980

ACADEMIC PRESS

A Subsidiary of Harcourt Brace Jovanovich, Publishers

London · New York · Toronto · Sydney · San Francisco

ACADEMIC PRESS INC. (LONDON) LTD.
24/28 Oval Road,
London NW1 7DX

United States Edition published by
ACADEMIC PRESS INC.
111 Fifth Avenue,
New York, New York 10003

British Library Cataloguing in Publication Data
McLaren, Donald Stewart
  Nutritional ophthalmology. – 2nd ed. – (Nutrition:
  basic and applied science).
  1. Eye – Diseases and defects
  2. Malnutrition
  I. Title   II. Malnutrition, and the eye
  617.7′1   RE65   80–40539

  ISBN 0–12–484240–2

Text set in 11/12 pt VIP Garamond, printed and bound
in Great Britain at The Pitman Press, Bath

Foreword

Vision and food intake are interrelated in two ways: (1) the acceptance or rejection of food is, in part, determined by its visual appeal; (2) foods consumed are the sources of nutrients to meet the nutritional needs of the eye during its embryogenesis and, subsequently, for maintenance and functioning. It is the second of these relationships that is treated in this excellent monograph, which updates the significant advances in understanding of nutritional influences on the structure and function of the eye.

Many of these influences are of primary importance to the ophthalmologist, internist and paediatrician because of their significance in daily practice; others are basic measures in preventive and public health medicine. The alert nutrition investigator, whether involved in research at the laboratory or clinical level, is presented with remarkable opportunities to observe and study newly identified physiologic roles of nutrients in the eye, a readily accessible and uniquely important organ. Dr. McLaren's book provides an interesting, authoritative background for those concerned with experimental or clinical problems pertaining to nutrition and the eye.

During the 17 years since the publication of his earlier comprehensive book, "Malnutrition and the Eye", there has been a great resurgence of interest in vitamin A deficiency xerophthalmia, its epidemiology and prevention. Medical and public health authorities, bilateral and international assistance agencies and officials in many developing regions have become aware of this severely injurious, preventable condition. The lament of Professor Oomen concerning neglect of the subject of vitamin A deficiency and xerophthalmia, and attention to its prevention, which I quoted in 1963 in the Foreword to Dr. McLaren's earlier work, no longer applies, although his moving expression of concern for the recently blinded child pertains. This lament, however, is worthy of repeated quotation:

"Xerophthalmia has been the most bitter pill for me to swallow during 18 years of doctor's work in Indonesia. The over and over repeated experience of discovering a child, recently blinded, in the arms of the mother; having to tell her that I now could do nothing more to save its eyesight; remembering that I could have done so with a few spoonfuls of cod-liver oil some days ago; these things still enter my nightmares. They belong to the most vivid examples of what disprivileged people in underdeveloped regions sometimes miss.

"Now what do I find in textbooks and scientific publications if I want to have real information about this horrible, though easily curable condition? Textbooks on tropical diseases tell you everything about Rift Valley fever, melioidosis and blastomycosis, but they sometimes do not spend one word on xerophthalmia. Every nutrition journal flows over with vitamin A, for instance, in heifers, turkeys and ducks which are eaten by the best-fed people in the world. More printing space nowadays is devoted to a few cases of hypervitaminosis A, induced by an irresponsible vitamin racket, than to the thousands of small children who die or get blind every year due to the lack of a handful of vitamin A units. What on earth is nutritional science good for, if, even in the atom age, it is not capable to counteract one of the foulest consequences of bad nutrition? Do you realize, that since the days of Mori, 60 years ago, not in Japan, but in countries like Indonesia, not one step forward has been taken, in spite of a mountain of thoughtful attention paid by doctors?"

The progress in the potential for institution of effective public health measures to prevent vitamin A deficiency blindness is leading to considered attacks in many countries through programs of intervention, guided by the World Health Organization (WHO), USAID, UNICEF and the International Vitamin A Consultative Group (IVACG). The Nutrition Foundation serves as the Secretariat, convener, editorial office, managing publisher and distributor for IVACG, the Chairman of which is Dr. E. M. DeMaeyer of WHO. Dr. McLaren is a member of the IVACG and has participated importantly in the preparation of reports, both of IVACG and WHO. He initially suggested the potential use of large doses of vitamin A for infants "at risk" in a lead article in *Nutrition Reviews* (D. S. McLaren. "Xerophthalmia: A Neglected Problem," *Nutrition Reviews*, Volume 22 (October), 1964, pp. 289–291) — a procedure now demonstrated to be practical and efficacious. Public health personnel responsible for or involved in such programs and clinicians and health workers at many levels will find a wealth of useful materials in the references appended to this foreword.

Such immediately applicable, effective public health nutrition measures using other nutrients for prevention of visual defects have not yet been devised. However, the advances in understanding of the nutritional biochemistry of many forms of cataract, especially diabetic, are leading to improved clinical management of patients whose visual functions are "at risk" from disease and can be influenced by appropriate nutritional or dietary management. We may, with confidence, predict that awareness of many of the nutritional considerations identified in this book will significantly decrease visual impairment and blindness of individuals affected with metabolic disorders and nutrient deficiencies that place them "at risk" of functional or structural defects in the visual organ. Of especial importance in this regard is the increasingly identified number of nutrient deficiencies and metabolic aberrations that, occurring during pregnancy, may result in fetal defects, either of structure or function of the eye or the nervous system.

I am confident that ophthalmologists, nutrition scientists and physicians generally will share with me a sense of indebtedness to Dr. McLaren for his timely compilation and critique of the literature of nutrition and ophthalmology relevant to "Nutritional Ophthalmology."

May 5th, 1980   William J. Darby, M.D., Ph.D.
                                       President, The Nutrition Foundation

References

1. A Report of the International Vitamin A Consultative Group (IVACG), "Guidelines for the Eradication of Vitamin A Deficiency and Xerophthalmia," The Nutrition Foundation, New York, 1977.
2. A Report of the International Vitamin A Consultative Group (IVACG), "Guidelines for the Eradication of Vitamin A Deficiency and Xerophthalmia: VI. Recent Advances in the Metabolism and Function of Vitamin A and Their Relationship to Applied Nutrition," The Nutrition Foundation, New York, 1979.
3. Report of a Joint WHO/USAID Meeting, "Vitamin A Deficiency and Xerophthalmia," Technical Report Series No. 590, World Health Organization, Geneva, 1976.

Preface

More than fifteen years after "Malnutrition and the Eye" was published it continues to sell, suggesting that no younger rival has risen to supplant it as the definitive reference text in this specialized area. That this is so is suggested by the fact that I have over the years scanned in vain the secondhand-book catalogues and shelves for a copy. It would appear to have been a book worth holding onto. However, a great deal has happened since the early 1960s when it was written and it has clearly become out of date. During this time, in addition to considerable advances having been made in our understanding of the nature of the classical nutritional deficiency ocular lesions, there has been a broadening of interest in the part that diet and nutrition play in a host of diseases in which the eye is affected. This has resulted in an entirely fresh approach being adopted in the present work and warrants the change in title that has been made.

Much has also happened to the writer in this period. My interest in the subject dates from the early 1950s when I encountered the problem of keratomalacia in the Khond Hills of Orissa in India. I started writing "Malnutrition and the Eye" some years later when I was investigating eye disease in the African population as a medical research officer at the East African Institute for Medical Research in Tanzania. It was completed shortly after my appointment as Director of the Nutrition Research Program and Professor of Clinical Nutrition at the American University of Beirut in 1962. The fourteen very happy, if turbulent, years spent there brought many opportunities for continuing research on nutritional eye problems in the Middle East and assignments to many developing countries in other parts of the world. I now find myself back in my old medical school and at a fairly advanced age undergoing adaptation to life as a clinician.

Ever since writing "Malnutrition and the Eye" I have kept a record of new contributions in the field, but it was not until shortly after returning to Edinburgh in 1976 when Academic Press agreed to publish a new edition of the book and I began to write seriously that I realized that an entirely new book was called for. This decision results not only from the large volume of new material published on topics previously covered but also from new findings, especially in areas of great clinical interest that did not receive attention in the earlier book. Notable among these are many metabolic disorders affecting the eye in which dietary management plays an important role, and prenatal influences on the development of the eye.

As I became engaged with rewriting the book rather than merely revising the text it also became evident to me that it would be more logical and far more convenient for the reader to have the material from animal studies and clinical experience on related subjects together, rather than separated in two sections of the book as previously. Many new figures and some additional tables have been included, and my only regret is that the original material was lost as a result of the civil war in Lebanon and some of the reproductions may lack clarity as a result.

My hope is that this work in its new guise will extend the service I have sought to provide to experimentalists and clinicians alike in this important borderland of knowledge for some years to come.

Edinburgh   DONALD STEWART McLAREN
January 1980.

Contents

Starvation   *Chapter 1*

Vitamin A   *Chapter 2*

Vitamins of the B Complex   *Chapter 3*

Other Vitamins

Chapter 4

Essential Elements

Chapter 5

Proteins and Amino Acids

Chapter 6

Carbohydrates

Chapter 7

Lipids   *Chapter 8*

Pre-natal Influences   *Chapter 9*

Dietary Toxins   *Chapter 10*

Miscellaneous Human Eye Conditions   *Chapter 11*

Starvation

I. Animal Studies

In the introduction to his classical work on the subject of malnutrition Jackson (1925) has summarized the various types of lack of nourishment that may be encountered. By total inanition is meant the absence or insufficiency of all nutriment and this may be either complete, when there is entire absence of food, or incomplete, when the diet is insufficient in quantity in all respects. In complete total inanition the subject would normally be subsisting on water alone, unless there were also aqueous deficiency inanition, in which case no nutriment of any kind whatsoever would be ingested.

The earlier work of Jackson, incorporated in his monograph referred to above, was contemporaneous with the discovery of the vitamins and the emergence of the concept of specific nutritional deficiency states in man and experimental animals. Subsequent work of this and other investigators tended to concentrate upon the effects of partial inanition resulting from deprivation of specific nutrients and little attention has been paid to this subject since, as far as the effects upon the eyes are concerned. The changes which have been observed have been in growth, as indicated by a change in weight, and in structure.

A. Total Inanition

1. *Growth of the Eye*

Manassein (1869) is credited with the first observation of the increase in weight of the eyeballs during inanition. He observed an apparent average increase of 12% in the weight of the eyeballs during inanition in three young rabbits, aged about 20 days, and of 24% in eight others somewhat older. The corresponding decrease in body weight was about 30–35%. Many other similar early observations are quoted by Jackson (1925), and this worker himself (Jackson, 1915) found that the eye had an intensity of growth greater than that of any other organ in the body. This amounted to about a 50% increase in weight in albino rats held at constant body weight by underfeeding for from 3 to 10 weeks. The relative intensity was greater when underfeeding was commenced even earlier (Stewart, 1918, 1919). For instance, a maximum increase of 143% occurred in rats held at birth weight by underfeeding for an average of 16 days. In newborn offspring retarded by maternal underfeeding Barry (1920, 1921) found that there was a similar, although rather smaller, increase in weight of the eye. The eyeballs, together with the spleen, had considerably larger increases in weight than any of the other organs. In some of the groups of rats studied in this way the numbers were small in both control and experimental groups. This may account for the apparent irregularity in the recovery of normal proportionate size of the eye after underfeeding noted by Jackson (1925). In adult animals there was either a slight loss in weight, or sometimes an actual increase as a result of total inanition (Jackson, 1915, 1925).

In one of the last experiments he carried out Jackson (1937) investigated the recovery of rats upon refeeding after their growth had been suppressed for long periods by underfeeding. He noted that the general appearance of the test animals was similar to that of others suffering from protein deficiency (Jackson, 1936) (see Chapter 6, Section IA). The most notable features were the humped back, the extrusion of the penis, and the prominence of the eyeballs. Kudo (1921a) in a comparison of the effects of total inanition and aqueous inanition on the rat found practically identical changes in body weight and eyeball weight under the two conditions. The body weight loss was 47% in both cases and the eyeball weight loss only 13.0% in total inanition and 13.3% in aqueous inanition (Section B1, below). Jackson attributed this continued growth of the eyeball in the rat, when the rest of the body is at a standstill, to the high water content of the eye as compared with other organs and cited some data of Lowrey (1913). However, that the increase in weight of the eye in total inanition is due to imbibition of water is very unlikely, for in the similar condition of severe protein deficiency, as will be seen in detail later (Chapter 6, Section IA), the water content of the eye was measured (McLaren, 1958) and found not to be changed, showing that tissue growth continues during inanition.

Results similar to those reported for the rat were obtained in a study of the growth of the pig (McMeekan, 1940). This worker carried out an exhaustive investigation into the effects of the influence of the plane of nutrition on the growth and development of various parts of the body. Those organs that are essential to the life processes and body functions were relatively well developed at birth and made a smaller proportional growth in postnatal life as compared with the body as a whole. Thus the eyes and the brain, as compared with the ears and the skull—one of the earliest developing bones—normally had but slight postnatal growth. In his low plane pigs the eye was the least affected of all organs and this was also true in subsequent experiments in which the plane of nutrition was altered in a variety of ways. McMeekan concluded that age was the dominant factor in the development of the eyes, this being hardly at all affected by nutrition. He attributed this to the essential role the eye has in the maintenance of life, thus being able to claim a proportionately large share of an inadequate food supply than later developing and less essential body tissues. Unfortunately the terminology of animal husbandry with regard to nutritional value of a diet cannot be readily interpreted into the language of the laboratory worker. It would seem however that McMeekan's pigs were not on the grossly deficient diets fed to the rat by Jackson and the present writer. His general conclusions concerning the eye however remain true although his explanation savours of the teleological.

Kauffman et al. (1967) have shown for the pig that the growth of the lens, as measured by total nitrogen content, is proportional to chronological age. This relationship is little influenced by variations in diet, although these result in marked changes in body size and weight.

2. Structural Changes

In the early literature there is a number of references to structural damage to the eye in malnourished animals but it is not possible to sort out the aetiological factors responsible for the various lesions. Thus Bourgeois (1870) reported that the cornea was flaccid and opaque and that corneal wounds healed imperfectly in starved mammals. Atrophic changes were also described in the eyes of fasting dogs (Carville and Bochefontaine, 1874, 1875; Falck, 1875). Von Bechterew (1895) made the interesting observation that the opening of the eyelids is delayed in newborn puppies and kittens and Stewart (1918) confirmed this in albino rats. By varying the number of rats suckled by a single mother from the first day of their lives Widdowson and McCance (1960) produced an acceleration of the growth rate of animals in the small litters so that by 21 days of age they were from two to four times heavier than those in the large litters. They found that some functions, such as sexual maturity, were closely linked to the attainment of a certain size, while others, including opening of the eyes and eruption of the teeth, were determined mainly by chronological age. The day of opening of the eyes was recorded for 483 rats and it was found that the peak incidence of this phenomenon for fast-growing animals came on the 13th and 14th days, when they weighed 32 g on the average, while the peak for the slow-growing animals was only one day later on the 14th and 15th days, despite the fact that they averaged only 13 g at the time. This subject will be taken up further in Chapter 9, where some evidence will be given for the role of protein (Section IL). Acceleration of lid separation in zinc deficiency is mentioned in Chapter 5, Section IC.

The dog was used by Bich (1895) and Lodato (1898a,b) in careful histological studies of the changes in the eyes during inanition. Water was given to some animals and withheld from others but neither worker described any difference between the eyes of the two groups. Both agreed that the main changes were in the retina. These consisted of cloudy swelling of the ganglion cells and chromatolysis was evident with Nissl's stain. These degenerative changes were progressive. Apart from the retina the rest of the eye showed no striking changes. Lodato made mention of a partial loss of the "epithelium behind Descemet's membrane", i.e. the corneal endothelium. This calls to mind the damage to this structure reported in a vitamin A-deficient monkey (Chapter 2, Section IB2) and also the possible importance such a lesion may have in a corneal condition frequently seen in malnourished Bantu children (Chapter 11, Section E). In the weanling guinea pig complete total inanition for varying periods up to 3 days failed to produce histological changes in any part of the eye (McLaren, unpublished observations).

Kammerer (1912) found that fasting resulted in the absorption of the eye pigment in *Proteus anguinus*, a change that also occurs in certain invertebrates (planarians and nemertine worms) according to Jackson (1925). Kornfeld (1922) demonstrated the depressing effect inanition has on mitosis in the corneal cells of *Salamandra maculosa* larvae. Upon refeeding there is no change in the number of counts per cornea until 4 or 5 days later when it rapidly rises, to reach about 100-fold increase after 6–14 days refeeding.

Jackson (1932) carried out a single study employing histological techniques to demonstrate the structural changes in the undernourished albino rat. The rats were held almost at birth weight for 16 days and the eye more or less doubled its weight while the body weight fell to a mean of only 7 g. The greatest changes were observed in the retina (Fig. 1). In the test rat the retina has not increased in thickness but has undergone remarkable differentiation. In the newborn control the layer of rods and cones is rudimentary, the two nuclear layers are still combined, and the nerve fibre layer is thin. In the test rat the layer of rods and cones has developed, the outer reticular layer separates the two nuclear layers, and a thin but distinct nerve fibre layer is apparent. Thus it may be seen that increase in size and development are by no means the same thing. This experiment would seem to indicate that as far as the retina is concerned development and differentiation are less affected

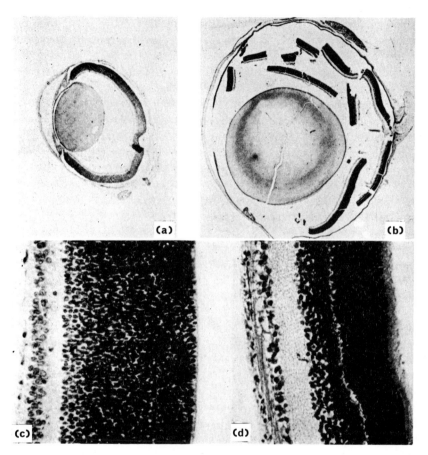

FIG. 1. Upper: Photomicrographs (×15) of sections of the entire eyeball in a normal newborn control rat (a) and a test rat (b) held nearly at birth weight for 16 days with final body weight of 7.0 g. The fragmentation of the retina in the test rat is an artefact. Lower: Photomicrographs (×260) of sections of the retina in the same rats. Note increased differentiation of the retina in the test rat (d). From Jackson (1932).

than actual cell multiplication and increase in size. That structural damage is less likely to occur in the eye than in many other organs of the body was shown by the work of Addis *et al.* (1936), who measured in albino rats the quantities of protein lost by various organs during a fast. The only organs that failed to lose protein were the eyes, the testicles, and the adrenals.

Lee *et al.* (1974) reported fine, punctate opacities in the cortex, a few water vacuoles and prominent Y sutures in the porcine lens following severe starvation. These changes disappeared on a normal diet. No biochemical changes were found in the protein fractions of the lens.

In a certain strain of mice, known as the Bruckner strain, degeneration of the outer nuclear layer of the retina occurs as a simple recessive character, appearing at about 11 days of age. Lucas and Newhouse (1957) failed to find any effect of various vitamins on the incidence or course of this condition but it was noticed that some female mice which were considerably underweight had litters in which the development of the retinal lesion was retarded. A group of seven females was restricted during pregnancy to about two thirds of the amount of food eaten by a control group. Of 17 young produced, eight had lesions within the expected range of severity but in nine it was less severe than expected. There was some inverse correlation between body weight and preservation of the outer nuclear layer. Thus it would seem that in this instance total inanition during intrauterine life had a mitigating effect upon the development of a genetically controlled lesion.

The mouse was also used in a study by Hellström (1956) of the influence of the state of nutrition on the effects of oxygen on the eye as an experimental approach to the problem of retrolental fibroplasia. Underfeeding was effected by separating the young from the mother every third day and by increasing the number of young suckled by the mother. Overfeeding was also produced by reducing the number suckled by a mother. The proliferation of hyaloid vessels was not influenced by the state of nutrition. Underfeeding did however slightly retard the outgrowth of vessels in the retina. The hyperplasia of vessels of the nerve fibre layer which occurs when animals exposed to oxygen are transferred to air, was greater in those underfed during exposure to oxygen than in those overfed during exposure to oxygen, and was greater in the latter than in animals underfed both during exposure to oxygen and during their subsequent stay in the air. These results suggest the importance of factors other than oxygen tension, some of which may be nutritional, in the aetiology of retrolental fibroplasia in premature infants (see also Chapter 9, Section IIA).

The effect of partial starvation on the development of cataract in the diabetic rat was studied by Patterson (1954). Animals starved on alternate days for a total period of 40 hours each week were protected against the development of cataract to a degree corresponding to the reduction of the blood sugar. When the non-fasting blood sugar level was 450 mg/100 ml or less cataract did not develop (see also Chapter 7, Section ID).

B. Aqueous Inanition

1. Growth of the Eye

The results of the few experiments carried out in which the effect of thirst on the visual apparatus has been investigated all indicate that, as in the case of total inanition, the eye loses considerably less weight than the body as a whole. In pigeons fed on a dry barley diet, Schuchardt (1847) noted an apparent loss of 4% in the weight of the eyeballs accompanying a loss of 44% in body weight. Falck and Scheffer (1854) fed a dog on a diet of dry biscuit for 4 weeks, at the end of which period it had lost 20% in body weight compared with a normal control. There was an apparent increase of 19.7% in the weight of the eyeballs, with only a very slight increase in their water content (from 89.8 to 90.9%). In the adult albino rat, Kudo (1921a), as mentioned already (see above, Section AI), found a similarly greater loss of body weight than eyeball weight in those animals submitted to acute thirst, as he also found in those with total inanition. In the young rat he further found (Kudo, 1921b) that after a period of from 9 to 13 weeks on a relatively dry diet there was a progressive increase in the weight of the eyeballs amounting to about 71%. Thus, as was the case for total inanition, in aqueous inanition the eyeballs of the adult rat lose weight slightly, but in the young rat they increase remarkably in weight.

2. Structural Changes

Although prolonged thirst did not seem to have any additional adverse effect on the eyes of the starved dogs studied by Bich (1895) and Lodato (1898a,b) it has been reported (Kudo, 1921a) in the rat and the frog (Durig, 1901) that cataractous changes may occur in the lens as a result of water inanition. The interesting observation was made by Smith (1932) that rats deprived of water, but given food ad libitum, developed what was called "bloodstained" wrists, together with staining of the mouth, nose, and eyes. Total inanition, with water given ad libitum, had no such effect. A similar phenomenon called "bloody tears" or, better, chromodacryorrhœa, in which there is a profuse outpouring of a dark red material around the eyes, was induced by injections of acetylcholine by Tashiro et al. (1940) and suggested by them as a new criterion for the biological assay of this substance. It had been shown by Derrien and Turchini (1924) that the secretion of the Harderian gland contains porphyrin and that this substance was responsible for the brick-red fluorescence which this gland exhibits when viewed in ultraviolet light.

In the rat, Figge and Atkinson (1941) failed to produce porphyrin incrustation of the nose and fur of rats subjected to total aqueous inanition, but it occurred in animals only partially deprived of water. They suggested that complete dehydration prevented the production of the pigment. They further noted that the porphyrin incrustation produced in this way was identical with that occurring in pantothenic acid deficiency (see Chapter 3, Section IA2).

II. Human Studies

A number of early observations on the changes undergone by the eye during periods of famine and starvation has been collected by Jackson (1925), but, as this author remarked, it is not always possible to disentangle those features attributable to total inanition or water inanition alone from those due to vitamin A deficiency and to infections. Thus in an individual fasting for 30 days it was reported that after the 28th day there was slight narrowing of the visual field and slight constriction of the retinal vessels, certainly difficult to measure and of doubtful significance. Not surprisingly the eyes have been reported to be deeply sunken, the periorbital fat to be depleted, and the eyeballs themselves soft in a man dying of starvation. Jackson (1925) compiled data on the weight of the eyeballs in marasmic infants and found that it was always above the normal weight at birth, 3.2 g, even in those infants that never reached a body weight of 3.2 kg. This persistent growth of the eye in the presence of generalized wasting recalls the similar results reported already in underfed young animals (Section IA1).

It was reported during the first world war that there was an increase of acute glaucoma, retinal hemorrhage, and thrombosis of the central vein, and a marked decrease in accommodative power. Just how real these reported changes were and what relation they might bear to malnutrition it is not possible now to say.

Many instances have been recorded (Palich-Szántó, 1924; Jess, 1930) of the occurrence of cataract following upon conditions in which there has been profound nutritional disturbance. Such diseases as typhus, malaria, meningitis, smallpox, scarlet fever, and encephalitis lethargica, and states of long-continued lactation, severe nutritional disease, hunger oedema, and marked loss of blood have all been incriminated. A case of bilateral subcapsular cataract complicating anorexia nervosa in a young woman was reported (Miller, 1958) in which it was thought that the extreme inanition might have been responsible. A 30-year old woman with anorexia nervosa had bilateral dense, irregular posterior cataracts for 4 years which necessitated operation (Stigmar, 1965). Interesting as such accounts are it has always proved impossible to establish any causal relationship between the impaired nutrition and the lens damage.

During and immediately after the second world war much greater attention was paid to the medical aspects of starvation and recovery therefrom. Generally speaking, disorders of the eye did not find a prominent place in these accounts. When the resistance shown by the eyes of experimental animals to total inanition is recalled (Section A) this is what might be expected. In their monumental work on experimental human starvation Keys and his colleagues (Keys *et al.*, 1950) noted no important deterioration in any sensory function after 6 months of semistarvation. They do however state that the sclera and conjunctiva were unusually devoid of blood vessels, the whites of the eyes resembling unglazed porcelain and failing to redden even when soap solution was applied.

Contrary to the general rule, however, there were reports appearing for the most part in the continental literature several years after the end of the second world war in which conspicuous damage to the eye was recorded. Some of the most interesting and distinctive of these have come from Greece. Djacos (1949; Eleftheriou and Djacos, 1950) has given clinical and histological accounts of what he termed "superficial polymorphous keratopathy" occurring in patients with nutritional oedema in Athens. These cases began to appear in November 1941, the daily caloric content of the diet distributed varying from 510 in the month of September to the lowest value of only 204 in February. In all, he examined the eyes of 107 cases among the large numbers of people found dying on the streets of Athens and brought into the State General Hospital. The eyes were negative on gross examination but the slit lamp revealed characteristic lesions staining with fluorescein. These took one of three forms. That associated with the mildest degree of generalized oedema consisted of numerous small round, oval, or bacillary-shaped spots which were either intra- or subepithelial in situation but not involving Bowman's membrane. In those cases showing more marked oedema there occurred what was termed the hydropic form of lesion, characterized by large circular opacities surrounded by halos. The third form, in the most severely ill cases, consisted of ulceration involving the epithelium only (Fig. 2a and b).

The rest of the cornea remained clear in all cases, with the exception that in the periphery in rare instances interstitial lesions of considerable size were seen. Djacos did not see any other abnormalities on clinical examination of the eyes but he refers to the descriptions of others in Greece to oedema of the retina in starvation (Spyratos, 1949; Petzetakis, 1950).

Six cases that came to autopsy gave Eleftheriou and Djacos (1950) the opportunity to study the histology of these lesions of the cornea. They were confined to the anterior epithelial and subepithelial layers, except at the

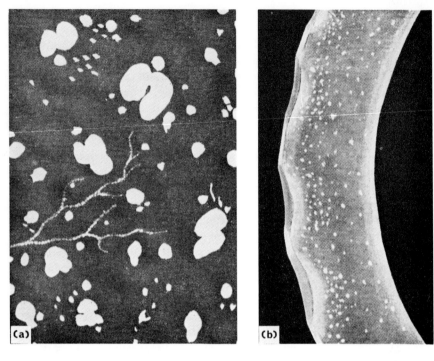

FIG. 2. (a) Granular appearance of corneal nerves. (b) The corneal corpuscles are very distinct, almost having the appearance of ulceration. From Djacos (1949).

periphery where the substantia propria was also involved and they extended to the neighbouring sclera. Microscopically the central lesions were seen to be formed by enlargement of the epithelial intercellular spaces which in frozen sections appeared to be filled with serous fluid. The surface epithelium sometimes ruptured in places, producing the small staining areas that appeared clinically. The peripheral changes were due to thickenings at the limbus where the connective tissue lamellae were destroyed and replaced by a homogeneous, formless, or finely granular substance.

The account of the anterior segment changes by Petzetakis (1950) included in the symptomatology oedema of the lids and chemosis, hypoaesthesia of the cornea, sluggish pupillary reflexes, diminution of lacrimal secretion, and irregularity and oedema of the superficial corneal layers. Histologically there was intracellular vacuolation and oedema of the epithelium closely resembling the changes described in rats fed on a cassava diet (see Fig. 83).

The description of night blindness and eye changes due to starvation in Greece during the years 1941–45 of Spyratos (1949) included in addition to the manifestations of vitamin A deficiency, ulceration and oedema of the corneal epithelium, oedema of the iris and ciliary body, and early paresis of accommodation. While oedema of the retina was especially common in those patients who died of starvation, seen most commonly in the region of the disc and the area of the macula, night blindness was not found in these fatal cases.

Several other accounts describe various retinal appearances which the authors consider to be characteristic of human starvation. They lack the histological description of the nature of the lesions that the corneal changes had, but together they do constitute a considerable body of evidence in favour of the involvement of the retina also.

In long-term prisoners of war in Germany, Siegert (1956)—in addition to nutritional amblyopia, impairment of dark adaptation, and xerosis of the conjunctiva and keratomalacia, all of which are dealt with in full else-where—described stippled lesions of the retinal tissue together with oedema in the central part secondary to vascular disturbances of the capillaries. Heinsius (1950) found the fundi of undernourished patients to be abnormally pale, with oedema of the optic disc and retina, spasm of the arteries, and retinitis consisting of white dots. Three especially severe cases, prisoners of war in Russia who were released and two of whom subsequently died, showed all these changes in a marked form. The arteries were sometimes so greatly contracted that they were only one quarter or one fifth the width of the veins, and one patient had ectasia of the arterioles.

As many as 800 patients suffering from inanition had fundoscopic examination carried out by Scholtyssek (1950). In 50 of these, and especially in those with the oedematous form of general dystrophy, abnormal appearances were found. These were narrowing of the retinal arteries, haziness of the macula and optic disc, and small yellowish-pink specks in the region of the macula. This report was confirmed by Obal (1950), and in two patients from a Russian prison camp with famine oedema Winkler (1948) also found yellowish well-defined spots in the central part of the fundus in both patients, and in one case they also extended to the peripheral fundus. In 81 patients with what was described as "alimentary dystrophy" Živkov and Teoharov (1958) found oedema of the retina in many. Eight of these patients died and all their eyes were examined histologically. Oedema of the retina, sometimes in limited areas and especially near the disc, was a constant finding. The white spots on the retina, a prominent feature in most of the other accounts, were not mentioned by these workers.

Others reported negative findings from the second world war in Europe. Edge (1945) made a study of 300 prisoners of war in a heavy labour camp in Germany, Leyton (1946) reported on other prisoners of war, and Lamy et al. (1948) from France. Fajgenblat (1946) found no deterioration in visual acuity or fields in daylight or under low illumination with white or coloured targets in 20 women in a ghetto in 1941–42. Small premature lenticular opacities were noted in all and intraocular pressures were only about 50% of normal.

This then would seem to be the extent of our knowledge about the ocular lesions of human starvation. Two comments may be made in conclusion concerning the significance of what has been reported. Firstly, it is clear that the eyes remain unaffected, at least as far as structural damage is concerned, until the terminal stages have been reached. Secondly, there must be some doubt as to whether both corneal and retinal lesions are truly due to starvation. It is possible that the cornea, especially in its devitalized state, was the seat of infection by one of the viruses known to cause a keratoconjunctivitis (see Chapter 3, Section IIA2a, and Chapter 11, Section C). The retinal spots may conceivably be identical with those reported in vitamin A deficiency (Chapter 2, Section III, 4i).

Chapter 2

Vitamin A

I. Animal Studies of Vitamin A Deficiency

A. Historical Background

In the absence of vitamin A many epithelial tissues in the body undergo keratinization, including the conjuctiva and cornea, and death eventually results. Increased susceptibility to infection, partly as a result of the breakdown of tissue barriers, with impaired cellular immunity probably contributing, enhances these destructive changes. Vitamin A has been shown to be essential for glycoprotein synthesis. Sterility also results.

Only one function of vitamin A has been well defined biochemically, namely its interaction in the photoreceptor rods and cones of the retina with proteins called opsins. On exposure to light the 11-*cis* form of retinol is isomerized to the all-*trans* form which triggers off a series of chromophoric changes in the complex. Concomitantly, ion transport and membrane potentials are affected and in some incompletely understood way nerve impulses result which are sensed in the brain as vision.

Various carotenoids in plants, of which the most important is β-carotene, are the ultimate source of vitamin A, conversion taking place in the small intestinal mucosa. Vitamin A (retinol) is absorbed as retinyl esters and transported in chylomicrons to the liver, where it is stored, mainly in parasinusoidal stellate cells: After passage to liver parenchymal cells retinol is coupled to a specific binding protein, retinol-binding protein (RBP), for transport to the tissues. It is found in plasma in this form, coupled also to pre-albumin (Kanai *et al.*, 1968).

Most tissues possess another distinct protein that binds retinol, known as cellular retinol-binding protein (CRBP) (Bashor *et al.*, 1973). Eye, brain, testis, ovary and uterus also have a retinoic acid-binding protein (CRABP)

(Ong *et al.*, 1975). Heller and Bok (1976) reported membrane proteins which specifically bind retinol and which may have a role in transporting retinol across membranes. There is evidence for the presence of specific high affinity receptor sites for retinol-RBP in retinal pigment epithelial cells (Heller, 1975). The greater affinity of these sites for retinol-RBP than for apo-RBP suggests that the control of delivery of retinol to target cells might be mediated by the relative plasma concentrations of apo and retinol-RBP. Similar receptors to those described above in the retina and other tissues have been identified in corneal epithelium, stroma and endothelium (Wiggert *et al.*, 1977).

All photosynthetic cells appear to contain carotenoids; the classic constituents of the chloroplast. All green terrestrial plants synthesis carotenes, as do certain yeasts, bacteria and fungi. The lower invertebrates do not appear to have been investigated, but from the first appearance of image-forming eyes, in mollusca and arthropods, all retinas contain, and directly depend for their function upon, a special group of derived carotenoids, the vitamins A. In invertebrates either vitamin A_1 (rhodopsin system) or vitamin A_2 (porphyropsin system) is highly concentrated in the eyes and appears to serve no function elsewhere (Wald, 1943). Most contain vitamin A_1, but the retinas of all freshwater fish examined have only vitamin A_2, and many saltwater fish and amphibians have both (Bridges, 1975). Higher vertebrates, including man, have only vitamin A_1 and, in contrast, most of this, usually amounting to 90% of the body content, is in the liver.

Magendie (1816), the noted French physiologist, would seem to have been the first to produce xerophthalmia experimentally, making him also the first to describe a symptom of a dietary deficiency in an experimental animal (McCollum, 1957). He restricted dogs to a diet of wheat gluten, starch, and sugar or olive oil and mentioned that on this regime ulcers developed on the corneae. There is little reason to doubt that these animals suffered from xerophthalmia. Almost 100 years later Falta and Noeggerath (1905) and Knapp (1908) also produced xerophthalmia, this time in rats fed on a diet obviously deficient in the as then undiscovered vitamin A. Knapp noted that the responsible factor was destroyed by sunlight and seems to have realized the resemblance between the experimentally produced eye condition and that affecting young children living on inadequate diets. The relationship between the experimental and the human condition was also recognized by Goldschmidt (1915) and McCollum and Davis (1913), the latter applying the term "xerophthalmia" to the eye changes in rats. Freise, Goldschmidt, and Frank (1915) showed that the condition in animals was not contagious and that the advanced changes known as keratomalacia were identical with those already described in man (Leber, 1883; see Section IIIA2 *b*). They were able to prevent it by adding 2 cm³ of milk daily to the artificial diet, and

Goldschmidt (1915) concluded that the efficacy of milk was due to its content of "noch unbekannten, aber für das Leben notwendiger Substanzen".

B. The Anterior Segment

Vitamin A deficiency was first, and has been most extensively, studied in the rat, and the eye lesions are particularly easy to produce and marked in this animal. The changes in other species are strictly comparable in nature although frequently much less pronounced. They commence in the rat with swelling of the eyelids and signs of conjunctival inflammation. Yudkin

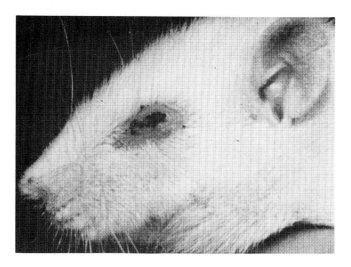

FIG. 3. "Spectacle eye" in a vitamin A-deficient rat. From D. S. McLaren (1960a).

(1922) described the typical sleepy appearance of the facies due in part to the recession of the eyeballs which Collins (1930) suggested was due to atrophy and necrosis of the secreting epithelium of the Harderian glands. The secretion of this gland becomes more and more viscid and patches of fatty material accumulate in the fornices. The rat tends to rub its oedematous eyelids with its front paws and the hair of the lids falls out, producing what has been described as "spectacle eye" (Fig. 3). This appearance of the eyelids is by no means specific to vitamin A deficiency and occurs also in a variety of other deficiency states (see Chapter 3, Section IA1 and Chapter 6, Section I

B). Porphyrin pigment from the Harderian gland becomes encrusted around the eyes, and the lids frequently stick together (Fig. 4).

The anterior segment of the eye in vitamin A deficiency has a characteristic xerotic or dry appearance due to the pathological changes taking place (see below). These affect the bulbar conjunctiva and then the cornea, but in the rat only in the latter site are they evident, for almost the whole of the

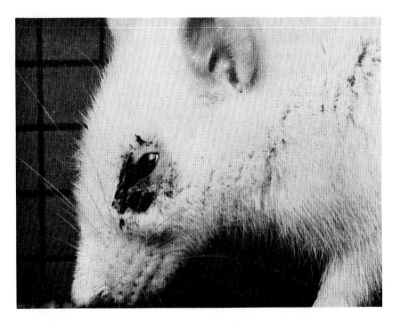

FIG. 4. Porphyrin incrustation of lids of a vitamin A-deficient rat. From D. S. McLaren (1960a).

externally visible eye consists of cornea, the conjunctiva being a mere narrow rim of tissue.

The histological appearances in experimental animals were first described by Freise *et al.* (1915). In the rat they found early cornification of the corneal epithelium, swelling and decreased staining power of the middle epithelial cells, and inflammatory infiltration of the lower epithelial cells. The substantia propria was oedematous with vascular invasion and local areas of cellular infiltration. Severe cases developed a perforating ulcer. Wason (1921) described hyalinization or necrosis of the outer layer of the corneal epithelium, exudation of serum and cells into the epithelium and stroma, a proliferation of blood vessels and fibroblasts, and in advanced cases invasion of the anterior or, occasionally, the posterior chamber. It was concluded by

Mori (1922a,b) that the xerosis or dryness of the conjunctiva and cornea was the essential change in the eyes of rats produced by vitamin A deficiency, secondary to atrophy and drying up of the secretion of the paraocular glands, and that the corneal ulceration and keratomalacia resulted from secondary infection. He was the first to describe in the experimental condition the formation of keratohyalin granules in the second layer of the epithelial cells in the conjunctiva but did not find them in the cornea, except at the limbus. Mori (1923) further found that xerophthalmia and keratomalacia could be produced in rats consuming diets containing an abundance of vitamin A but with certain unfavourable salt mixtures, and the specificity of these lesions to vitamin A deficiency was at one time questioned (McCollum et al., 1922). Subsequently (McCollum et al., 1926–27; Jones, 1927; Simmonds et al., 1927a,b) it was shown that the substitution of ferrous sulphate for ferric citrate in the diet was responsible. Jones suggested that the vitamin was destroyed by an oxidation catalysed by the ferrous salt.

To return to the pathogenesis of the conjunctival and corneal lesions; at about the same time it was reported (Yudkin and Lambert, 1922a,b; Lambert and Yudkin, 1923; Yudkin and Lambert, 1923) that the earliest lesions consisted of focal inflammatory changes in the conjunctivae of the lids and nictitating membrane. They regarded the involvement of the cornea as a secondary phenomenon, the rapidity of development and the degree of destruction depending mainly on the type of bacterial infection. Findlay (1925) found a diminution in the concentration of the enzyme lysozyme in the ocular glands of vitamin A-deficient rabbits and that treatment with normal tears prevented keratomalacia.

Things had reached this rather confused state when doubts as to the primary role of vitamin A deficiency in not only the ocular changes but also lesions in many other parts of the body were dispelled by the classic study of Wolbach and Howe in the rat (1925) and extended shortly afterward to the guinea pig (Wolbach and Howe 1928). They fed rats a diet of casein, starch, salt mixture, lard, and brewer's yeast which, although lacking in vitamins D and E as well as A, produced lesions which were undoubtedly predominantly due to vitamin A deficiency. These changes have been reproduced many times since then with highly purified vitamin A deficient diets; see Pfister and Renner, 1978 (Fig. 5). The essential change was a substitution of the normal epithelium by stratified keratinizing epithelium not only in conjunctiva, cornea, and paraocular glands but also in parts of the respiratory, alimentary, and genitourinary tracts. This process in which the character of the epithelium changes, becoming thickened and horny like the skin, was called keratinizing metaplasia by these workers (Fig. 6). Wolbach and Howe commented upon the marked atrophy of the Harderian gland, which they regarded as being non-specific to vitamin A deficiency. Along with the

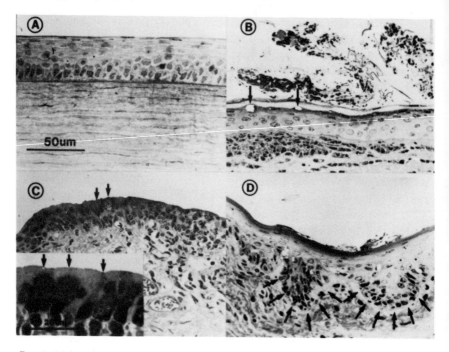

FIG. 5. Light microscopic comparisons between control and vitamin A-deficient cornea and conjunctiva reveal changes in epithelial and stromal cytology and morphology. All micrographs represent the same magnification except where noted. (A) Typical control cornea shows the normal appearance of basal, wing and squamous epithelial cells. Many keratocytes are found in the anterior stroma. (B) In the 6-week vitamin A-deficient cornea the columnar appearance of the basal epithelium was lost with keratinizing epithelium at the surface. Although most epithelia were slightly thinner than normal, this specimen shows a large accumulation of keratin, inflammatory cells, and amorphous cellular debris. Many inflammatory cells are found in the anterior stroma. Two cysts (arrows) are located in the superficial epithelial layers. (C) Epithelium from control conjunctiva shows three or four layers of cells with goblet cells (arrows) interspersed (see inset). (D) Six-week vitamin A-deficient conjunctiva shows epithelium with superficial keratinization and rite peg formation (arrows) where the thickness is twice normal. From Pfister and Renner (1978).

keratinization of the conjunctiva and cornea they noted the same process going on in the ducts of the Meibomian glands, the lacrimal glands, Harderian glands, and extraorbital (lacrimal) glands. The formation of mucus continued in the epithelium in which many foci of keratinization were established. The mucus cells of the conjunctiva persisted after keratinization had occurred and they were to be seen overlaid with keratinized cells, but they eventually atrophied and disappeared. In only one of Wolbach's 18 rats was there histological evidence of an infectious process in the eye. They did not believe that the vascularization of the cornea was due to infection for the substantia propria only became oedematous and vascularized after keratinization was established.

Later (Bessey and Wolbach, 1938) it was shown that the replacement of normal by keratinizing epithelium is a late effect and follows epithelial atrophy, which in turn is followed by proliferation on the part of the basal layer cells. In epithelia of the stratified and transitional types, such as those of the cornea, conjunctiva, bladder, ureter, and renal pelvis, the basal cells engaged in reparative proliferation tend to produce a continuous layer from

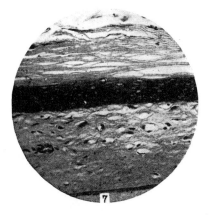

FIG. 6. Histological appearance of keratomalacia in the rat. From Wolbach and Howe (1925).

the beginning and the process appears to be true metaplasia. However, in other epithelia, such as those of ducts and glands, the respiratory mucosa, and the uterus, where proliferative ability is limited to a few scattered basal cells, focal areas of new cells appear. By their continued growth these groups of new cells undermine and replace the original epithelium by a stratified keratinizing epithelium. For a period an atrophic epithelium may remain above the replacement epithelium which at first consists of only one or two layers of flat cells. The epidermis-like tissue is soon formed and the original atrophic epithelium is shed. Regardless of its origin this replacement epithelium is comparable in all its layers to epidermis. It returns to normal when vitamin A is administered, showing that the cells of the basal layer retain their innate ability to produce once more the appropriate epithelium. A very careful study of the effects of vitamin A deficiency on the eye of the rabbit was made by Mann et al. (1946). The first sign of any effect from the deficient diet was failure to gain weight at the same rate as the litter-mate control. Later on, the conjunctival and corneal epithelium keratinized. There was no green staining of the cornea with fluorescein, indicating no loss of surface. Of the area of metaplasia, only the central part stained faintly pink with eosin showing that these cells were keratinizing. The second eye change detected was an outward migration of chromatophores of the limbal pigment ring in pigmented rabbits. It was definitely a migration and not the development of new chromatophores. The substantia propria, endothelium, and corneal nerve fibres showed no abnormality on slit lamp examination. It is noteworthy that in these animals there was no corneal vascularization or infiltration but this may have been because the deficiency was rather chronic and mild. A final change observed was keratinization of the conjunctiva especially in the lower fornix. In this experiment the conjunctival change was preceded by that in the cornea, the reverse of the normal process in man, but probably attributable, as the authors suggested, to the way in which the conjunctiva of the rabbit is protected. In the rabbit and also the monkey deficient in vitamin A, Hetler (1934) claimed to have produced Bitot's spot-like lesions. She states that there were Bitot's spots of the right eye of one monkey and that they appeared in the eyes of all ten of the experimental rabbits. Unfortunately no description is given of what is meant by a Bitot's spot, nor is any evidence provided to assure the reader that the investigator was familiar with this lesion in man. More satisfactory evidence for the experimental production of Bitot's spots is that of Ramalingaswami et al. (1955), who found them in two out of three deficient monkeys. The first author is a clinician working in India and has had experience of human xerophthalmia (personal communication). The evidence for the view that these lesions are not always a sign of vitamin A deficiency and that they may occur in the absence of any demonstrable deficiency of this vitamin is given in Section IIIA3b.

When the xerosis has involved both cornea and conjunctiva (xerosis conjunctivae et corneae), xerophthalmia may be said to be present. It is probably as a result of the impairment of corneal nutrition brought about by keratinization of the epithelium that an ingrowth of new vessels takes place from the limbic plexus. Stephenson and Clark (1920) first described this, the first account of corneal vascularization due to a nutritional deficiency in the literature. Wolbach and Howe (1925) noted that the ingrowth of capillaries took place at the same time as the epithelial changes. They did not regard the vascularization as being secondary to infection for it was present in their rats before there was any considerable accumulation of desquamated cells and before more than early histological signs of inflammatory reaction in the limbus. Bowles et al. (1946) compared the nature of the corneal vascularization occurring in vitamin A deficiency with that due to riboflavin deficiency in the rat. The appearance of the cornea in riboflavin deficiency is described in Chapter 3, Section IBl. In both states in about 60% of animals the first visible invading capillaries seemed to stem from the circumferential artery in the superior nasal quadrant, in 20% from the 12 o'clock position and in the remaining 20% in the superior temporal quadrant. In vitamin A deficiency this invasion of vessels took place about 3–7 days after the corneal changes of xerosis had appeared. The vessels were usually dendritic in type, contrasting with the usual terminal loop type of riboflavin deficiency, and formed a dense collar of vascularity extending one half or three quarters around the cornea.

Following imperceptibly but rapidly upon the drying and haziness of the cornea comes the softening and deformity of the corneal substance characterizing the final stage known as keratomalacia (Fig. 7). Invasion of

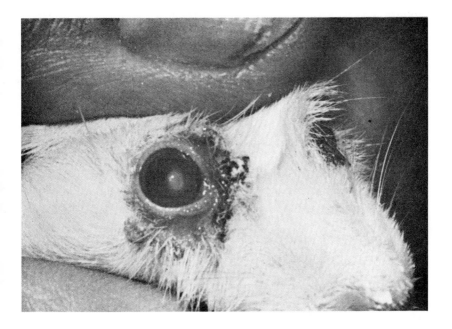

FIG. 7. Keratomalacia in the rat.

the cornea by pyogenic organisms usually plays a part in this process but it is always a secondary one due to the breach in the continuity of the corneal surface epithelium and not, as was once thought, of primary aetiologic significance (see below). As a result of the softening of the cornea it gives way under the pressure of intraocular tension.

If the process is arrested before perforation of the cornea has taken place it will remain ballooned forward as a "bell-shaped" or "nipple-like" deformity or what is known to the ophthalmologist as ectasia of the cornea. By means of heavy dosing of vitamin A-deficient rats at this stage Mutch and Richards (1939) were able to produce a marked cone-shaped deformity of the cornea resembling the clinical condition called keratoconus. There is, however, no evidence that vitamin A deficiency plays any part in the production of this condition in man and the experimental situation was a highly artificial one. If the cornea ruptures as a result of softening then the usual sequelae are prolapse of the iris, loss of vitreous, and extrusion of the lens. Generalized secondary infection of the eye at this stage is almost inevitable and the resulting panophthalmitis leads on to a shrunken globe (phthisis bulbi) if the animal survives.

Several factors determine the time of onset of the ocular lesions and the rapidity with which they progress. The amount of vitamin A or carotene in the experimental diet was one of the most important factors accounting for the variability of ease with which the earlier workers were able to produce the deficiency state. The age of the animal when the deficiency regime is commenced is of great importance, young animals being much more susceptible than older ones. The vitamin A status of the mother animal is also significant in this respect for this will determine whether or not the newborn animal has adequate stores of the vitamin in its liver. There is finally very considerable variation between different species in the suscepti-bility to vitamin A deficiency and indeed in the ease with which the various features of the deficiency develop. Young rats fed on a diet devoid of vitamin A usually begin to show a slowing of the rate of growth and to develop the earliest eye signs after about 6 weeks on the diet. Puppies must be born from bitches themselves rendered deficient if they are to show deficiency signs. In the pigeon the hyperkeratosis of the lids is so marked that it prevents the lids opening although there is no xerosis of the underlying cornea (Mouriquand *et al.*, 1949).

The early accounts of the condition in the rat were soon confirmed for other species; thus the reports of xerophthalmia in the chick (Guerrero and Conception, 1920), the young rabbit (Nelson and Lamb, 1920), the dog (Steenbock *et al.*, 1921), the duck (Rumbaur, 1922), and the pigeon (McCarrison, 1923) are among the earliest.

The list has been considerably extended since (see below). Mellanby (1934) concluded from studies on the rabbit and the rat that the xerophthal-mia of vitamin A deficiency might be secondary to a loss of neurotropic control by the ophthalmic division of the trigeminal nerve. While confirm-ing the occurrence together of xerophthalmia and myelin degeneration of the afferent nerves, later workers found no causal relationship to exist (see below). From the work of Studer and Frey (1949) and Sabella *et al.* (1951) in which changes in the skin were brought about by oral dosing or local application of high concentrations of vitamin A, and from the tissue culture work which Mellanby himself initiated (Fell and Mellanby, 1953) we now know that the vitamin has a direct action on epithelium without the mediation of nervous tissue, although the precise function of vitamin A in epithelial structures is still unknown.

One anterior segment change reported fairly early on in the young of rats deprived of vitamin A, namely that of typical zonular cataract by von Szily and Eckstein (1923), has not been generally confirmed. This received a certain amount of credence by having been coupled with apparent clinical support for this from Pillat (1929) (see Section IIIA3*h*). It is evident that the diet employed by von Szily was not deficient solely in vitamin A. Vitamin D was almost certainly also deficient and although a deficiency of this vitamin per se has not been shown to cause cataract, the consequent derangement of calcium metabolism has. This subject is discussed fully in Chapter 5, Section IA. Lahiri (1938) claimed that cataracts accompanied night blindness in bullocks fed a diet deficient in carotene, and Moore (1939) noted wrinkling of the lens capsule in carotene-deficient calves. However, in a recent careful study by Pirie and Overall (1972) in the rat, although cataract did not result, there was observed reduplication of cylindrical cells at the anterior pole, with disruption of nuclei and cells in mitosis in the lens epithelium (Fig. 8).

Subsequently the conjunctival and corneal changes have been demonstrated in numerous other species including man, monkey, pig, cattle, dog, fox, rabbit, guinea pig, mouse, and fowl (Wolbach, 1954), as well as cat (Gershoff *et al.*, 1957), pigeon (Mouriquand *et al.*, 1955), which is very resistant, and hamster (Salley and Bryson, 1957). Typical keratinization has been noted in terrapins in many tissues including conjunctiva and cornea (Zwart, 1966; Elkan and Zwart, 1967; Hime, 1972). This species is prone to develop vitamin A deficiency in captivity.

An interesting and extreme example of the transformation wrought in the epithelium by the keratinizing process of vitamin A deficiency is the account of the presence of a patch of thick hair in the centre of one cornea of a calf born to a vitamin A-deficient cow (Schmidt, 1941). A further example, in which anophthalmos was also present (see Chapter 9, Section IA*l*) may well have been the case reported by Haigh *et al.* (1920) in which a Jersey heifer, which had been on a calcium-deficient ration of silage and corn, almost certainly also low in vitamin A, gave birth to an undersized and maldeveloped calf, with no eyes and with hair growing from the "eye sockets".

A relationship between the epithelial lesions and damage to nerves was suggested by the work of Mellanby (1934) in rabbits, rats, and a dog. In animals with xerophthalmia degenerative changes were found in the myelin sheaths of the ophthalmic division of the trigeminal nerve and in the cells of the Gasserian ganglion. He claimed that the degree of nerve damage paralleled the severity of the corneal lesions. In India, Rao (1936) made an

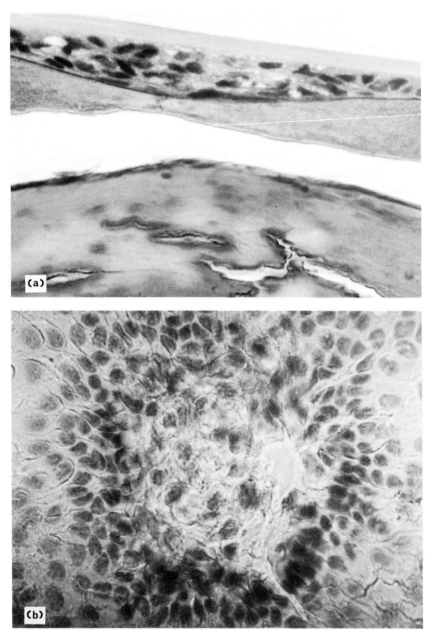

FIG. 8. Photomicrographs showing early keratinization of the lens epithelium. From Pirie and Overall (1972).

extensive study of this problem using rabbits, rats, and fowls and although often finding myelin degeneration in the afferent nerves of the eye he failed to correlate the degeneration with the onset and course of the ocular lesions. Xerophthalmia healed following the administration of vitamin A but was not accompanied by recovery of the nerve changes. Mellanby had claimed that coarse cereals aggravated the nervous system damage, but Rao had been able to produce it using a "synthetic" diet consisting of casein, starch, olive oil, dried yeast, and minerals. Furthermore, Sauer (1939) was able to demonstrate that nerves actually grow into the metaplasing corneal epithelium in vitamin A deficiency and concluded that degeneration of nerve fibres could not be a primary cause of the epithelial damage.

The metabolic activity of the cornea in both vitamin A and riboflavin deficiency was studied by Lee and Hart (1944). They found that normally the epithelium has a much higher metabolism than the stroma. In the xerotic cornea of vitamin A deficiency the activity was normal or slightly higher than normal. They offered in explanation for this, that the processes of metaplasia and hyperplasia with increase in energy demands might predominate over that of cellular destruction.

Mann *et al.* (1946) in their careful study of vitamin A deficiency in the rabbit noted no change in the cornea's basal cell layer apart from a slight increase in the number of dividing cells and no alteration of the substantia propria. The lids became keratinized but showed no infiltration and both Meibomian and Harderian glands were normal. These results contrasted with those in the rat, but the lacrimal gland showed the same changes of keratinization as had been reported in that animal. The conjunctiva of the bulb was also keratinized with pigment present in the cells of the basal layer. No mucous cells could be found. The symptoms seem to be altogether milder in the rabbit as compared with the rat, and the grosser corneal changes never appeared.

Mitotic activity and wound healing in the corneal epithelium of vitamin A-deficient rats were studied by Friedenwald *et al.* (1945). They found that the overall mitotic rate per 1000 basal cells was reduced by about 30% and the speed of the mitotic cycle similarly reduced in the deficient group. In some of the experimental animals the epithelial cells were considerably enlarged in their horizontal diameters and it was concluded from this that the inhibition of mitosis was not due to a failure in growth of individual cells. The post-traumatic cell movements in the healing of small wounds of the coreal epithelium were found not to be significantly delayed. Agarwal and Adhaulia (1954) claimed that superficial and deep wounds of the cornea in the nutritionally normal rabbit healed more quickly and with less scarring with vitamin A therapy. Only six animals in all were used. The writer found no delay in the healing of corneal burns in vitamin A-deficient rats, but only in those deficient also in protein (see Chapter 6, Section IF).

Descemet's endothelium has received little attention in histological studies of the eye in vitamin A deficiency. Ramalingaswami *et al.* (1955)

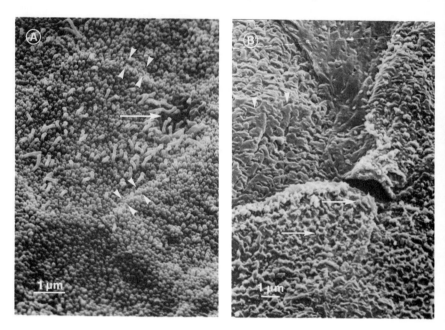

FIG. 9. (A) Corneal conjunctiva. A fine carpet of microprojections, primarily microvilli, texture the flat, polygonal cells of the epithelial sheet, the numerous microvilli obscure the junctions (arrowheads) between cells, the orifice (arrow) probably representing an opening to a resting goblet cell. (B) Six-week vitamin A-deficient conjunctiva. Smaller numbers of stubby, mound-like, irregular microprojections (arrows) are common on the surface cells. Broad, reticulate microplicae (arrowheads) are common. The cell margins are readily apparent, often separated from contiguous cells. From Pfister and Renner (1978).

found mild degenerative changes in the corneal endothelium of one eye of one monkey out of three deficient in the vitamin. Mori (1922a,b) had been able to demonstrate keratohyalin granules in vitamin A deficiency in the conjunctiva, but they also occur in the cells of the intermediate and superficial regions of the cornea, and their origin was studied in the mouse with the electron microscope (Sheldon and Zetterqvist, 1956a,b). The cells of the basal layer contained numerous and apparently normal mitochondria but in the intermediate layers where keratinization was in progress the mitochondria, although numerous, were distorted with dense areas within the matrix. These dense areas appeared to be identical with the keratohyalin granules seen by light microscopy and it was suggested that they arise in vitamin A deficiency from interference with the normal metabolism of the mitochondria. An interesting electron microscopic study of the changes in

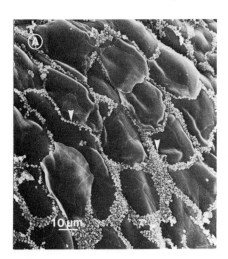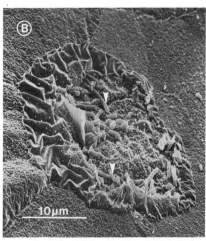

FIG. 10. Distribution of presumed bacterial forms in 6-week vitamin A-deficient eyes. (A) Conjunctiva. Cocci (arrowheads) in this specimen formed a net-like distribution in the valleys of fine wrinkles of the surface. (B) Cornea. Bacilli (arrowheads) in this specimen were largely confined to severely degenerated cells which were distributed randomly over the cornea. From Pfister and Renner (1978).

the surface of conjunctiva and cornea in vitamin A-deficient guinea pigs has recently been made by Pfister and Renner (1978) (Figs. 9, 10, 11).

Before leaving the pathological aspects of vitamin A deficiency as it affects the anterior segment of the eye, attention may be drawn to the fact that the nature of keratomalacia is still little understood. The colliquative necrosis which the cornea undergoes in the advanced stage of vitamin A deficiency appears to be a unique process with no precise parallel in any other tissue or any other disease state in the rest of the body. Infection from outside, in both man and animals, undoubtedly plays a part but just what that part is has not been fully elucidated. Johnson (1943) applied liquid paraffin and metaphen ointment to the eyes of rats with severe xerophthalmia and prevented corneal ulceration, probably partly as a mechanical and partly as an anti-infective effect. The precarious nutrition of the cornea might be expected to make that structure susceptible, but that this alone cannot be responsible is shown by the fact that the lens, which has a poorer supply still, is not affected in vitamin A deficiency.

It has long been suspected that vitamin A deficiency is a necessary factor, but not sufficient to cause keratomalacia. In the germ-free rat (Beaver, 1961; Rogers *et al.*, 1971) corneal liquefaction does not occur. The lacrimal and orbital glands undergo squamous metaplasia with almost no inflammatory changes. The cornea has a thin superficial layer of keratinized cells, but inflammation and vascularization are absent. Beitch (1970) compared the effects of extirpation of the lacrimal gland on the corneal epithelium of

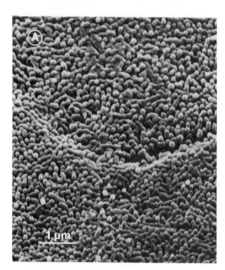 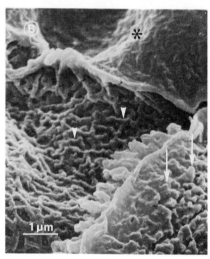

FIG. 11. (A) High magnification view of the control cornea surface discloses the high density of fine microprojections, tightness of intercellular junctions, and plasmalemmal integrity. (B) In comparison, this micrograph of a vitamin A-deficient cornea shows three abnormal surface morphologies. Sparse numbers of moundlike, mis-shapen microprojections (arrows) are noted on the irregular surfaces. Netlike, broad microplicae (arrowheads) or no surface microprojections (asterisk) are present in two other cells. Surface cells frequently were separated from one another and lifting off the epithelial sheet. From Pfister and Renner (1978).

the rat with those of vitamin A deficiency. Extirpation resulted in changes similar to those seen in man in the condition keratoconjunctivitis sicca, but keratinization was less extensive than in vitamin A-deficient animals, and there was neither oedema nor vascularization in extirpation.

Kreger and Griffin (1975) demonstrated that the organism *Serratia marcesceus* produced extracellular proteases *in vitro* that were capable of causing rapid and extensive damage in the rabbit cornea. Collagenase (EC 3.4.24.3) is secreted during culture of the normal cornea in several species, including man, and more of this enzyme than normal is secreted during ulceration. Pirie *et al.* (1975) have shown that proteolytic and specific collagenolytic activity is greater in media from retinol-deficient rat corneas than in the normal. The level of hydroxyproline was increased in parallel with the increase in enzyme activity.

Studies on the pathogenesis of ulceration in the alkali-burned cornea (Brown *et al.*, 1970) may shed some light on the nature of the not-dissimilar liquefaction of keratomalacia. These workers showed that collagenase from ulcerated tissues of the alkali-burned cornea produced full thickness ulcers in intact alkali-burned corneas when injected intralamellarly. The enzyme is produced by the epithelial and cellular elements of the stroma. In vitamin A deficiency lack of mucus in the tear film predisposes to instability of the precorneal film and to dryness of the cornea. This dryness leads to epithelial damage and corneal ulceration. Disruption of the integrity of this anatomical barrier may activate collagenases of the corneal epithelium and stroma. In addition, secondary infection is facilitated and this could cause corneal damage directly and also by the activation of corneal collagenases. Kessler *et al.* (1977) reported that *Pseudomonas aeruginosa*, a leading cause of severe central ulcers of the cornea, produces a very active protease. The host response produces collagenolytic and proteoglycanolytic enzymes which may further the process of dissolution. Smolin *et al.* (1979) produced amelioration of herpes simplex keratitis in rabbits with a large systemic dose of vitamin A.

There have been suggestions that corneal liquefaction is not just the final stage of vitamin A deficiency, but that it supervenes only if additional deficiency is present. Protein malnutrition is usually invoked. The confusion has arisen because of the almost invariable joint occurrence of both states in human xerophthalmia (see Section IIIA7a). In well-controlled pair-fed animal studies vitamin A deficiency alone produces keratomalacia. It also results when animals fed vitamin A only in the form of retinoic acid have this withheld and develop an acute deficiency in which anorexia and low protein intake play no part. Furthermore, protein deficiency has been shown actually to delay the onset of eye lesions in the vitamin A-deficient rat (McLaren, 1959), probably by decreasing growth and consequently vitamin A requirement. The only sure role of protein deficiency is its effect in diminishing circulating RBP, as does vitamin A deficiency, and impairing delivery of retinol to the tissues. It may be concluded that local corneal damage plays a decisive part in keratomalacia, and this is consistent with observations in animals and man that the two eyes are frequently affected to different degrees.

C. The Posterior Segment

As early as 1907 Hess observed the eating habits of hens before and after a period spent in the dark. He found that the exposure to darkness enabled them to go on eating in a less intense light than when they had no such period in darkness. In this way he demonstrated the phenomenon of dark adaptation. Although it had been known for centuries that night blindness was a feature of a certain kind of malnutrition the experimental work in the earlier years of this century on changes produced in the eye was dominated by the gross blinding effects on the anterior segment. It was not until 1925 that Holm showed that rats deficient in vitamin A suffered from night blindness. An ingenious method was devised to do this. The animals were taught to jump across a gap to the safety of their cages. Those deficient in vitamin A would only behave normally when the intensity of light was increased or after they were given the vitamin. The night blindness occurred before there was any other evidence of avitaminosis. In passing it may be noted that hemeralopia (which strictly speaking means impairment of day vision) and nyctalopia are terms which are both used for night blindness but for the sake of clarity will not be used here. In Holm's deficient rats night blindness did not develop unless the animals had been previously exposed to bright light for considerable periods. We know now that this was due to the bleaching of visual purple in bright light, and it was the same worker (Fridericia and Holm, 1925) who showed that these deficient animals showed a subnormal rate of regeneration of visual purple. In 1931 Tansley confirmed these results and found that the retinas of vitamin A-deficient rats contained subnormal amounts of visual purple. The visual purple was extracted from the retinas by a dilute solution of digitonin and quantitatively measured by a photographic method. These results were confirmed for the rabbit by Scullica and Fulchignoni (1937). De Leonibus (1939) showed that the curve of retinal glycolysis was lowered more slowly in deficient rats than in normal.

Up until this time there was no evidence to show that vitamin A was involved directly in the visual processes, but only that it had an influence on the formation of visual purple. The first step toward providing this proof was taken by Holm (1929) with the detection of the vitamin in the retina of the calf, and this was confirmed for the pig by Yudkin (1931). The concentrations detected were low and it was quite possible that the retina contained no more than other tissues.

The first description of the histological changes in the retina in vitamin A deficiency was given by Tansley (1934) in the rat. They consisted of degeneration of the rods and the nuclear layers. (Ishikawa (1921) had previously briefly mentioned alterations in the rods in the rat.) Johnson (1939) confirmed this work with a more detailed study, showing the progression of the degeneration beginning with the visual cells and affecting in order the outer nuclear layer, the pigmented epithelial layer, the outer molecular and inner nuclear layers. The rods stained palely in their outer segments, being thinned at their junction with the inner segments and showing final degeneration. The external limiting membrane disappeared and the nuclei of the outer nuclear layer took on an "untidy" appearance, being pushed apart, and there was a characteristic detachment of the layer from the outer pigmented layer. The outer nuclear and molecular layers became greatly reduced and this change finally affected the inner nuclear layer.

However, the classical research of Wald several years later proved that vitamin A directly participates in dark adaptation. In studies using the frog, pig, sheep, and cattle he found vitamin A in the retinas and combined pigment epithelia and choroid layers (Wald, 1935a). The absorption of the vitamin in ultraviolet light at 328 and at 620 nm by the antimony trichloride test, and its antixerophthalmic and growth-promoting properties were all used for its identification. The participation of the vitamin in the changes accompanying dark adaptation was shown (Wald, 1935b) by experiments on the retina of the bullfrog, *Rana catesbiana*. Wald found that the dark- adapted retina contained only a trace of vitamin A which could be extracted in the dark without affecting the visual purple. After exposure to light for a short time a further extraction produced a yellow pigment which he called retinene. The final stage in the story was completed by allowing retinas bleached by light to stand for about an hour at 25 °C either in the dark or in the light and observing that the yellow colour seen immediately after light adaptation was lost, that extraction produced no retinene, and that in its place substantial amounts of vitamin A were present. On the basis of these experiments Wald devised a cycle which, despite the fact that modifications have had to be made subsequently, remains of fundamental importance in both the field of visual research and of research on the function of vitamin A. We know now that vitamin A does not combine directly with protein to form visual purple and that visual yellow is more complicated than represented there. That vitamin A deficiency affects the visual thresholds of both cones and rods will be mentioned further in Section IIIA4.

When light falls on the retina a change of potential is produced. A record of the changes occurring in this way is known as an electroretinogram (ERG). Electroretinography of experimental animals has proved to be more reliable and informative in the assessment of vitamin A status than have photometric determinations of visual response under conditions of dark adaptation. Charpentier (1936) measured the curve of dark adaptation in normal and deficient rats by using a constant light stimulus and plotting the height of the b-wave at intervals after preliminary light adaptation. He found that there was some reduction in the size of the b-wave in vitamin A deficiency. Waters (1950) showed that the sensitivity of the retina in seven rabbits gradually decreased as the vitamin A deficiency state progressed. A rise in the final rod threshold measured in this way could be detected before there were any corneal changes. The ERG was restored to normal by the administration of vitamin A. Waters (1952) also examined the dark adaptation of pigeons deficient in vitamin A by this method. The pigeon retina has almost no rods. In a pigeon with very little vitamin A in the liver there was no impairment of dark adaptation. In view of the fact that vitamin A, in the form of its aldehyde retinal, plays a part in cone as well as rod vision it may be concluded from this that the requirements of the pigeon for this function are much less than those of the rabbit.

Mann *et al.* (1946) failed to find any evidence of retinal damage in their vitamin A-deficient rabbits, and pointed out the occurrence of retinal degeneration in stocks of inbred rats as a possible pitfall in interpretation when this animal is used. However, it may be that the deficiency was not sufficiently severe in these rabbits to affect the retina. In the monkey, Ramalingaswami *et al.* (1955) also found atrophy of the visual cells and degeneration of the pigment epithelium. One animal had retinal damage without involvement of the cornea and they conclude from this that the retina may be affected more frequently than would be indicated by the occurrence of xerophthalmia.

Sorsby *et al.* (1966) fed rabbits a diet free of vitamin A but containing retinoic acid. After about 10 months white dots appeared in the fundus, first at the periphery, with the central area below the optic disc affected last. These changes were irreversible. Histologically the white dots appeared to be aggregates of eosinophilic debris. As in Uyemura's disease and retinitis albi punctatus (Section IIIA4i) only the pigment epithelium showed substantial changes, with the rods little affected. This differs from the rat (see below) in which the changes occur first in the rod outer segment, there is a fairly rapid decrease in the number of visual cells and the pigment epithelium remains normal.

Retinal degenerative changes have been reported in the cat (Scott and Greaves, 1964) but from other studies in this species it is evident that vitamin A deficiency was not responsible (See Chapter 6, Section IE).

Hayes (1974) produced typical xerophthalmia and keratomalacia in New World cebus and Old World cynomolgus monkeys. Accompanying these anterior segment changes was retinal degeneration, most marked in the macula area and less in the periphery. Structural disruption was more advanced in cones than in rods (Fig. 12). This is surprising when it is recalled that cone visual pigments are synthesized more rapidly than those of the rods and cones have a much greater affinity for retinal.

Dowling and Wald (1958) showed that a consistent series of events takes place, starting with depletion of liver stores, then fall in blood level, and followed shortly afterward by evidence of tissue deprivation. The first of

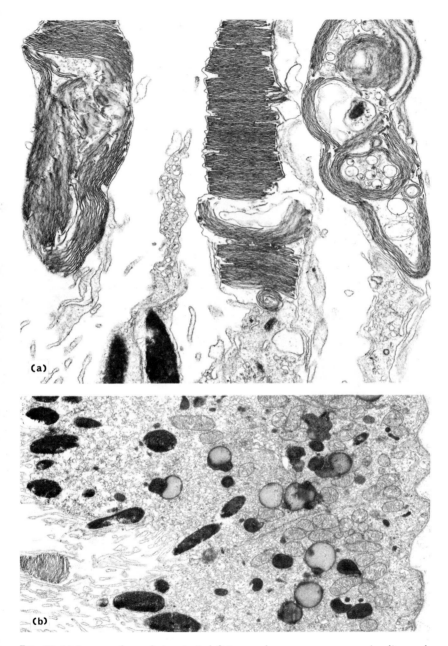

FIG. 12. (a) In more advanced vitamin A deficiency rod outer segments were also disrupted, as evidenced by these tips from three outer segments adjoining the pigment epithelium (*PE*) in the paramacular retina (×12 700). (b) Pigment epithelium from the same vitamin A deficient monkeys contains an abnormal number of lipid-laden lysosomes (×8700). From Hayes (1974).

these is night blindness with changes in the ERG, the visual pigments losing their prosthetic group, retinal. The protein components of the visual pigments, the opsins, decline later but only when there are other signs of general tissue disintegration in the eye and elsewhere.

In a further series of experiments (Dowling, 1960) the fact that retinoic acid prevents the general tissue deterioration in vitamin A deficiency but is not reduced *in vivo* to either retinal or the vitamin itself was used to study the effects of the deficiency over a longer period. Rats dosed with retinoic acid and fed a vitamin A-deficient diet became extremely night blind and eventually completely blind but did not succumb to the systemic effects of vitamin A deficiency. It was shown that together with the decline in rhodopsin content of the eye there was a rise of the logarithm of the electroretinographic threshold. Light adaptation also decreases the rhodopsin content of the eye and raises the ERG threshold. During dark adaptation the rhodopsin content of the eye increases in parallel with the fall of the logarithm of the ERG. It was shown that the potentials of the ERG arise in the visual and the bipolar cell layers (Brown and Wiesel, 1958; Noell, 1958). The loss of the a-wave of the ERG accompanies the degeneration of the outer segments, and when later the remaining part of the visual cell degenerates the rest of the ERG disappears (Fig. 13).

Normally the rat after about 8 weeks on a vitamin A-deficient diet becomes sick and rapidly dies, at about the same time as the retina is beginning to degenerate. By taking advantage of the fact that retinoic acid prevents general tissue degeneration and death, without being reduced *in vivo* to retinol or the vitamin, which are necessary for vision, the Harvard workers (Dowling, 1960) have been able to follow the changes in the retina for as long as 10 months. Figure 14 shows the progressive changes in these animals. In (a) the retina is perfectly normal. It belonged to a rat fed the vitamin A-free diet for 10 months but supplemented with vitamin A. After 2 months on the deficient diet supplemented with retinoic acid the retina has begun to degenerate (b), the first change being in the outer segments with the rods staining less intensely than normal. In (c), after 6 months on the diet, only scattered fragments of the outer segments remain and the inner segments and visual cell nuclei are reduced to about half their number. At 10 months (d) no inner or outer segments are visible and the layer of visual cell nuclei is reduced to a single incomplete row.

These workers have also shown that a surprising degree of regeneration may take place with vitamin A therapy, provided degeneration has not progressed too far. In Fig. 15 the histological changes and those in the ERG are shown following vitamin A. In Fig. 15a is shown the normal retina of a rat fed vitamin A for $6\frac{1}{2}$ months. The changes in the retina of a litter-mate fed the same vitamin A-free diet for the same period are shown in

Fig. 15b and are seen to be strictly comparable with those in Fig. 14c. In Fig. 15c is shown the retina of a third litter-mate fed a large dose (1 mg) of vitamin A 16 days before the end of the experiment and further supplements before being killed. This third animal has regenerated new outer segments

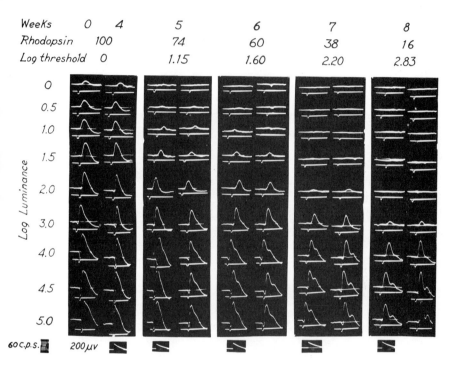

Weeks	0	4	5	6	7	8
Rhodopsin		100	74	60	38	16
Log threshold	0		1.15	1.60	2.20	2.83

FIG. 13. Effects of vitamin A deficiency on the electroretinogram. The top three lines show the number of weeks on the deficient diet; the rhodopsin content of the retina expressed as percentage of normal and the logarithm of the threshold, the lowest luminance needed to evoke a perceptible electroretinogram. The average threshold is set arbitrarily at 1, therefore log threshold = 0. As the rhodopsin declines, the electroretinographic threshold rises and the electroretinogram changes characteristically in form. From Dowling (1960).

which are quite normal in appearance. The number of outer segments remains about half the normal as there has been no multiplication of visual cells. There is a remarkable correspondence between the permanent rise in threshold of the ERG and the loss in the number of visual cells.

With the aid of the electron microscope it has further been shown that while the outer segments undergo marked internal changes, none occur in the inner segments, the visual cell nuclei, or the synapses before they

Months of diet

Control   2   6   10

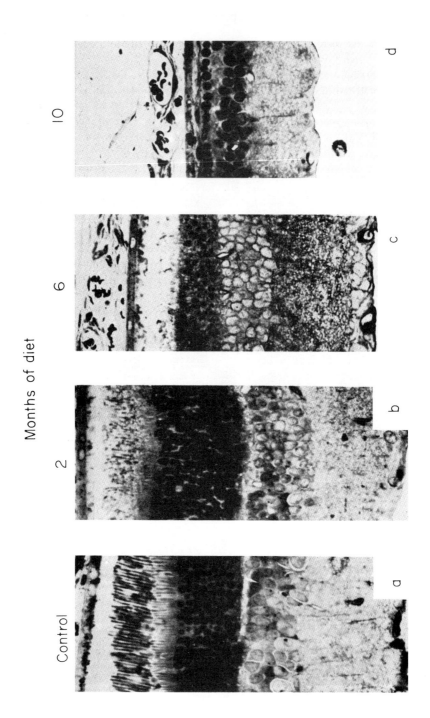

a   b   c   d

disappear, which they only do after the outer segments are almost gone (Dowling and Gibbons, 1961).

Noell *et al.* (1971) demonstrated the dependence on light of the effect of vitamin A deficiency on the retina. Depleted rats kept in the dark had a virtually normal ERG and rhodopsin for 5–6 months, but those kept in weak cyclic light lost rhodopsin continuously. It was further shown (Noell and Albrecht, 1971) that diffuse retinal irradiation by visible light ordinarily encountered (1500 lx fluorescent light through a green filter) causes severe retinal damage in 40 hours in rats, especially albino, and some other species. There is death of visual cells, degeneration of pigment epithelium and irreversibly low ERG. Vitamin A deficiency protects against this damage. The normal protection depends on a long-term state of cell adaptation to light. The normal diurnal cycle of light and dark seems to be the essential factor in controlling visual cell viability and susceptibility.

Schneider *et al.* (1977) found that in the vitamin A-deficient rat visual sensitivity (measured behaviourally) declined with rhodopsin loss and as a function of rhodopsin depletion was more similar to the loss measured electrophysiologically by Dowling and Wald (1958) than to the loss (measured behaviourally) during dark adaptation following intense light in man. This would seem to conflict with the results obtained by Sauberlich *et al.* (1974) in their human deprivation study (Section IIIA4a).

Decrease in the number of intramembrane particles in the discs of rod outer segments has been visualized by freeze-fracture electron microscopy and there is evidence that these particles are rhodopsin molecules (Hong and Hubbell, 1972; Jan and Revel, 1974).

Vitamin A deficiency has been induced in *Xenopus laevis* embryos, larvae and adults to study photoreceptor thresholds and visual pigments (Witkovsky *et al.*, 1976; Bridges, 1977).

Of special interest is the report of Berson (1973) in which vitamin A

FIG. 14. Retinal histology of rats raised on vitamin A-free diets and supplemented with retinoic acid. (a) The retina from a control animal that had been raised for 10 months on a vitamin A-free diet supplemented with vitamin A. The structure is entirely normal. (b) The retina of an animal raised for 2 months on vitamin A-free diet supplemented with retinoic acid. The primary change has occurred in the outer segments which are disorientated and stain less intensely. The rest of the visual cell appears normal, as do the other layers of the retina. (c) After 6 months, the outer segments have almost entirely disappeared. The inner segments and visual cell nuclei are reduced to about half the normal number. The rest of the retina and the pigment epithelium appear normal. (d) Retina from an animal maintained for 10 months on the diet supplemented with retinoic acid. The visual cells have disappeared, except for one irregular row of visual cell nuclei. Other parts of the retina appear normal. From Dowling (1960).

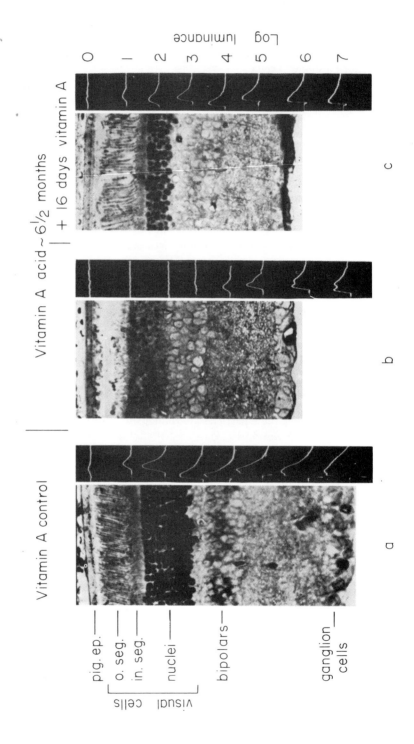

Vitamin A control

Vitamin A acid ~ 6½ months + 16 days vitamin A

pig. ep.
o. seg.
in. seg.
nuclei
bipolars
ganglion cells

visual cells

Log luminance

0
1
2
3
4
5
6
7

a

b

c

I. ANIMAL STUDIES OF VITAMIN A DEFICIENCY

deficiency was shown to alter cone structure and function in the cone-dominant retina of the ground squirrel. In this species Remé and Young (1977) found that hibernation led to degeneration of the cones with rapid recovery following arousal.

Retinal dystrophy occurs in the rat as an autosomal recessive trait: 12–15 days after birth there is degeneration of photoreceptor cells. At this time there is an increase above normal in retinol content of the pigment epithelium with abnormally low concentration of retinyl esters. A defect in esterification has been postulated (Nicotra *et al.*, 1976). In dystrophic rats the normal phagocytic removal of displaced outer segment material by the pigment epithelium is impaired (Herron *et al.*, 1969). Delmelle *et al.* (1975) maintained two strains of rat with hereditary retinal dystrophy in the dark. From day 20 of the experiment there was progressive decrease in width of the outer nuclear layer, increase in rhodopsin content, failure to transfer retinol into the pigment epithelium after photopic bleaching, and decreased ability to convert retinal to retinol after light exposure. In animals made vitamin A-deficient these changes were enhanced.

The final subject to be considered in this section on the ocular manifestations of vitamin A deficiency involving the posterior segment is the occurrence of degenerative changes in the optic nerve. In the expectation of producing xerophthalmia in pigs Hughes *et al.* (1929) fed these animals at weaning a diet of white maize and tankage and they were allowed access to a sunlit yard to prevent rickets. At first only a slight watering of the eyes was produced but after 6–10 months all the 27 animals developed a marked nervous disorder with blindness, incoordination, and spasms. The condition was fatal in those animals that were not killed for study or treated by rich sources of vitamin A with recovery.

In 1935 Moore *et al.* published the results of 12 years' work in which they had been investigating the effect of the quality of hay on the health of dairy

---

FIG. 15. Recovery from night blindness. Three animals were kept for $6\frac{1}{2}$ months on a vitamin A-deficient diet supplemented with retinol (control) and retinoic acid. The retinal histology and electroretinograms of the control (a) are normal. Sixteen days prior to the end of the experiment one of the other animals was fed a large dose of vitamin A. Its electroretinograms before being fed vitamin A are shown (b) along with a retinal section from the third animal, similarly night blind. The electroretinograms show a high degree of night blindness. The retina shows an almost complete loss of outer segments and reduction of nuclei to about half the normal number. After recovery (c) the remaining cells have regenerated new outer segments. But there has been no increase of visual cell number. The electroretinograms closely resemble the normal in threshold level and form, but remain much reduced in size. The reduction in size is permanent and probably due to the loss of visual cells. From Dowling (1960).

cows and calves. Some calves born of mothers given a poor roughage diet or calves receiving this diet during the first few months of life were found to be blind, not from xerophthalmia, but with clear corneae, dilated pupils, and sometimes accompanied by other nervous system signs such as partial paralysis of the front quarters, spasms, and a peculiar position of the head. The blindness was shown to be due to pressure by bone on the optic nerve (see below). Further work by Moore (1939) showed that calves became night blind with papilloedema and constriction of the optic nerve leading to total blindness on a diet low in carotene and that all these changes could be prevented by the administration of crystalline carotene. He had suggested that a rise in intracranial pressure might be responsible for these lesions in view of accompanying syncope, spasms, and incoordination. That there was a rise in spinal fluid pressure in vitamin A-deficient calves was shown shortly afterward (Moore and Sykes, 1941). The severity of papilloedema, incoordination, and liability to syncope and convulsions directly paralleled the degree of increase in cerebrospinal fluid pressure. The same worker (Moore, 1941) demonstrated night blindness and a mottled appearance of the tapetum nigrum and lucidum in mature cows on a low carotene ration. The latter changes are well illustrated by colour drawings of the fundus. Histological evidence of degeneration in various nerves and nervous tracts, including the optic thalamus and optic nerves, was found by Hughes *et al.* (1929) in their vitamin A-deficient pigs. The relationship between bone and these nerve lesions was next brought out by the demonstration in dairy cows and calves deficient in vitamin A of injury to the optic nerve precisely at the optic foramen, which was greatly diminished in relation to the size of the nerve (Moore *et al.*, 1935) (Fig. 16a,b). The possible part played by an increase in intracranial pressure is mentioned in the preceding paragraphs. In addition to this the role of vitamin A in regulating the modelling of bone was especially emphasized by Mellanby (1943, 1944, 1947). He was able to show that in vitamin A deficiency there was an increased and disorganized activity of both osteoblasts and osteoclasts, and although the end result was not without order it always caused a thickening and dysplasia of bone. There was a tendency for the formation of soft cancellous bone rather than that of the hard compact type. Mellanby showed that vitamin A deficiency had no effect on the main factor in growth, the laying down by osteoblasts of bone. Support for the hypothesis that an elevated spinal fluid pressure is brought about principally by bone growth abnormalities came from a study in the vitamin A-deficient baby pig using radioactive sulphur (Frape *et al.*, 1959). They found that the severity of the deficiency was paralleled by the accumulation of ^{35}S at the costochondral junction, growth of bone, and the

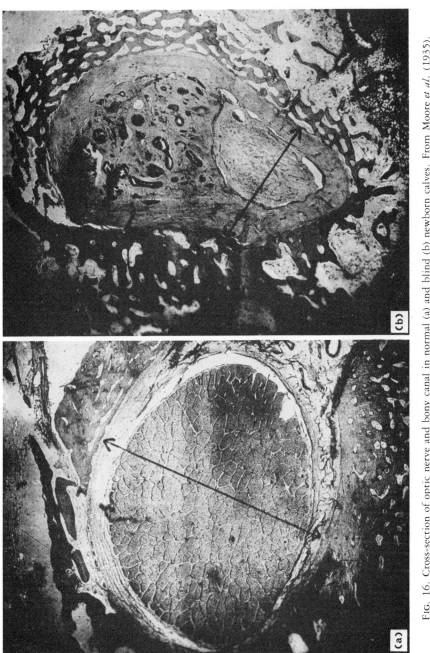

Fig. 16. Cross-section of optic nerve and bony canal in normal (a) and blind (b) newborn calves. From Moore *et al.* (1935).

cerebrospinal fluid pressure. Thus in severe deficiency there was a maximum accumulation of radioactive sulphur, minimum bone growth, and maximum cerebrospinal fluid pressure.

It was the demonstration by Mellanby of the continuing growth of bone that weakened the alternative and rival theory of Wolbach and Bessey (1941). However, we still do not know enough to be in a position to reconcile the differing views and provide a unifying theory (Moore, 1957b). Wolbach and Bessey produced signs of nerve damage in young rats deficient in vitamin A. Histological examination showed that the underlying pathology was an overcrowding of the bony cavities and foramina of the body resulting from an apparent retardation of the growth of bone accompanied by the normal, and therefore relatively greater, growth of nerve. Seemingly of a similar nature is the explanation of Blakemore *et al.* (1957) for the optic nerve lesion in their calves deficient in vitamin A. They found no evidence of direct pressure on the optic nerve by the surrounding bone but a greater relative growth of the nerve as compared with bone, that caused the nerve to become unduly long, to kink, and finally to break. That the picture here too was complex is shown by the evidence presented of disproportionate growth of bones of the skull, a malformation without any actual narrowing of the optic foramen and a rise in intracranial pressure.

The interesting possibility that vitamin A might have a hitherto unsuspected function in controlling the formation of the cerebrospinal fluid was suggested by the work of Millen *et al.* (1953, 1954). They first of all showed that there was a very high incidence (about 80%) of hydrocephalus in young rabbits born to dams receiving a vitamin A-free diet for many weeks before mating. Among other features of pressure of bone on nerves was constriction of the optic nerves at the optic foramina (Fig. 17). They found no evidence of disordered bone growth in these animals and although in their first report they considered stenosis of the cerebral aqueduct to be the cause of the hydrocephalus they later thought that this, if present, was not sufficient alone to account for the rise in pressure. The absence of dilatation of the aqueduct together with the wide expansion of the lateral and third ventricles which they found suggested that the cause might be sought at the point of production of the cerebrospinal fluid in the choroid plexus. There is some evidence that overproduction of fluid may be one of the causes of human hydrocephalus but in the few cases of hydrocephalus in man associated with vitamin A deficiency the mechanism was not evident.

Dehority *et al.*, 1960 investigated this point in the vitamin A-deficient calf. The calves were depleted initially of vitamin A and were then maintained at one of three levels of plasma vitamin A by rations differing in carotene content. Those on the two lower levels showed a marked increase in the cerebrospinal fluid pressure but there was very little change in the composition of the fluid. It was concluded that the rise in pressure resulted from an increase in volume of fluid due to increased formation, decreased absorption, or perhaps both. The slight increase in intraocular pressure was

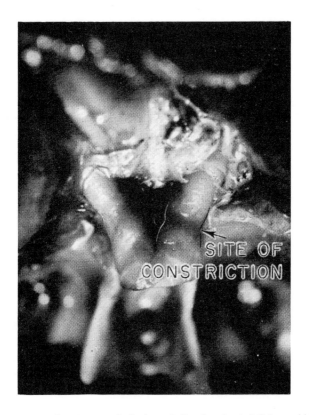

Fig. 17. Constriction of optic nerve in hydrocephalic vitamin A-deficient rabbit ($\times$ 7.5). From Millen *et al.* (1953).

not significant but the composition changed, the potassium level decreasing accompanied by an increase in chloride content. The significance of these changes is not known.

D. Invertebrates

Vitamin A deficiency in an invertebrate was first demonstrated by Goldsmith *et al.* (1964) using house flies (*Musca domestica*). Reared under sterile conditions and deprived of carotenoids or retinol, the visual receptor sensitivities of the flies by ERG were more than 2 log units on average subnormal, in the near violet (340 nm) and visible (500 nm) wavelengths. β-Carotene added to the larval food prevented this effect. Several generations reared under carotene-free but not sterile conditions showed no further loss in sensitivity. This suggests that carotene stored in the eyes (or elsewhere) prevents commencing blindness in the first generation and that micro-organisms can supply small amounts and prevent complete blindness in later generations.

The effect of vitamin A deficiency on the retina of the compound eye of a moth (*Manduca sexta*) was studied by Carlson *et al.* (1967). They reported extensive degeneration in the retinal epithelium and underlying nervous and connective tissues, although normal growth, metamorphosis and reproduction occurred. The changes were reversed when the moths were reared on tobacco, their usual diet. This group (Boëthius *et al.*, 1972) later found that despite these structural abnormalities, receptor potential was normal in configuration, amplitude and spectral sensitivity.

In the eye of mosquitos Brammer and White (1969) found both severe impairment of electrical response and ultrastructural damage, consisting of absence of multivesicular bodies and the presence of masses of smooth membrane lamellae near the nucleus.

The fruit fly (*Drosophila melanogaster*) has been used to study the effects of vitamin A deprivation on the fine structure, photopigment content and sensitivity of invertebrate receptors (Stark and Zitzmann, 1976). In common with those of vertebrates these have similar 8-nm intramembrane particles in the stacked microvilli which form their light-sensitive rhabdomeres. The number of particles is comparable to the number of pigment molecules present and is dependent upon the state of light adaptation (Brandenburger *et al.*, 1975). There is strong evidence that most of these particles, like those in vertebrate photoreceptors (see Section IC), are rhodopsin molecules (Harris *et al.*, 1977).

E. Sex Differences

It has been shown that in vitamin A deficiency in the rat there are more fatalities among males than females (Coward, 1942) and Mayer and Krehl (1948) found that males developed signs of deficiency before females. In a study in which the effect of both sex and protein level on the development of xerophthalmia was investigated in the rat the writer (McLaren, 1959) found in those animals that lived long enough to develop the eye signs that females lived significantly longer and developed xerophthalmia in a significantly longer time than males. The reason for this marked susceptibility of the male, which is also true in man (Section II7e), is not known. In this last experiment it was found that this effect of sex was reversed, as far as survival time was concerned, in those animals receiving only 4 and 6% protein. The body weight of these animals was stationary and males survived considerably longer than females. It may be that the greater growth of the male under conditions where it can occur accounts for the using up of the stores of vitamin A more quickly and the consequent earlier onset of signs of deficiency and death.

II. Animal Studies of Hypervitaminosis A

The toxic effects of large doses of vitamin A are now well recognized both in experimental animals and in man. Congenital anomalies have been produced in this way in the rat, and among the organs affected has been the eye. These ocular changes are described, together with other congenital eye lesions, due to nutritional deficiency, in Chapter 9, Section IA2.

Early experiments with large doses of vitamin A concentrates caused death in mice and rats, the animals becoming progressively emaciated, with paralysis of the hind limbs and alopecia of the head. The liver, kidneys, and heart were found to be the seat of degenerative changes and the lungs and digestive tract showed hyperaemia and haemorrhages. With more refined concentrates it was later shown that the bones became very fragile. Moore and Wang (1945) demonstrated the toxicity of a sample of crystalline vitamin A acetate, giving a dose of 25 000 to 40 000 i.u. (international units) daily to rats. Growth was checked, many bones became fractured, there were subcutaneous and intramuscular haemorrhages, and death resulted in about 3 weeks. One notable feature of this syndrome was pronounced exophthalmos. It is probable that this unusual prominence of the eyeballs resulted from intraorbital haemorrhage together with the general depression of growth affecting the bony orbit more than the tissues of the eye. Exophthalmos was also a feature of hypervitaminosis A in the fox and mink (Helgebostad, 1955).

It will be recalled that deficiency of vitamin A causes a rise in cerebrospinal fluid pressure in several animal species but that in the one instance where the intraocular pressure was also measured there was no significant rise in the latter (Section IC, above). The effect of vitamin A excess has been studied on the ocular tension in the rabbit (Hartmann and Saraux, 1957). These authors claimed that the tension fell 48 hours after the ingestion of 300 000 i.u. of vitamin A and that this was accompanied by an increased elimination of ascorbic acid in the urine.

III. Human Studies of Vitamin A Deficiency

A. Primary Vitamin A Deficiency, Xerophthalmia

1. Nomenclature

Deficiency disease has perhaps been dogged more than most branches of medicine by problems of nomenclature. Some names have doubtful origins in the distant past—such as pellagra (Italian, *pelle* skin; *agro* rough), beriberi (Singhalese, extreme weakness), and rickets (English, "wrick" to twist)—while that of scurvy is altogether obscure. Despite our increased knowledge today we seem to be able to do little better in this respect, for the most recent nutritional disease entity to emerge has a host of local and several aetiological names, but the most generally popular—"kwashiorkor"—is borrowed from the Ga language of Ghana, and means "the sickness the older child gets when the next baby is born".

The terms which have been applied to vitamin A deficiency eye disease have been no exception to the rule. Difficulty in seeing at night is simply referred to here as night blindness. "Nyctalopia" means the same thing but is pedantic. "Hemeralopia," however, means precisely the opposite (Greek, *hemera* day) and although in general use on the continent, should be avoided. The names given to the disease as it affects the conjunctiva and cornea have been numerous. Oomen (1961) culled many of these from the older literature and discussed in some detail their varied merits. As he points out, they tend to fall into one of three groups as they refer chiefly to the aetiology of the disease, describe the eye changes, or the general symptoms. Oomen argues very convincingly for the retention of the term "xerophthalmia" to indicate the clinical syndrome as a whole. The use of xerophthalmia in this way has received the blessing of the World Health Organization (McLaren *et al.*, 1966; WHO, 1976) and this practice will also be followed here. Other terms such as "night blindness," "Bitot's spot," and "keratomalacia" will be used when reference is made particularly to some definite aspect of the condition of the eye to which these terms apply. "Xerophthalmia" will generally be replaced by the terms "xerosis of the conjunctiva" and "xerosis of the cornea" when specific changes in these structures only are referred to without any implication as to the general nutritional state.

In the two WHO publications mentioned above, the characteristic ocular manifestations have been described and pictured in colour, in most instances from cases in which the vitamin A deficiency state has been substantiated with markedly depressed serum and liver vitamin A levels. The first Technical Report of WHO (1976) on the subject was a milestone along the hard road leading towards the eradication of xerophthalmia. Most importantly, at this meeting world expert opinion reached a consensus on the method of reporting the ocular lesions, known as the WHO Xerophthalmia Classification (Table I). In addition, a tentative set of criteria were proposed

TABLE I. *WHO Xerophthalmia Classification*

Classification	Signs
	Primary[a]
X1A	Conjunctival xerosis
X1B	Bitot's spot with conjunctival xerosis
X2	Corneal xerosis
X3A	Corneal ulceration with xerosis
X3B	Keratomalacia
	Secondary[b]
XN	Night blindness
XF	Xerophthalmia fundus
XS	Corneal scars

[a] Indicative of clinically active vitamin A deficiency and relatively easily detected in the hospital and field.
[b] Either difficult to assess, less specific, or unrelated to active disease.

for community diagnosis of a xerophthalmia and vitamin A deficiency problem of public health magnitude (Table II). Both of these may require modification in the light of further experience.

TABLE II. *WHO Proposed Criteria for Community Diagnosis*

Clinical
1. X1B in more than 2.0% of the population at risk
2. X2 + X3A + X3B in more than 0.01% of the population at risk
3. XS (attributable to vitamin A deficiency) in more than 0.1% of the population at risk

Biochemical
4. Plasma vitamin A level of less than $10\,\mu g/100\,ml$ in more than 5% of the population at risk.

2. Historical Background

a. Early References

It is widely held that the ancients recognized the effectiveness of liver in curing night blindness. The Ebers papyrus, written about 1600 B.C. in

Egypt, is usually quoted as the source. At about the same time the physicians in China reputedly were giving liver, dung of the flying fox, and tortoise shell for the cure of night blindness (Mar and Read, 1936).

There is, however, complete doubt, which cannot be resolved at this distance in time, as to the identity of the eye disease for which liver was prescribed. Ebbell (1924) made a thorough study of the original texts. He found that Papyrus Ebers 57.11 and the London Medical Papyrus 11.8–12.14 refer to a disease with the vocalized transcription "shaw", or "sharw". It was clearly an eye disease because the prescription in the London Papyrus reads:" Ox-liver cooked on a fire of splet- and barley-stalks, . . . squeeze out the juice of it onto the eyes." In addition there is something about the "steam of the ox-liver" which was also to be used. The Papyrus Ebers says much the same: "Put ox-liver, roast and pressed out, on it." The nature of the eye complaint is not referred to. The London Papyrus ends with," Rub it into his eyes—of the one suffering from "shaw"—with your hand, then he will see immediately."

It is clearly quite specific therapy and not used by the Egyptians for any other illness. Ebbell (1924) stated that the London Papyrus prescribes magical spells which must be used to drive out demons, so the Egyptians evidently thought the disease had magical origins.

It was Dioskurides (De Mat. Med. II.45) and later Greek physicians who used the juice and the steam of roast, or boiled, liver, clearly borrowed from the Egyptians, for a single eye disease which they called "nuktalòpía"—night blindness.

Wolf (1978) has recently reviewed the subject, including early Greek accounts of night blindness, but missed the point that the original condition for which the Egyptians prescribed liver is quite obscure. He reasonably suggested that some of the vitamin A from the liver juice may have entered the lacrimal ducts and reached the throat via the nose, thus being absorbed and ultimately reaching the retina. Accompanying xerophthalmia might have been relieved directly by local application. It is believed that Celsus (25 B.C. to A.D. 50) first used the term xerophthalmia.

It has been suggested that the "white films" of the eyes that affected Tobit as recounted in the Apocryphal book of that name were due to xerophthalmia. There is really nothing in the account to suggest this. We are told that being polluted he slept by the wall of his courtyard and "mine eyes being open the sparrows muted warm dung into mine eyes"—a chemical keratitis. He was 58 years old at the time, prosperous, and celebrating the 7 weeks' feast of Pentecost. After 8 years of blindness he was cured by the local application of bile from a fish. None of this suggests nutritional deficiency. The contention of Etzine (1968) that Tobit suffered from band-shaped nodular dystrophy of the cornea, common in hot and dry climates, is quite fanciful.

Similarly the view of Taylor (1944), that the condition affecting the eyesight and skin of St Hilarion as recorded by St Jerome was due to vitamin A deficiency, must be contested. The only clinical details in the account refer merely to increasing dimness of vision and roughening of the skin and are too vague for any conclusions to be drawn. The saint lived for 3 years on a daily ration of 6 ounces of barley bread and vegetables cooked without oil until the symptoms developed, when he used a cooking oil. Taylor suggests that this was olive oil, but, if this was so it would not have cured a deficiency of vitamin A containing only 20–30 i.u./100 g. This and other vegetable oils are fairly rich in essential fatty acids and the skin condition if it were indeed hyperfollicular keratosis might well have been relieved in this way.

There are two brief references from the time of the Crusades that suggest that night blindness may have been common during sieges. Keys *et al.* (1950) quote the "Historia Damiatina" by Oliverius Scholasticus, which states that in 1221 the crusaders at Damiette were "stricken by blindness at night, although their eyes were open they could not see anything". At Montreal the garrison was reported to have gone blind "for lack of salt" (Fedden and Thomson, 1950).

What appears to be the first reference to what we now term Bitot's spots is given by Grassus Benvenutus of Jerusalem about the same period in his "De oculis": "The second form of paniculus appears on the eye tunics like an opacity or speckled like a fish scale" (Wood, 1929). It is remarkable that some present-day communities also liken the appearance to fish scales.

It would seem that night blindness was widespread in Europe in mediaeval times, for we find a fourteenth century poet in Holland, Jacob van Maerland, referring to the disease and its cure in this way (Bicknell and Prescott, 1953):

He who cannot see at night
Must eat the liver of the goat.
Then he can see all right.

Bayly, who was Queen Elizabeth I's physician, wrote a book on eye diseases in which he recommended "rawe herbes" among which was "eie bright". References were made to mists and films over the eyes but whether these were due to night blindness, or early xerophthalmia, or even conditions not associated with malnutrition is not clear (Drummond and Wilbraham, 1939).

An accurate description of xerophthalmia was given by the French physician Jacques Guillemeau (1585), who also recommended for night blindness "le foye de bouc rosti, estant salé et le manger."

b. The Pre-vitamin Era

With increasing attention on the part of physicians to careful description of disease and a more precise consideration of the related circumstances, the clinical picture began to emerge. Bergen and Weise (1754) seem to have been the first to write about the relationship between dietary deficiency and night blindness and they also noted the association with excessive exposure to sunlight. An English naval surgeon, Bampfield (1814), from his experience with lascars in East India Company ships distinguished two forms of night blindness; the first he called "idiopathic" and the second "scorbutic" because of its occurrence in patients with scurvy. The latter form did not improve with lemon juice, but disappeared when a balanced diet was given.

In 1827 the following interesting letter, published here in full, appeared in the *Edinburgh Journal of Medical Science.* The rapidity of the course of untreated keratomalacia, the important role of diet, and the gravity of the general condition of the patient are all clearly recognized.

> Case of Ulcerated Cornea, from inanition. In a letter to the Editor, from Joseph Brown, M.D., Sunderland.
>
> On going yesterday to visit a poor babe which you know I was attending at ———, I found that both corneae had become opake over a considerable portion of their surface and that ulceration had commenced; and, on repeating my visit today, I found that this ulceration had proceeded so rapidly, that, should the little patient live four and twenty hours longer, I am convinced that the content of the eyes will be discharged. The child, which is six months' old, is as much emaciated as possible, the movement of the intestines being visible through the parietes of the abdomen. It was born prematurely, and never had the breast-milk. Since my attendance, which began ten days ago, its diet has consisted of asses' milk, sugar, and biscuit-powder. But, from the feebleness of the digestive function, it never seems to have derived sufficient nourishment from any food that has been given to it, and has been harassed ever since its birth with bowel complaints. Compare this case with Magendie's account of the dogs fed, or rather starved, on sugar.

The Royal Oculist in Scotland, William Mackenzie, in 1830 published "A Practical Treatise on the Diseases of the Eye" in which he gave an account of xerophthalmia under the name of "conjunctiva arida". He also gave the appropriately descriptive name of "myocephalon", literally "head of a fly", to that stage of keratomalacia in which a small knuckle of iris has prolapsed through the cornea. Also in 1830 von Ammon applied the term "xerosis conjunctivae" to the earliest stage of the condition, a name still in common use. One of the best early descriptions of xerophthalmia and keratomalacia was given by Arlt (1851).

Although the Bordeaux oculist Bitot (1863) is usually given the credit for the first description of the conjunctival spot that bears his name traditionally (see below, Section 3b), this rightfully belongs to Hubbenet (1860), chief medical officer of the small French force in the Crimean War.

He recorded in soldiers and prisoners of war a dry patch of epithelial degeneration situated on the exposed area of the bulb from which small waxy scales sloughed off. Hubbenet, like Bitot after him, noted an association of this lesion with night blindness and further that the more severe cases had loss of the normal lustre of the cornea. There seems little doubt that, as has happened so frequently in the history of medicine, this condition has received the wrong eponym.

Bitot attributed the night blindness that accompanied the conjunctival xerosis in his cases to some corneal disturbance interfering with the passage of light to the retina. However, Netter (1870) rightly disputed this explanation, for his hemeralopes had no xerosis. The true nature of the disturbance was suspected by Parinaud (1881), when he connected night blindness with a retardation in the regeneration of retinal pigment.

The great German ophthalmologist von Graefe (1866) gave a clear description of keratomalacia and in his practice in Berlin saw three or four cases a month. At this time the first account of the condition from a tropical country was given by Gama Lobo (1866), in malnourished children of black slaves on coffee plantations in Brazil. As Oomen (1961) points out, it was not until the turn of the century that the next report from the tropics came from Indonesia (Ouwehand, 1900), where the disease has ever since continued to take tremendous toll of life and sight (Section 8b below).

Therapeutic value was claimed for cod liver oil in the cure of Bitot's spots (Snell, 1881) and night blindness (Kubli, 1887). The former reported 10 cases of "nyctalopia with peculiar appearances on the conjunctiva"; the oldest being 10 years. He noted that most cases occurred in the spring (when dietary intake would have been at a minimum for some time). Other notable papers about this time include those of Evetzki (1890), who described circumscribed epithelial xerosis of the conjunctiva in glass workers who did not complain of night blindness, a recognition of the important role of local irritation, and of Herbert (1897), who reported from India pigmentation of the lower fornix and exposed conjunctiva. Stephenson (1898) demonstrated from Bitot's spot material colonies of xerosis bacilli by culture on blood agar. He also emphasized the variability of the association of spots and night blindness.

When one recalls the relatively advanced state of knowledge in which ophthalmology was during the latter half of the nineteenth century, in comparison with some other medical specialties, it is not surprising that the pathological basis of xerophthalmia was soon established. Saemisch (1876) used the term "epithelial xerosis" to describe the diffuse lesion now known as xerophthalmia. Leber (1883) described the later changes of keratinization and xerosis. He found a thickening of the whole conjunctival and corneal epithelium, a flattening of the superficial cells with disappearance of their nuclei, and a separation of the prickle cells in the deeper layers by leucocytes. The superficial cells were frequently arranged in irregular, wavy bands with the most superficial of all staining diffusely as keratohyalin. Those immediately underneath showed granules of the same material and in these respects these layers exactly resembled the stratum granulosum of the epidermis. In both superficial and deeper cells fatty globules staining deeply with osmic acid were common. A constant feature was the desquamation of degenerated superficial cells and it was noted that the xerosis bacillus (*Corynebacterium xerosis*) was invariably present, both intra- and extracellularly.

It was at this time considered by some that the xerosis bacillus played a causative role in conjunctival xerosis. Its presence on keratinizing conjunctival epithelium has been repeatedly confirmed and it is especially prolific in Bitot's spot material, where its gas-forming properties may possibly account for the foamy nature of these lesions. An account of the histological appearances of the xerotic conjunctiva in six human cases was given by Mayou (1904). He regarded Bitot's spots as being formed from modified secretion from the Meibomian glands.

The relationship to poor general health and infectious disease was noted frequently in early accounts of xerophthalmia with special attention paid to intestinal disorders (Teuscher, 1867; de Gouvêa, 1883). Baas (1894) described both night blindness and xerophthalmia in patients with liver disease and there have been many confirmatory accounts since. There is now reason to believe that impairment of dark adaptation in patients with disease of the liver may not always be due to deficiency of vitamin A (Section B, and Chapter 5, Section IIC).

Early writers recognized the predilection of xerophthalmia for young children. They were frequently infants of the poorer classes or they had been subjected to special nutritional or social stress. It remains true today that the most severe damage that deficiency of vitamin A causes is still in the youngest members of the community, especially among the "toddler" age group, who have broken free from the protective care of the mother but are still not really old enough to fend for themselves.

Although the cure for night blindness had been known since time immemorial, it was not until the last century that the dietary deficiency nature of the condition was recognized. I am indebted to Dr W. J. Darby for drawing my attention to an account of night blindness in the Confederate Army (Hicks, 1867) in which this fact was noted. The author mentions that a constant feature was the failure of the pupil to contract in the light of a single candle, and goes on to attribute the condition to the "meagre diet, absence of vegetables and vegetable oils, and other depressing influences of a soldier's life." Kollock (1890), working among the blacks of South Carolina, was one of the first to recognize the dietary origin of xerophthalmia.

With the turn of the century several further steps forward were taken in the understanding of the nature of the disease. Jensen (1903) was the first to show that xerophthalmia could be cured by an adequate diet and for this purpose used raw cow's milk. It is interesting to note that he observed a rapid improvement on this regime not only as judged by the condition of the eyes and gain in weight but particularly by the disappearance of what he called the "characteristic psychic indifference". This recognition of the profound systemic effects of vitamin A deficiency has not always persisted since this time and the high mortality attributable to the disease in its severest form has also been lost sight of at times.

In 1904 the important observation was made by Mori that the disease known as "hikam", characterized by conjunctival xerosis and keratomalacia and widely prevalent among children aged 2–5 years in Japan, was most common in the children of people living largely on rice, barley and other cereals, beans, and vegetables. It did not occur among fisher folk, and cod liver oil, chicken liver, and eel fat were all effective remedies.

This report of 1400 cases of the condition aroused considerable interest and showed that although xerophthalmia occurred rather sporadically and under special circumstances in Europe, in Japan, and as was shown later in other parts of Asia particularly, the disease was often endemic and affected quite a high proportion of the younger members of the population.

The association of xerophthalmia with an excessive intake of carbohydrate in the diet in infancy was recorded by Czerny and Keller (1906) in their classical monograph on the syndrome they termed *Mehlnährschaden*. It is now recognized that this condition is identical in all basic features with what has been called "the most serious and widespread nutritional disorder known to medical and nutritional science" (Brock and Autret, 1952) and due in essence to a deficiency of protein and excess of carbohydrate in the diet. Many local and other names have been applied to this disease but it will be necessary here to use one, and that chosen, "kwashiorkor", has found wide acceptance. Since Czerny's day there has been a great number of other accounts in which ocular involvement has been described (McLaren, 1958), providing good evidence for the contention that a deficiency of vitamin A is the most common of all vitamin deficiencies associated with protein-energy malnutrition. The worldwide occurrence of this association (Section A9, below) and the ways in which it may arise (Section A7a, below) are dealt with later.

3. The Anterior Segment

a. Xerosis of the Conjunctiva

Dryness of the conjunctiva accompanied by loss of transparency, thickening and wrinkling usually precedes any changes in the cornea and is itself normally preceded by a fall in plasma vitamin A concentration and by deterioration of dark adaptation, although there may be no complaint of night blindness (Fig. 18). None of the 23 volunteers in the experiment

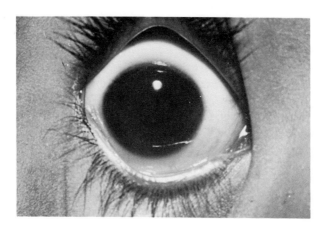

FIG. 18. Early conjunctival xerosis (XIA) in a 4-year-old child. Dryness, wrinkling and pigmentation are confined to the lower half of the bulbar conjunctiva. Plasma vitamin A was low (9μg/100 ml).

carried out by the Medical Research Council in Sheffield, England (Hume and Krebs, 1949) who received a diet deficient in vitamin A for periods ranging from $6\frac{1}{2}$ to 25 months developed any change in the conjunctiva. This was also true in the experiment carried out on eight male volunteers by Sauberlich et al. (1974). In adults and older children, therefore, in whom the deficiency progresses slowly, conjunctival xerosis is not an early sign and for this reason plasma levels and the dark adaptation test, which may be readily carried out in these subjects, are of more value but have their own distinct limitations. Furthermore after a number of years of exposure to smoke, dust, glare, and eye infections—all part of the common lot in those parts of the world where xerophthalmia is frequent—the bulbar conjunctiva of even the well nourished becomes thickened, wrinkled, and pigmented. Patches of dryness, best seen on oblique illumination, almost always involving the interpalpebral area of the temporal quadrant, and often the nasal quadrant as well, must be regarded as the diagnostic appearance of the condition at this early stage. The presence of thickening, wrinkling and pigmentation, sometimes together with Bitot's spot which can no longer be regarded as pathognomonic of vitamin A deficiency (Section A3*b*, below), has been repeatedly and erroneously taken as evidence of xerophthalmia in an adult population. The practice of the superficial examination of the conjunctiva by the inexperienced without supporting evidence from blood chemistry and night vision testing cannot be too strongly deprecated.

In the preschool child the position is rather different. Here there have not yet been the long years of exposure to local trauma to affect the bulbar conjunctiva and if it shows a dry, wrinkled, thickened, and muddy appearance then xerophthalmia is by far the most likely cause. This is fortunate also because satisfactory testing of night vision is hardly possible and blood may not be easy to obtain. In practice, however, another factor altogether may vitiate the results of any examination of the conjunctiva in this age group. Even from the neonatal period conjunctivitis of one kind or another will probably occur in a very high proportion, masking the changes of xerosis.

John (1931), working with Pillat in Peiping (Peking), appears to have been the first to demonstrate diminished sensitivity of conjunctiva and cornea. In 20 patients with varying degrees of "ocular vitamin A deficiency" he found almost no diminution if Bitot's spot alone was present, but distinct depression in the more advanced stages with corneal involvement. It is possible that those with isolated Bitot's spots did not have vitamin A deficiency. This might form a useful field test to help to distinguish between the types of spot, but has not been tried as far as the writer is aware.

Oomen (1961) has emphasized the way in which the xerotic bulbar conjunctiva is not wetted by tears and this is an important characteristic. The reason for this is not fully understood but it is probably connected with keratinization of superficial epithelial cells, absence of goblet cell secretion, and formation of a greasy layer on the conjunctiva in this condition that sometimes forms into a Bitot's spot. Infants with xerophthalmia certainly produce tears on occasion although their general weakness sometimes means that they are fretful and whimpering, lacking the energy for a good cry.

Lemp (1973) has shown that vitamin A deficiency and other causes of the "dry eye syndrome" (e.g. ocular pemphigus, Stevens-Johnson syndrome, severe trachoma and chemical burns) have in common mucin deficiency associated with marked decrease in conjunctival goblet cells.

Vital stains such as rose Bengal and Lissamine Green stain degenerate cells, dead cells and mucus (Norn, 1974). Sauter (1976) has advocated their use in the detection of conjunctival and corneal xerosis. However, recent experience (Emran and Sommer, 1979; Kusin *et al.,* 1979) has shown the stains not to be sufficiently specific, with about 10% positive staining in normal children and 20–50% of those with vitamin A deficiency and related night blindness, conjunctival xerosis or corneal destruction not staining at all.

It is in the young child that Bitot's spots are most frequently accompanied by conjunctival and corneal xerosis and therefore under these circumstances a much surer indication of xerophthalmia than in older children and adults. I stated some years ago (McLaren, 1956) that Bitot's spots are extremely rare under the age of 4, but this is not so and I have seen them subsequently frequently in infants in the first and second years of life.

b. Bitot's Spot

This lesion, although an integral part of the conjunctival pathology already mentioned, deserves to be considered separately. The French oculist Bitot (1863) in his paper entitled "Sur une lesion conjonctivale non encore décrite coincidant avec l'héméralopie" gave his first account of the conjunctival spots that bear his name. His subjects were 29 debilitated orphans in an institution at Bordeaux. Bitot's original description bears repetition, in translation, after nearly 120 years.

> It is triangular, its tip external; its base adjacent to the cornea is a little concave. In some cases it is circular or oval; in others, singly linear. Most often the particles which compose it are agglomerated to produce a punctate, granular surface; at other times these particles are arranged in series of wavy parallel lines, which give the lesion the appearance of an undulating or rippled surface.

The Bitot's spot is easily visible grossly when large but one or two bubbles of foam may sometimes be seen under magnification in subjects who would otherwise be passed as normal. Various shapes are seen; the triangular form, although classical, is exceptional in practice. The situation is very variable. It may be anywhere on the bulbar conjunctiva but is much more frequently temporal than nasal (Fig. 19), very occasionally both nasal and temporal, and usually confined to the interpalpebral fissure especially near the temporal limbus where, for anatomical reasons, there is the least lid pressure on the bulbar conjunctiva. The importance of exposure as a factor in the production of Bitot's spots is exemplified by a case of unilateral coloboma of the upper lid with a Bitot's spot on the exposed part of the globe (Appelmans et al., 1957), another instance overlying a pinguecula (Levine and Rabb, 1971), and the case of the writer in a Gogo boy associated with cicatricial ectropion of one lower lid (Fig. 20).

The usual form taken by the Bitot's spot is a larger or smaller, more or less compact refractile mass of a silvery-grey hue with a foamy surface (Fig. 21). Most of the spots seen in Ethiopian schoolchildren were of this nature (Paton and McLaren, 1960) as were those in the cases of Roels et al. (1958a). The spot is raised above the general level of the conjunctiva and is quite superficial,

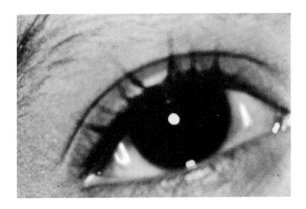

FIG. 19. Small Bitot's spots on both nasal and temporal aspects; an unusual occurrence.

being confined to the conjunctival epithelium. It is not usually altered by rubbing over the closed eyelid but, if scraped directly with a spatula, most of the foam can be removed, leaving a chalky conjunctival bed with a wrinkled surface. Less frequently, the surface of the spots lacks a foamy appearance and the lesion may consist of a compact plaque or resemble vegetations (Fig. 22).

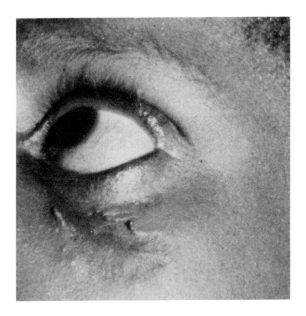

FIG. 20. Bitot's spot of the lower temporal aspect of the left eye associated with ectropion of the lower lid, indicating the influence of local exposure.

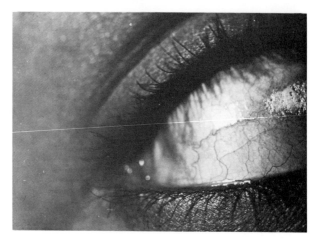

FIG. 21. Bitot's spot of characteristic foamy appearance (XIB).

Nicholls and Nimalasuriya (1939) suggested that foamy spots are produced when the xerotic changes in the conjunctiva take place relatively rapidly, and that the denser accumulations of desquamated epithelium are the result of a more chronic process.

Many workers have reported the presence of *Corynebacterium xerosis* in the Bitot spot material and although the suggestion that it had an aetiological role was short lived, it is a gas-forming organism and is probably responsible for the foamy appearance. The suggestion by Kreiker (1930) that movement of the eyeball and lids whips the material into foam is certainly fanciful

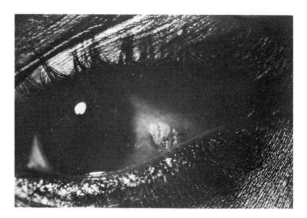

FIG. 22. Bitot's spot with exuberant frond-like growth and "cheesy" appearance, lacking a foamy surface.

although this may have a moulding effect on the spots. This movement will result at times in compression and compaction of epithelial debris into a single small mass, and at others in a corrugated effect like that arising from the pounding of heavy traffic on a dirt road. Rodger *et al.* (1963) on a morphological basis divided Bitot's spots into (a) pearly, with many *Corynebacterium xerosis* present, and (b) mucoid, free from organisms.

The appearance of the rest of the conjunctiva varies considerably. In Ethiopia (Paton and McLaren, 1960) one of us (D.P.) carried out macroscopic and slit lamp examinations on 34 children with Bitot's spots and on 183 children in the same schools without spots. Conjunctival scrapings were also taken from some in each group. Compared with healthy American schoolchildren the bulbar conjunctiva of all these children showed some alteration but there was no difference at all between the two groups with or without the spots. This mild degree of conjunctival wrinkling, roughness, and dryness might be termed conjunctival xerosis by some and has been regarded as indicative of early vitamin A deficiency. However, this conclusion, without supporting biochemical and dark adaptation data, should be scrupulously avoided for in these particular children the vitamin A status was shown to be satisfactory (see below).

Sometimes there is a prominent vessel running to the area of conjunctiva beneath the Bitot's spot and frequently there is a stippling of melanin pigment around the spot. It may be surmised that if more were known about the changes going on in the neighbouring conjunctiva then the aetiology of the spots themselves might be clearer. Bitot's spots, consisting as they do of keratinized epithelial debris, are indicative of a chronic process in the conjunctival epithelium and when associated with a true vitamin A deficiency are much more commonly seen accompanying xerosis of the conjunctiva than the more severe and rapidly progressing changes of xerophthalmia and keratomalacia.

Males are more commonly affected than females (Section A7e, below) and although it is possible that the former may be exposed to more local trauma the reasons for this sex difference are not understood.

These spots do not interfere with vision and are of no significance in themselves. Their importance lies in the interpretation that may be put on their presence. In trying to clarify this confused subject certain initial statements may help to pave the way for later discussion. The precise aetiology of these spots is not known. While some instances show every evidence of being due to vitamin A deficiency, in that they occur in subjects with definite signs of this deficiency and respond to treatment with the vitamin, others are negative in these respects. Their common occurrence in a community is always an indication of poor nutrition in a general sense, but isolated instances may occur in healthy individuals.

Sie Boen Lian (1938) was perhaps the first to bring evidence of the absence of vitamin A deficiency in patients with Bitot's spots. Nineteen cases without night blindness or xerophthalmia with normal serum vitamin A levels, all but one of whom were males ranging in age from 11 to 44 years, all showed no response to vitamin A therapy. Similar results were reported by Basu and De (1941) and Métivier (1941), the latter mentioning accounts from many parts of the world with failure of response to therapy. Ascher (1954) found 20 cases in white Americans among 642 patients with malnutrition in Birmingham, Alabama. He concluded from the presence of the spots and their lack of response to specific vitamin therapy that they indicated poor nutrition in general but deficiency of no vitamin in particular.

Recent studies have produced the same conclusions (Yourish, 1953; Gorduren and Ören, 1958; Bouzas, 1959). Although Roels et al. (1958a) found a positive correlation between low serum vitamin A levels and the incidence of Bitot's spots it does not follow that these were causally related; they may both have been indications of general poor nutrition.

An extensive investigation of the relationship of Bitot's spots and vitamin A deficiency took place in Addis Ababa in connection with the Interdepartmental Committee on Nutrition for National Defense (ICNND) Survey in 1958–59 (Darby et al., 1960; Paton and McLaren, 1960). Among 6417 schoolchildren (average age 12 years), 157 (2.4%) had Bitot's spots. Dark adaptation was tested, using a modified radium plaque device (American Optical Instrument Company, US Navy specifications). Of 244 of these children, including 28 with Bitot's spots, not one was found to have any impairment as judged by the final rod threshold. Mean serum vitamin A and carotene levels did not differ for the two groups, and repeated estimations revealed no response of the Bitot's spots to vitamin A therapy or to the skimmed milk that some were receiving in addition. Similar lack of response to therapy, normal dark adaptation, and serum levels were also found in a group of lepers with Bitot's spots studied in Tanganyika (McLaren et al., 1961). Bagchi et al. (1959) in India claimed a rapid response of Bitot's spots to treatment with 50 000 i.u. vitamin A daily and 30 g protein as skimmed milk powder. They found a positive correlation between serum vitamin A and serum albumin levels in their cases, who were mostly quite young children between the ages of 4 and 6 years.

In those infants who have Bitot's spots that accompany xerophthalmia or even keratomalacia and who have the marked systemic disturbance of nutrition evinced by marasmus or kwashiorkor, the Bitot's spots together with the other eye and systemic signs usually respond to vitamin A therapy and a balanced diet. It may well be that protein as well as vitamin A plays a part in reversing the localized defect in the conjunctiva responsible for the abnormal keratinization of cells. In older schoolchildren and young adults with no evidence of nutritional disease it is probable that the spots have a quite different aetiology in which exposure plays a prominent part. Although the long-term studies over many years to prove the point have never been carried out, there is a strong suspicion that many of the Bitot's spots seen in older subjects are persisting stigmata of vitamin A deficiency that occurred in earlier life.

It has been stated that the best cure for Bitot's spots is a few drops of zinc sulphate in the eye. By this is meant that any local treatment will remove the

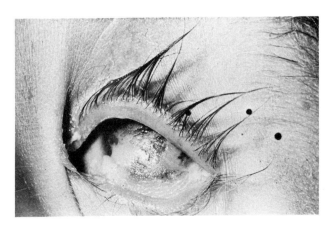

FIG.. 23. Massive accumulation of Bitot's spot material of a "cheesy" character involving both cornea and conjunctiva.

material. One has had the experience more than once of demonstrating a case to students and finding that the spots had been rubbed away before the last students could observe them. The underlying surface remains roughened, of course, and more material will form in a few days. Some maintain that the surface is permanently altered even though no more material forms after treatment. In any case it should be evident that the apparent effect of treatment on such an ephemeral lesion must be observed with caution.

Occasionally, in advanced xerosis there is *accumulation of debris* on the surface of the bulbar conjunctiva which may spread onto the adjacent part of the cornea. The material is creamy white, glistening, non-foamy and easily becomes detached to lie in the canthi, the lower fornix, or on the borders of the eyelid (Fig. 23).

c. Pigmentation

In prolonged xerosis the lower fornix first becomes yellowish, then light grey and finally dark brown due to the presence of chromatophores in the basal cell layer of the epithelium. This characteristic "gutter" pigmentation responds slowly, over a period of weeks or months, to treatment. The only form of pigmentation likely to be wrongly attributed to vitamin A deficiency is the diffuse deposition of melanin throughout the exposed area of the bulbar conjunctiva found in the eyes of most dark-skinned peoples. This pigmentation is so common that it may be regarded as normal rather than exceptional among these races. It does, however, take a number of years to develop and is not seen to any extent in very young children. If there is this kind of pigmentation of the conjunctiva in an infant, accompanied by the changes of xerosis, then xerophthalmia may be suspected. If truly nutritional in origin it should slowly disappear with vitamin A therapy.

Considerable prominence was given to conjunctival pigmentation as a sign of vitamin A deficiency by the early accounts of Pillat (1933, 1939) of long-standing instances of xerophthalmia in young adults. Pillat himself stressed that it took a long time to develop and was therefore seldom seen in children. Under treatment it was the last sign to disappear.

d. Xerosis of the Cornea

This is a later stage than that described above when xerosis was confined to the conjunctiva. Nevertheless, slit-lamp examination of the fluorescein-stained cornea has revealed punctate epithelial keratopathy in many children with night blindness and normal conjunctiva of cornea to naked eye examination alone (Sommer *et al.*, 1979). By the time the cornea has become hazy the conjunctiva usually shows marked xerosis (Fig. 24). In the young

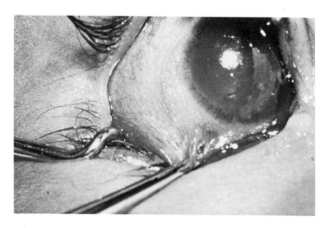

FIG. 24. Marked conjunctival xerosis with corneal xerosis (XIA and X2). The conjunctiva is very dry, thickened and thrown into numerous folds. The cornea is also dry, has lost its normal lustre and the stroma is infiltrated with white cells. There is early neovascularization and a small, superficial erosion. Plasma vitamin A was only 3 μg/100 ml.

infant, however, in whom the deficiency tends to progress with particular rapidity, the cornea may become involved early on with the development of keratomalacia before there has been time for the conjunctiva to be affected. Only rarely is bilateral xerosis of the cornea seen in a symptomless child (Fig.

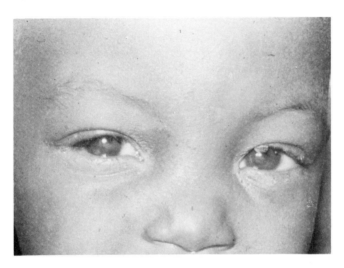

FIG. 25. Bilateral corneal xerosis (X2). The subject was symptomless and was identified during a survey in Tanganyika.

25). The clinical features of xerosis corneae in man are very similar to those seen in the severely deficient animal (Section IB).

In health the cornea is protected by the pre-corneal tear film, spread and maintained continuously over the corneal surface. Conjunctival mucus is spread by action of the lids and adsorbed at the corneal surface, and is thought to be the principal factor in maintaining the pre-corneal film (Lemp et al., 1970). This process is impaired in xerosis, and its presence may be detected clinically by measuring the BUT (break-up time) interval; it is less than the normal 10 seconds in xerosis of the cornea. This interval is shortened by many factors, including reduced tear secretion, impaired tear flow, increased viscosity and surface active forces.

The dull, hazy, lack-lustre appearance of the cornea results from the same changes described in xerosis of the conjunctiva. Infiltration of the stroma adds to the haziness, and neovascularization, usually minimal, may occur. Exfoliation of the epithelium and hypopyon are inconstant features.

e. Corneal Ulceration with Xerosis
This is the earliest change in which an irreversible element occurs; there is

bound to be some residual defect, and vision will be affected. "Ulceration" is not an ideal term but it is the best available (Fig. 26). Ulceration of the

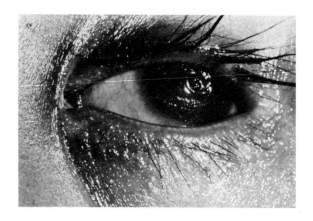

FIG. 26. Corneal xerosis with "ulceration" (X3A). This is the earliest change in which an irreversible element occurs; some degree of scarring is inevitable. "Ulceration" does not imply infection in this context.

cornea may result, of course, from many causes. It is only the ulceration that accompanies corneal xerosis X2 that is referred to here. It involves loss of substance of a part or of the whole of the corneal thickness. Minimal denudation of the epithelial surface (erosion) without transgression of Bowman's membrane leaves no permanent damage and is not included here. There are only mild signs of reaction or inflammation unless there is accompanying secondary infection. When the ulcer progresses to advanced stromal loss it may result in descemetocele and complete perforation with iris prolapse. These lesions are most common in the lower half of the cornea.

f. Keratomalacia

This consists of a characteristic softening (colliquative necrosis) of the entire thickness of a part, or frequently the whole, of the cornea, invariably leading to deformation or destruction of the eyeball (Fig. 27). The process is a rapid one, the corneal structure melting into a cloudy gelatinous mass that may be dead white or dirty yellow in colour (Fig. 28). Extrusion of the lens and loss of vitreous may occur (Fig. 29). In untreated cases endophthalmitis not infrequently supervenes. Particularly in very young children, keratomalacia may rapidly develop in the absence of the characteristic changes, described earlier, in the conjunctiva. A striking feature of the condition is that it is initially accompanied by very little reaction of the surrounding structures.

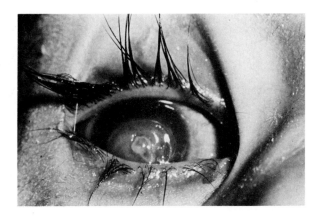

FIG. 27. Typical keratomalacia (X3B) involving part of the corneal surface.

From descriptions of the ways in which keratomalacia develops it is clear that considerable stretches of the corneal surface are immediately affected. Sometimes the central origin is stressed; sometimes the origin is peripheral, crescentic, or quadrant-like. The term "perforation" is often used in keratomalacia. This is an understatement: after malacia, the cornea, or the majority of it, no longer exists. There is apparently no demarcation, as in local destruction, but infection and eventually panophthalmitis are always close at hand.

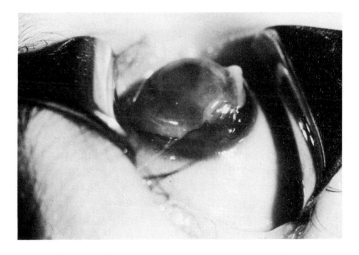

FIG. 28. Total keratomalacia (X3B) with melting and sloughing off of the entire cornea.

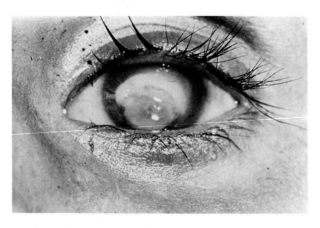

FIG. 29. Keratomalacia with prolapse of the lens (X3B).

Recent work offers a possible explanation for the changes seen in keratomalacia and also some possibility for improved treatment. Lack of mucus in the tear film owing to vitamin A deficiency will predispose to instability of the film resulting in dryness of the cornea (Section IIIA3*d*). This dryness will lead to epithelial damage and corneal ulceration. It has been shown that corneal collagenases can be activated by a variety of corneal diseases associated with corneal ulceration (Section IB). Disruption of the integrity of this anatomical barrier may activate the collagenases of the corneal epithelium and stroma and/or invite secondary infection, which would produce corneal damage by direct invasion as well as by activation of the corneal collagenases.

g. Corneal Scars

This is a better term than sequelae because the latter presupposes that corneal scars are definitely known to follow upon xerophthalmia, whereas this is rarely the case. There are many possible causes of corneal scars, but when the clinical picture is compatible with healed corneal ulcer and/or keratomalacia and onset between the ages of two months and five years seems probable, when there is association with severe generalized malnutrition with or without an acute decompensating event (diarrhoea, tuberculosis, urinary infections, etc.) and when there is no known trauma, prolonged purulent discharge, or severe trachoma, the scars are likely to be the result of vitamin A deficiency. Only these cases should be classified XS (Fig. 30).

Corneal scars result from the healing of the irreversible corneal changes mentioned above. Vision is least seriously affected by nebulae and small leucomata situated away from the pupillary area, usually in the lower central part of the cornea (Fig. 31). If the iris has prolapsed there will be leucoma

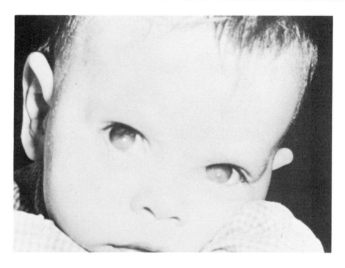

FIG. 30. Corneal scars (XS) in a Syrian infant, consisting of leucomata situated in the characteristic lower central position.

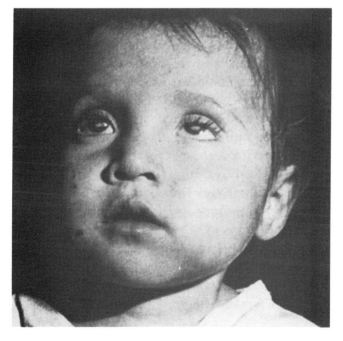

FIG. 31. Corneal scars (XS) in a child in El Salvador recovering from kwashiorkor.

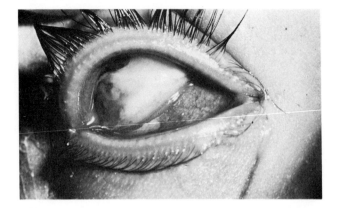

FIG. 32. Corneal scars (XS) with total disorganization of the eyes—phthisis bulbi.

adherens with distortion of the pupil. Large, often heavily vascularized and pigmented, total or subtotal leucomata cause loss of vision, fortunately often affecting only one eye with minimal changes in the other.

Keratomalacia, on healing, results in ectasia of the cornea and anterior staphyloma composed of the scarred remnant of the cornea and incorporated

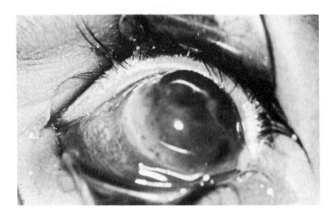

FIG. 33. Corneal scars (XS) in which the cornea has bulged forwards under increased ocular pressure due to blockage of the anterior chamber angle—corneal ectasia.

elements of the uvea bulging forwards under the influence of the intraocular pressure (Fig. 32). If the damaged cornea ruptures rather than bulges then the contents are extruded, and a shrunken globe—phthisis bulbi—is the result (Fig. 33).

h. Some Debatable Matters

The precise role of secondary bacterial infection in relation to the production of keratomalacia has not been elucidated. That it would be largely responsible for the unequal degree to which the two corneae are frequently affected seems reasonable. Frankly pathogenic and potentially pathogenia organisms are usually present (Valenton and Tan, 1975) but the part they may play is not clear and no particular culprit has emerged.

While it is true that the lids and their associated structures often appear unhealthy in severe cases of xerophthalmia, there is no evidence that the changes are specific and they are not helpful in diagnosis. The eyelashes are often fine, dry, and straight (Oomen, 1955), but this is most likely to be related to protein lack as in kwashiorkor. The hair of the head shows even more remarkable changes in this condition. No special alterations have been noted in the palpebral conjunctiva but the skin of the lids is often dry and there may be a mild heaping up of keratinized cells between the lash follicles.

Pillat (1929) described the most severe skin changes unique to his adult cases of keratomalacia and possibly quite unrelated to deficiency of vitamin A itself. The colour of the skin ranged from a peculiar faded grey to greyish yellow—this in Chinese patients. The surface was rough, dry, and earthy to the touch. In severe cases the skin gave the impression of having been dusted with coarse powder and in some there was marked scaling. The skin was slack and heavily lined with folds, giving an aged appearance to the face. The skin of the face and neck was sometimes covered with scores of comedones, indicating the lack of activity of sebaceous and sweat glands.

Attention has been called to the prominence of the orifices of the Meibomian glands as indicating vitamin A deficiency but Oomen (1961) now seems to doubt the specificity of this sign. Certainly in Africans one may find all degrees of prominence quite apart from malnutrition. Several workers have commented upon the frequent occurrence of chalazion in xerophthalmia.

In general Pillat's views on xerophthalmia have been amply confirmed when others have had the opportunity to investigate comparable material. Two points he made, however, have not been substantiated. Decrease in lustre and increase in shagreen of the surface of the lens and thickening of the corneal nerves at an early stage of the disease have not been reported by others.

Pillat also had rather special views on what he termed pre-xerosis and mummification of the cornea. The first of these he regarded as being characterized (Pillat, 1930) by loss of lustre and drying of the cornea when the eyelids are held open for 30 seconds, by reduced sensitivity, and by the presence of xerosis bacilli in degenerated epithelial cells of the cornea. Whether all these signs can be present in the absence of actual structural change is doubtful and most would regard them as features of xerosis corneae. Mummification of the cornea seems to have been described by Pillat (1932) in a single case as a kind of dry gangrene or slow desiccation of the parenchyma resulting in a scab-like disc of tissue. This is quite different from keratomalacia and whether it is really due to deficiency of vitamin A is hard to say.

The status of discrete colliquative keratopathy (DCK) (see Chapter 11) is in doubt at present but Sommer (personal communication) believes that similar cases seen in Indonesia may be related to vitamin A deficiency with accompanying protein deficiency.

4. The Posterior Segment

All that we know about the function of vitamin A in the posterior segment of the eye, and that is quite considerable in comparison with our knowledge of what it does elsewhere in the body, is confined to the retina. Even there it is its role in scotopic vision with which we will be mainly concerned. Night vision is a highly complex function and it will only be necessary to go into those aspects of the subject upon which malnutrition has some bearing. Reference should be made back where necessary for relevant experimental animal information (Section IC).

a. Dark Adaptation

Impairment of dark adaptation, resulting in night blindness, is the first symptom of the vitamin A depletion syndrome. Scotopic vision, tests of its function, and its abnormalities have been the subjects of many papers and reviews and at least one monograph (Jayle and Ourgaud, 1950). This latter work may be consulted for descriptions of the instruments in use for measuring dark adaptation and a discussion of their merits. Rod function is affected by many conditions other than vitamin A deficiency and these also receive adequate attention in this work.

Before entering into a description of the many instrumental methods that have been employed in the testing of retinal function it is appropriate to discuss the value of the indirect assessment of night vision, as this is usually the only means readily available in the field and applicable to the young child.

Many communities where vitamin A deficiency is endemic have their own names for poor night vision; usually translating as "night eyes", or "chicken eyes". These people are usually quick to notice if an individual's movements are hesistant in the dusk. Undoubtedly a positive diagnosis has frequently been made on the basis of casual and leading questioning.

Recently evidence has been provided that thorough questioning concerning night blindness can be a simple and reliable screening test for xerophthalmia in a community. Sommer *et al.* (1980) in rural Indonesia accepted a history of night blindness from a guardian or relative accompanying the child in the study if the response was definite, a difference had already been noted between the child's behaviour and that of its peers, and where this represented a recognized change in the child's behaviour. Among 321 preschool-age children such a history (XN in the WHO classification) was found to be as specific a determinant of vitamin A deficiency as was the presence of conjunctival xerosis with Bitot's spots (X1B), the presently accepted clinical criterion (mean serum vitamin A levels were 13.4 and 12.6 μg/dl respectively). It was far more sensitive; over twice as many children had a history of XN than had X1B, and it was easier to diagnose.

The broad principles of dark adaptation testing are common to the use of all instruments. The subject is first exposed to a bright light for about 5 minutes to ensure bleaching of all the rhodopsin in the retina. Then in total darkness lights of known intensities are flashed before his eyes and his ability to see them is recorded. As the eyes become increasingly adapted to the dark the intensity of illumination may be reduced without the lights becoming invisible. From the different degrees of illumination in relation to time of testing a curve of dark adaptation can be constructed (Fig. 34). In the first few minutes adaptation proceeds rapidly and is probably due to adaptation of the cones. This is followed by a plateau, known as the cone-rod transition time when the visual function is in the process of being taken over by the rods. Thereafter vision is predominantly due to rod activity. It is normally found that no further change occurs after about half an hour by which time the maximum dark adaptation of which the retinae of the subject are capable has been achieved. Methods vary with regard to such factors as length of time for initial bleaching, use of a fixation point, distance of the eyes from the test object, size and nature of the test object, and whether the whole dark adaptation curve is plotted or only the final rod threshold.

The ordinary dark adaptometers can only be used with intelligent and cooperative subjects. In an attempt to detect vitamin A deficiency in children under 2 years of age by determining their ability to see a dim light under conditions of dark adaptation Friderichsen and Edmund (1937) measured what they called the "minimum reflexible"—the reflex irritability of the eye to light. They did this by placing a lamp 10 cm from a screen which presented a diffusely illuminated ellipsoid appearance measuring 12 by 14 cm. Various light-absorbing glasses were used and the "minimum reflexible" was indicated by the number of the glass. Careful observation of the reactions of the child was necessary but results before and after treatment were consistent with plasma vitamin A levels. Although tedious and requiring a totally dark room the apparatus is simple for this test and it might well be applied in the field to detect early signs of vitamin A deficiency in infants.

Much interest was shown in the testing of rod function about 40 years ago. The onset of the second world war and the importance of night vision for both military, especially air force, and civilian personnel enhanced this. Most

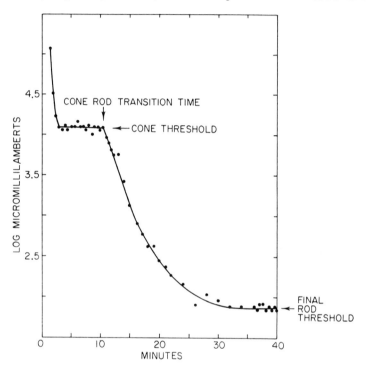

FIG. 34. Normal curve of dark adaptation showing cone threshold, cone–rod transition time, and final rod threshold. From Hume and Krebs (1949).

of the confusion and discrepancies of the earlier work can be attributed to the wide variety of instruments used, lack of attention to the evaluation of the nutritional status of the subjects, and failure to appreciate the very variable responses to be obtained from apparently healthy subjects (Jayle and Ourgaud, 1950). In most studies in which subjects have been taken at random, it has been possible to demonstrate a correlation between plasma vitamin A levels and retinal sensitivity only when large numbers have been used, the observations carried out over a considerable period of time, and then only considering mean and not individual values. These points are particularly well illustrated in the work of Chevallier (1946), who throughout the second world war studied the changes in diet, serum vitamin A, and threshold adaptometry in a homogeneous sample of 350 subjects in Marseilles.

A thorough experimental investigation of the effect of a vitamin A-deficient diet in man was undertaken by the British Medical Research Council (Hume and Krebs, 1949). In all, 23 subjects were studied for periods varying from 6½ to 25 months. On the average the blood vitamin A

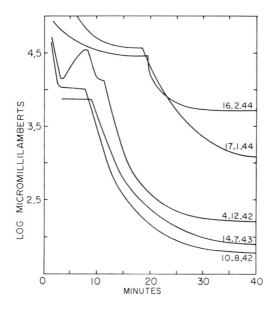

FIG. 35. Curves of dark adaptation for one deprived subject at different stages of depletion. The differences in the cone threshold curve are of doubtful significance. From Hume and Krebs (1949).

began to fall at the beginning of the eighth month and was progressive thereafter in those who continued on the experimental diet. Dark adaptation threshold levels showed unexpected seasonal fluctuations which appeared to be related to mean monthly temperature, but in addition several subjects showed significant changes which could be related to the deficient diet.

Comparison of successive curves of dark adaptation for one of the Sheffield experiment subjects deficient in vitamin A (Fig. 35) shows a progressive rise in the final rod threshold together with prolongation of the cone–rod transition time and lengthening of cone adaptation. These changes were preceded by a fall in plasma vitamin A from about 100 i.u./100 ml to less than 50 i.u./100 ml. Only three of the 16 subjects tested in this experiment showed impairment of dark adaptation, after 12, 13, and 20 months on the deficient diet. None complained of true night blindness. Plasma vitamin A levels and dark adaptation curves returned to normal over a period of weeks or months in three subjects treated daily with either 1300 i.u. vitamin A or 2500 i.u. carotene.

Sauberlich *et al.* (1974) studied retinal function in eight male volunteers on a vitamin A-deficient diet. In all but one subject dark adaptation was impaired after the plasma vitamin A level had fallen below 30 μg/100 ml; there was rapid return to normal with treatment. ERG abnormalities occurred in five subjects only after plasma vitamin A had fallen below 11 μg/100 ml, and correction took much longer once treatment had been instituted.

It should not be thought that there is always a simple relationship between the vitamin A status as judged by plasma level and dark adaptation, or that response to dietary deficiency or to therapy is prompt. The visual threshold has remained unchanged for periods ranging from several months (Hecht and Mandelbaum, 1940; Wald *et al.*, 1942) to 2 years in one of the Sheffield subjects. This discrepancy may probably be explained by the great variation in the concentration of vitamin A stored in the liver in health, in some instances large enough for several years' normal requirements.

Hecht *et al.* (1948) showed that exposure to bright sun for long periods raises thresholds for several hours afterwards. This is consistent with folklore (Section A5g) and has been demonstrated in experimental animals (Section IC).

All authors are agreed that the male is more susceptible to night blindness than the female (Birnbacher, 1928; Aykroyd, 1928; Pillat, 1929), although Bietti (1940) stated that this difference does not hold after the age of 45. The frequent occurrence of night blindness in pregnancy (Jayle and Ourgaud, 1950) is probably partly due to underlying disease and partly to increase in vitamin A requirements.

There has also been great variation found in the response of the deficient subject to vitamin A supplementation. In some studies night blindness was cured only after months of treatment (Hecht and Mandelbaum, 1938, 1939, 1940). In this connection Dowling and Wald (1958) suggested that too much attention has been concentrated upon vitamin A in the past and that it is possible that deficiency of other rod and cone constituents, particularly the specific proteins, the "opsins," might be responsible. Their experimental work in the rat (Section IC) suggests, however, that the opsins are not affected until the stage of general tissue disintegration has been reached, and that so long as the prosthetic group retinal is present the protein moiety remains stable. In severe protein and vitamin A deficiency, as seen in infantile kwashiorkor and xerophthalmia, it is quite possible that rod and cone function is impaired and that permanent structural changes may result, although this would be difficult to investigate.

Rather in keeping with the idea that not all clinical night blindness is due to deficiency of vitamin A is the outbreak investigated by Someswara Rao *et al.* (1953) near Madras. The cases were confined to one village and the results of examination were compared with those in neighbouring villages who had no night blindness. Both groups of villagers were very poor and the main cereal consisted of sorghum in a diet providing only about 1000 calories daily per consumption unit. Dark adaptation studies showed that this function was impaired in 40% of the population complaining of night blindness as compared with 5% in the other village. The vitamin A intake, chiefly as carotene, was 2600 i.u. and 1000 i.u., respectively. There was a relationship between night blindness and degree of anaemia. In subjects with haemoglobin levels below 7.4 g/100 ml, 66% had impaired dark adaptation; in those between 7.5 and 10.4 g/100 ml the incidence was 46.9%, and for levels of 10.5–14.8 g/100 ml it was 36.6%. The incidence of anaemia and hookworm infestation was higher in the village with night blindness than in the other one.

The same workers carried out a therapeutic trial in which 71 patients with impaired dark adaptation were divided into three groups, receiving daily either 130 to 260 mg of ferrous iron, 1 ml shark liver oil containing 12 000 i.u. vitamin A, or a placebo. All three groups were given 8 ounces of rice daily in addition to their normal diet. After 1 month improvement in dark adaptation occurred in 83% of the first group, 100% of the second, and 73% of the third. The improvement in the first and last groups could not have been due to vitamin A, for rice contains no carotene, and is unlikely to have been due to iron in the second and third groups, for rice is poor in this element. It is possible that the protein of rice may have supplemented favourably that of sorghum in eliminating any amino acid deficiency. The results must remain inconclusive, for a seasonal improvement in the local diet might conceivably have been responsible.

Norden and Stigmar (1969) reported results in a vitamin A-deficient subject using the automatic dark adaptometer of Krakau and Öhman.

The possible role of zinc deficiency is mentioned later (Chapter 5, Section IIC).

b. Electroretinogram (ERG)

The electroretinogram consists of a record of the change in potential across the retina caused by light. Studies with experimental animals have shown that there is considerable alteration of the record in vitamin A deficiency (Section IC). Dhanda (1955, 1956) used this as a means of diagnosis of vitamin A deficiency and certain other eye diseases. From his results it seems that changes in the ERG do not arise before those detectable by the dark adaptometer. The apparatus for the ERG is expensive and involves problems of standardization. Young children may only be examined under general anaesthesia although the results obtained are interesting this method is unsuitable for use in the field or in the ordinary eye department of a hospital.

A preliminary report on the ERG in undernourished children in Indonesia and Thailand (Genest *et al.*, 1967), 33 aged between 5 and 9 years and 21 between 10 and 14 years, suggested that those with a history of previous clinical vitamin A deficiency had lower responses.

c. Rod Scotometry

This method of testing night vision was devised by Livingston (1944) and given its first trial in vitamin A deficiency in the Sheffield experiment (Hume and Krebs, 1949). In this test the field of vision is plotted on a modified tangent screen using test objects of known luminosity under conditions of dark adaptation. Rod scotometry was carried out on 13 of the volunteers at Sheffield during their 13th month on the vitamin A-deficient diet and on five subjects who were receiving protective supplements. In five of those on the unsupplemented diet there was considerable reduction of the fields of vision by this method at a time when examination by using a dark adaptometer showed defective night vision in only one. According to Livingston the first change to appear is enlargement of the blind spot, usually greater at the lower pole of the nerve head, combined with a reduction in sensitivity of the rod area to the temporal side of the blind spot whereby this scotomatous area enlarges to the limits of the field. An islet of deficiency may be found between the macula and the blind spot. At about the same time the normal central scotoma enlarges beyond physiological limits. Later still a concentric contraction of the peripheral fields occurs.

Figure 36 shows (a) the normal type of visual field chart compared with (b) one for a vitamin A-deficient subject. In the latter there is marked reduction of the field of vision with enlarged central scotoma and the peripheral scotoma merging with the blind spot. During a period of just over 1 year the examination was repeated several times in the Sheffield experiment, and it was found that although the areas varied somewhat in the same individual there was a consistent difference between the mean blind areas for the

---

FIG. 36. (a) Rod scotometry. Normal type of chart showing small central scotoma and large scotoma round the blind spot. (b) Abnormal chart showing field of vision reduced as a result of vitamin A deprivation, with central scotoma enlarged and peripheral scotoma merging with blind spot. From Hume and Krebs (1949).

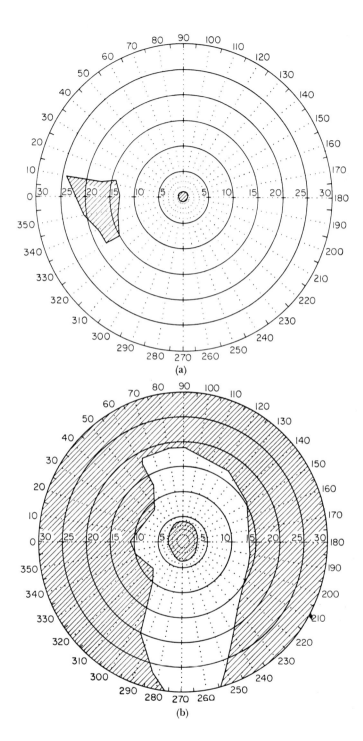

(a)

(b)

deprived and non-deprived groups. The former at one time or another in every subject exceeded 100 cm² while for the latter it was seldom greater than 50 cm². Relatively small doses of vitamin A (1300 i.u. vitamin A daily in one subject, and 1250–2600 i.u. β-carotene daily in another) produced striking improvement over a period of 6 months in two depleted subjects. Two others improved on similar regimes although not having signs of deficiency by any other criteria, and four other subjects showed less fluctuation in blind area value after dosing than before.

Weekers and Roussel (1945) also found that the extent of the visual fields during dark adaptation differed significantly in a group of malnourished patients from war prison camps in Europe as compared with that for a group of control subjects. The similar results reported by Sloan (1947) suggested the involvement of both rods and cones in vitamin A deficiency with concentric contraction of the visual fields.

From these studies it would seem that rod scotometry may prove to give an earlier indication of vitamin A deficiency than other methods of measuring rod function. It has not, however, been extensively tested for this purpose with standard target lights and modern equipment. It is doubtful if the method will ever prove of practical value in the field for the equipment is not readily transported and for consistent results intelligent cooperation is essential.

d. Differential Fundus Reflectometry

Sheorey (1976) has described an objective method for the clinical assessment of rhodopsin in the eye which appears capable of use under field conditions for detecting early vitamin A deficiency in young children. It is based on differential fundus reflectometry. Bleaching is produced by a short, intense flash of light. The fundus is subsequently photographed to record the flux reflected from the bleached area, the optogram and the surrounding unbleached area.

e. Electro-oculogram (EOG)

This depends on the measurement of a standing potential present between the cornea and the retina, which varies as the eyes are moved. It is measured by means of electrodes placed on the eyelids and reflects most accurately abnormalities in the retinal pigment epithelium.

The test does not appear to have been used in primary vitamin A deficiency, but changes were reported by Thaler et al. (1976) in a 30-year-old female with malabsorption, complaining of night blindness. There was impaired dark adaptation, lack of b-wave in the ERG and loss of dark response in the EOG. Cone function was unimpaired. Recovery occurred with vitamin A in 3 days.

f. Opticokinetic Reflex

This reflex consists of the nystagmus elicited by objects passing in succession through the visual field. The movements of the eye observed in a passenger gazing out of the window of a moving train are of this nature. Gorman *et al.* (1957) have shown that the majority of infants respond to this kind of stimulation within the first 5 days of life. In Poland, where there used to be a considerable vitamin A deficiency problem in infants (Section 9 below), Miś (1958) used this method under conditions of dark adaptation to test night vision objectively. If results could be satisfactorily standardized this might provide an answer to the need for a simple night vision test in the field for infants.

g. Cone Function and Colour Vision

Retinal combined with protein is present in cones as well as in rods. As early as 1909 Hess showed that the function of cones as well as of rods was affected in night blindness associated with chronic liver disease. Wald and Steven (1939) found that the visual thresholds of both rods and cones rose in two subjects deprived of vitamin A and that the thresholds of both returned to normal on the oral administration of vitamin A or carotene.

Cone adaptation was studied in 16 healthy persons aged 8 to 30 years by Reichel and Bleichert (1958). The time needed by the light-adapted eye to perceive an object at a low intensity of illumination and the width of the pupil in relation to light intensity after 15 minutes' dark adaptation were measured. Both tests were carried out several times both before and after doses of 50 000 i.u. vitamin A and more. There was no evidence of a learning effect of treatment, but there was clear evidence of shortening of the cone adaptation time as a result of treatment.

The concentric contraction of the visual fields demonstrated by Sloan (1947) in subjects deficient in vitamin A suggested cone as well as rod dysfunction. She cited numerous examples of workers who had found visual defects on routine perimetric examination in subjects with impaired dark adaptation.

Diminished retinal sensitivity for green and for red has been reported in association with night blindness. Stephenson (1898) described contraction of the visual fields for red and to a lesser extent for green.

Reddy and Vijayalaxmi (1977) found colour vision normal by pseudoiso-chromatic plates in 28 Indian children aged 4–12 years with conjunctival xerosis or Bitot's spots. Eighteen had night blindness. There was biochemical deficiency in all the children, as plasma vitamin A ranged from 4–20 μg/100 ml; in 16 it was less than 10 μg. All signs cleared with treatment. This is further evidence that dyschromatopsia is a late sign of vitamin A deficiency in man, but it has to be pointed out that the plates used were designed for detecting mainly red–green defects and those occurring in vitamin A deficiency are often for yellow and blue. There is a need for the development of suitable procedures for measuring thresholds of hue descrimination in young children.

h. Form Sense

Using Livingston's apparatus, Steadman (1942) investigated this visual function in more than 2000 personnel of anti-aircraft units in Britain during the second world war. There was an apparent improvement in the form sense of 68 subjects with impaired dark adaptation in response to 18 000 i.u. vitamin A daily for 3 weeks.

i. The Xerophthalmia Fundus

In clinical practice carried out in areas where the gross destructive lesions of the anterior segment of the eye are sadly commonplace little attention has been paid to the fundus. When the cornea is heavily infiltrated or undergoing liquefaction it is obvious that the fundus will not be visible. In the earlier stages of vitamin A deficiency, however, an unobstructed view may be obtained, although the fact that the subjects are usually quite young children necessitates a patient approach. The writer has to confess that he has not carried out a careful funduscopic examination in the many xerophthalmia cases he has seen in various parts of the world and regrets the passing by of this opportunity. In extenuation it may be said that this sign is not even mentioned in the standard texts on ophthalmology and nutrition and was not known to him when he had his best opportunity to study it in India and Indonesia. It is to try to atone for this omission, and because it is clear that there is good evidence for the existence of this important sign, that it is intended to give this subject the prominence it deserves here.

It is significant that all the descriptions of this condition have come from countries like Japan, where vitamin A deficiency used to be prevalent, or Indonesia where it is still one of the major paediatric problems. Although Fuchs (1959) coupled the syndrome with the name of Uyemura there seems little doubt that Mikamo also of Japan was the first to describe the condition (Elliot, 1920). He associated a collection of small white dots in the horizontal meridian of the fundus, resembling the appearance seen in retinitis punctata albescens, with conjunctival xerosis and night blindness. It was noted that the spots disappeared when the night blindness improved with vitamin A. Earlier workers had described pallor of the fundus in association with night blindness and this has also been seen by some in cases in which the spots were present.

Uyemura (1928), whom the writer had the privilege of discussing this with in Tokyo, gave the first detailed description of the condition, in two Japanese boys aged 10 and 14 years, both of whom also had Bitot's spots and night blindness. Medication with cod liver oil brought about disappearance of the white spots over a period of about 2 months in the one case that could be followed up. Fuchs (1959) subsequently reported details of 20 further cases seen by Professor Uyemura since 1928. All were young people from 4 to 18 years of age, and only two were girls, giving the condition the same male preponderance observed in some other aspects of vitamin A deficiency disease. All these cases were night blind and in addition all but three had Bitot's spots and all but two xerosis. Following the institution of cod liver oil treatment the retinal spots disappeared in 16 of the 19 cases that could be followed up satisfactorily. It would seem to be of significance, although Fuchs makes no comment, that the three cases failing to respond were the only ones in the group that did not have Bitot's spots and two of them were the only ones without xerosis. The disappearance of these retinal spots under treatment with vitamin A is the most helpful feature in the differentiation of this condition from retinitis punctata albescens and fundus albi punctatus, in both of which the fundus has a closely similar appearance. That the unresponsive cases in the series of Uyemura lacked other signs of vitamin A deficiency is very suggestive that they were in fact instances of one or other of these non-nutritional conditions.

Retinitis punctata albescens differs in that the rest of the visual field is affected, there is attenuation of retinal vessels, atrophy of the papilla, and usually slow but progressive deterioration. Fundus albi punctatus bears a closer resemblance to xerophthalmia fundus and differs only in that the spots do not involve the macula and there is progressive deterioration. Fundus albi punctatus was reported (Levy and Toskes, 1974) in a 51-year-old man following gastrectomy. Night vision improved 6 days after commencing vitamin A therapy, but the final rod threshold remained raised and the rod–cone break delayed. The vitamin A deficiency element in this case was probably due to the digestive defect (Section IIIB). Two recent reports failed to find any evidence of vitamin A deficiency in fundus albi punctatus (Carr et al., 1976; Marmor, 1977).

Confirmatory reports have come from Japan (Imai, 1930; Kuwahara, 1935), from China (Pillat, 1940), and from Indonesia (Teng Khoen Hing, 1959; Sie Boen Lian, 1960). Pillat observed "small glomerations in the external strata" of the retina in vitamin A deficiency and had what would still seem to be the only histological preparation of such an eye. The largest series is that of Teng Khoen Hing, who was able to collect no fewer than 54 cases during a period of 15 months, commencing in December 1956, at the eye hospital in Bandung. The fundus drawings (Fig. 37) of two of his cases

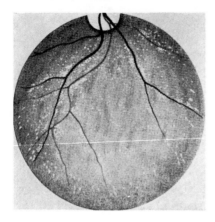 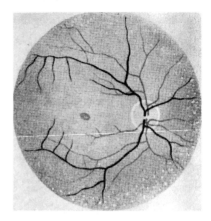

FIG. 37. Fundus changes in hypovitaminosis A. From Teng Khoen Hing (1959).

give a clear idea of the appearance of these lesions. They are sometimes glaring white, looking like sugared caraway seeds scattered profusely along the course of the vessels. When the spots are fewer in number they tend to have a yellowish appearance and the retina is a reddish brown in colour, like the skin of a spotted deer. The spots may fuse together and are usually in the periphery of the fundus, the macula remaining free. They are never seen on top of a vessel, but a vessel may run over them. Both eyes are always affected, but not necessarily to the same degree.

Nearly all of Teng's cases complained of night blindness and in 11 in whom the dark adaptation could be measured it was found to be markedly impaired. Xerosis of the conjunctiva and Bitot's spots were frequent accompaniments. The visual acuity was diminished in many instances, sometimes because of corneal change, but in 6 cases poor visual acuity was attributed to the fundus changes alone. In this series too there was a preponderance of males of about 4 to 1. Seventeen patients could be followed up for considerable periods, varying from 4 to 40 weeks with an average of 10. In 15 of these patients the lesions "seemed to have become less" during treatment with vitamin A, although in no instance did the spots actually disappear. The dosage of vitamin A was not stated and the period of observation was rather short in some cases.

Subsequently Teng Khoen Hing (1965) reported 208 cases of xerophthalmia fundus in children 5–14 years old. Serum vitamin A levels were lower than normal. There was usually night blindness but often no anterior segment changes. He stresses that it is not an early sign of vitamin A deficiency.

A unique and most informative case of a 25-year-old male who induced severe vitamin A deficiency in himself, has been described (Fells and Bors,

1969; Bors and Fells, 1971). This occurred because he read an article about the damage caused to cells by an excess of vitamin A. He deduced that the epilepsy from which he suffered would be benefited by putting himself on a diet virtually devoid of the vitamin. Over a period of 5 years plasma vitamin A fell to very low levels, dark adaptation and ERG became grossly abnormal and xerophthalmia occurred. Of especial interest were the white spots that developed on the retina. These are identical with the xerophthalmia fundus described above. At the point of blindness (perception of light in one eye and 4/60 vision in the other, absent ERGs, constricted fields and very severe

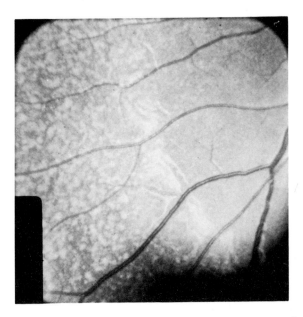

FIG. 38. Fundus photograph of right eye taken on ninth hospital day shows sharp transition, between normal and abnormal retina. Very bright crescentic banding is primarily artifactual light reflex, not pigmentary alteration. From Sommer, Tjakrasdjatma, Djunaldi and Green (1978).

conjunctival and corneal changes) and grave systemic disease, the patient agreed to be treated with vitamin A and made a remarkable recovery.

Another instructive case has recently been reported from Indonesia (Sommer *et al.*, 1978). The patient was a healthy 25-year-old female with conjunctival and corneal xerosis and early stromal oedema. There was constriction of the visual fields, corresponding to the lesions located in the retinal pigment epithelium by fluorescence angiography (Fig. 38). Treatment with vitamin A cleared the conjunctival, corneal and visual field changes within 2 weeks. Many of the retinal lesions had disappeared $1\frac{1}{2}$ months after treatment was started.

5. Pathology

It will be recalled that it was the demonstration by Wolbach and Howe in the rat that many other epithelia besides those of the eye undergo the process of keratinizing metaplasia in the absence of vitamin A that settled the controversy over the pathogenesis of the eye lesions (Section IB). Two years earlier Wilson and Dubois (1923) had carried out postmortem examination of an infant dying of vitamin A deficiency. A corneal ulcer had perforated 19 days before death and the ophthalmological appearances were characteristic of keratomalacia. There were inflammatory changes in the pancreas and lacrimal and salivary glands. Keratinization had occurred in the epithelia of the trachea, bronchi, uterine mucosa, and pancreatic and submaxillary ducts, resulting in pancreatic cysts and bronchiectasis.

Kreiker (1930) studied the earliest changes in the conjunctiva and found that before there was any evidence of keratosis the goblet cells had disappeared and that a hyaline degenerative change had occurred in the cells of the epithelium.

Blackfan and Wolbach (1933) reported 13 cases, eight boys and five girls, between the ages of 1 and 13 months, the majority being between 3 and 9 months old. The diagnosis was established clinically in six by the presence of keratomalacia but in the other children only at necropsy. All but one of the patients died and that one received permanent scarring of the cornea. Shortly afterwards Sweet and K'ang (1935) described 203 cases from China and in the 17 coming to postmortem they confirmed widespread epithelial keratinization.

Since that time it is remarkable that there have been no detailed studies of the pathology of endemic vitamin A deficiency in man. It is true that permission to conduct autopsy is difficult to obtain in most countries where the condition is common, but even a limited series of cases using the newer histochemical techniques would be a valuable contribution to knowledge of the subject.

6. The Age Spectrum

Age plays a very significant, although not entirely understood, part in determining the incidence and nature of the eye manifestations of vitamin A deficiency. In the account which follows, human life history is pictured as a continuous spectrum made up of bands of time which imperceptibly merge one into the other just as do the bands of coloured light in the visible spectrum. The different pathogenic factors at work at different periods and the results they have are summarized in Table III. Amid the complex array of

TABLE III. *The Age Spectrum of Vitamin A Deficiency*

Stage	Pathogenic factors	Manifestations
Pregnancy	Basic diet low in vitamin A (mostly carotene) Increased requirements Food taboos Strain of repeated pregnancies	Low plasma vitamin A Low liver stores Bitot's spots (occasional) Xerophthalmia (rare)
Fetus		Low liver stores Xerophthalmia (rare) ?Abortion ?Congenital malformations
First year of life	Breast milk: low concentration, diminished volume Artifical feeding Maternal neglect Infections	Lowering plasma vitamin A Depletion of liver stores Xerophthalmia and keratomalacia (relatively common) Xerosis conjunctivae and Bitot's spots (rare)
Aged 2–5 years	Prolonged breast feeding Supplementation with foods low in vitamin A Deposed child situation Infections	Peak incidence of xerophthalmia and keratomalacia Xerosis conjunctivae and Bitot's spots (not uncommon) Fundus changes
School age	Diet low in vitamin A (mostly carotene), fat, and protein Infections	Xerosis conjunctivae and Bitot's spots predominate Night blindness Fundus changes
Adult	As above plus special privation (famine, prison)	Night blindness predominates Bitot's spots (occasional) Keratomalacia (rare)

aetiological factors and predisposing circumstances the reader may at times lose track of the single basic and admittedly axiomatic fact that an inadequacy of vitamin A in the diet is of paramount importance at all ages. The risk has been run of labouring this point at the outset and perhaps stating the obvious to ensure that a balance of emphasis is preserved throughout.

a. General Status

In trying to elucidate the role that diet plays in the pathogenesis of xerophthalmia one has to begin before the conception of the individual under consideration, with the maternal status. It must be realized that in areas of the world where xerophthalmia is endemic the vitamin A status of all is low and the entire population is at risk although clinical evidence of deficiency is

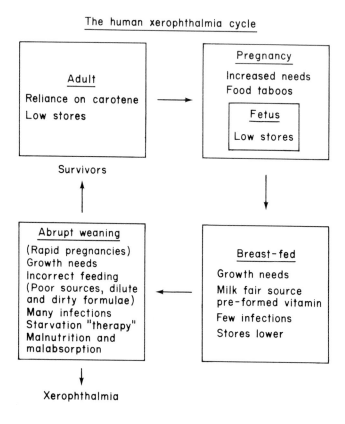

FIG. 39. The human xerophthalmia cycle.

seen in only few. Many investigators have shown that plasma vitamin A levels tend to be on the low side under these circumstances and liver stores are also probably low (Woo and Chu, 1940). In a community at risk the process may be visualized as a cycle (Fig. 39).

b. Pregnancy

Thus women enter upon pregnancy, when vitamin A requirements are increased to meet fetal needs and storage, with some degree of vitamin A impoverishment. Food taboos during pregnancy may play a part in some areas and usually apply to articles of diet such as eggs, fish, meat, and milk that are sources of the vitamin. The lack of family planning, with the consequent rapid succession of pregnancies and prolonged periods of lactation, undoubtedly make exhausting demands on the woman's low resources.

Night blindness is the commonest manifestation (Jayle and Ourgaud, 1950). Dixit (1966) in Poona district, India, found that 79 of 203 women had experienced night blindness and 29 had it at the time of examination.

c. The Fetus

Whether vitamin A deficiency may be responsible in man, as in animals, for abortion and congential malformations (Chapter 9, Section IIB) is unknown but it is certainly possible. Moore (1957c) presented the evidence for the influence maternal status has on fetal stores, and although not entirely consistent this evidence did suggest that in man it is considerable. Undoubtedly many infants born without any clinical evidence of vitamin A deficiency have very low stores of the vitamin and only escape developing signs subsequently by receiving satisfactory amounts in breast milk and supplementary foods. In endemic areas liver vitamin A has been found to be very low (Moore, 1957a; Suthutvoravoot and Olson, 1974). In 20 stillborn infants in Tanzania with no clinical evidence of deficiency (McLaren, 1963) no vitamin A was detectable in eight; in the remainder it ranged from 4–112 $\mu g/g$ fresh liver.

That the fetus may sometimes survive the effects of severe vitamin A malnutrition but carry stigmata until its dying day is shown by the occasional presence at birth of xerophthalmia or even keratomalacia (Rumbaur, 1922; Bouman and van Creveld, 1940—Germany; Maxwell, 1932—China; Katznelson, 1947—Russia; Houet and Lecomte-Ramioul, 1950—France; and Jensen, 1968—Scandinavia). However, in these exceptional cases it may be that there is some innate error of vitamin A metabolism; otherwise one might have expected more accounts from areas where the general problem is so great.

d. The Infant (First Year)

If this period be taken to include the first year of life then many babies in endemic areas will be breast-fed throughout. The vitamin A concentration in ordinary breast milk tends to be of the same order as that of the blood plasma (about 40 $\mu g/100$ ml). It is highest in colostrum and diminishes with duration of lactation. Meulemans and de Haas (1936) showed that the vitamin A content of the breast milk of Javanese and Chinese women in

Djakarta was significantly lower than that of European women in the same city. The milk of the mothers of two breast-fed cases of keratomalacia did not contain any vitamin A and in a third case was only 14 i.u./100 ml with 18 i.u. in the blood. Of equal importance as the concentration of vitamin A may be the volume of milk produced. This is known to diminish in prolonged lactation. Orientals tend to be short of stature and light in build, and if milk output is at all related to breast size many of them would seem to be inadequate in this respect (Darby and McLaren, 1957).

Even under quite adverse circumstances it is likely that breast milk will remain adequate as the only source of the vitamin at least during the first half or so of this period of life. In those babies that do develop xerophthalmia at this age there is usually a deviation from the normal pattern of infant feeding or some additional stress.

The dangers inherent in artificial feeding of infants, under conditions where there is ignorance of the infant's actual needs, cannot be overemphasized. Several instances will be cited to illustrate how xerophthalmia may arise in this way under totally different circumstances.

To Bloch (1921, 1924a,b) must largely go the credit for the demonstration that human xerophthalmia is due to deficiency of vitamin A. It was he who drew attention to the identity of the factor in liver which cures night blindness and to the then newly discovered vitamin A. During the years 1909–20 between 600 and 700 cases of xerophthalmia occurred in Denmark, more than 80% of them in infants under 1 year of age (Blegvad, 1924), in a population of less than 3 million. This was a truly notable and unprecedented epidemic for Europe in modern times, but may be compared with figures from the district of Jogjakarta, Indonesia (population just over 2 million), where in one hospital alone in the city of that name 2056 cases were admitted from the district during the six years 1952–53, 1955–58. As will be seen later (Section 9*aiii*, below), these figures are typical of the present-day position throughout Java and some other parts of Indonesia as well as certain other parts of Asia. When these data are compared it is seen that the experience at the single hospital in Java was 10 times greater than that of all the physicians in Denmark during the epidemic.

The situation which gave rise to xerophthalmia in Denmark is worth recounting because it has its parallel in more recent times but with a less fortunate sequel (see Singapore and Djakarta, below). Denmark is a dairy farming country and produces and exports butter. During the first world war most of the butter was shipped to Germany, where it brought a high price, and oleomargarine was substituted. In Denmark the price of butter and consequently that of fresh milk became prohibitive for the poor. They could obtain only separated milk or buttermilk which was practically free from fat and besides being pasteurized was again heated at home before being fed.

The other important constituents of the diet were oatmeal gruel and barley soup. It was not until 1918, when butter was rationed so that everybody, including the child, was entitled to 0.25 kg per week, as a result of the German blockade, that the disease was checked. When the war was over, butter was no longer rationed and xerophthalmia returned although with nothing approaching the former incidence and there were no severe cases. This was because the people and the Danish physicians had come to recognize the disease and had learned how to avoid and treat it.

An example of Bloch's painstaking observations may be cited. He found (1919) that xerophthalmia developed in eight of the 16 children in a ward of a children's home while none arose in a neighbouring ward. The only difference in the diets was that for breakfast the nurse in charge of the first ward gave a gruel of oats and biscuits while the one in charge of the second gave beer soup and whole milk. It was the whole milk that was protective in the second ward, being the only source of fat and vitamin A in the diet.

In Singapore before the Japanese occupation in the second world war keratomalacia was common among Chinese infants. This was attributed (Williamson, 1948; Williamson and Leong, 1949) to the popularity among this race of sweetened condensed milk as an infant food. During the occupation condensed milk was no longer available and the incidence of keratomalacia fell away to almost nothing. However, after the war, unlike the Danes, the Chinese did not learn a lesson from their captivity. Condensed milk came back again and its incorporation into the infant diet was paralleled by a short-lived recurrence of keratomalacia.

It is doubtful if purely racial factors have any influence upon the development of vitamin A deficiency. This is exemplified by a comparison of the situation among the Chinese of Singapore just described, and of the Chinese in Indonesia, where they rarely suffer, nearly all the cases being in the Javanese. The disease in Singapore was strictly related to the sale of dried and condensed milk which was largely to the Chinese community. In Djakarta, the capital city of Indonesia, de Haas, Posthuma, and Meulemans (1940) reported that among 353 cases of xerophthalmia seen by them in Javanese infants between 1935 and 1939 sweetened condensed and skimmed milk were incriminated as the major cause. Van Stockum (1938) reported similarly for other towns of Indonesia.

There exists a real danger associated with improper artificial feeding of infants over and above the basic cause which lies in poverty and population pressure. The coming of modern civilization to the developing countries has resulted in the possibility of alternative methods of infant feeding to the natural one of the breast. Welbourn (1958) studied the reasons for the adoption of artificial feeding and its harmful effects in African mothers in the large town of Kampala, Uganda. Supplementary feeding with very dilute milk tended actually to replace the breast milk and the consequent underfeeding lowered the child's reserves, predisposed to infection, and sometimes led on eventually to kwashiorkor. Signs of vitamin deficiencies were not seen in these children, probably because of the practice of the Baganda of giving relishes of green vegetables from about 6 months of age and the availability of fresh fruit. It must be remembered, however, that in the conurbations rapidly growing up all over the world the poorer people often have no land for growing their own food and may not be able to afford vitamin A-rich articles of diet which under these circumstances are frequently regarded as near-luxuries and the most readily dispensed with. While most physicians in Asia are aware of the problem of infant xerophthalmia, in other areas of the world where modern civilization is bringing this situation, together with many other evils, in its train, an alarm needs to be sounded.

An instance of this may be quoted from Durban, South Africa (Scragg and Rubidge, 1960), where 1565 cases of kwashiorkor were studied during a 2-year period in the paediatric unit of King Edward VIII Hospital. Many of these infants had not been breast-fed at all and their diet had consisted of a concoction of maize such as mealie-meal or corn starch and water, and added condensed milk. One of the more important complications in these children was keratomalacia, occurring usually in the most severely ill cases. All but one of the 14 children seen during this period with keratomalacia died. The authors noted that keratomalacia as a complication of kwashiorkor seemed to be on the increase. There were three cases in 1955; 11 in 1956; and 17 out of 1102 cases of kwashiorkor with 12 deaths during the year July 1958 to June 1959.

A fundamental point of difference should be noted here between the dietary factors that have given rise to xerophthalmia in the countries of Europe and North America, on the one hand, and in the lands of Asia, Africa, and Central and South America, on the other. It is doubtful if, even in the most primitive times in the distant past in Europe, there was ever food shortage coupled with pressure of population as is found in an ever increasing degree in so many parts of the world today. Generally speaking, the accounts of the sporadic occurrence of xerophthalmia that came from Europe and in white children in the United States during the nineteenth and early part of the twentieth centuries were associated with improper artificial feeding of infants among the poorer classes and unbalanced diets in orphanages. Examples of xerophthalmia arising in this way have been quoted above (Section IA).

A note of warning may be sounded at the present time concerning the potential dangers of anti-allergic diets for infants in countries like the United States where more emphasis is laid upon this form of therapy than elsewhere. The foods employed in replacing milk frequently consist of a soya bean preparation. Although they are usually adequate in protein, fat, carbohydrate, and mineral content they often contain no vitamins in the belief that these are specifically allergenic. Vitamins have to be obtained from other sources as prescribed by the physician, and vitamin A has been inadvertently omitted on occasion. Two cases reported from the San Francisco area of California by Vaughan (1954) and one from New Jersey (Wolf, 1958) may serve as typical examples. The children of parents who are food fadists may also be at risk.

During a lecture tour throughout the United States in 1960 the writer was informed in several of the paediatric and ophthalmological centres he visited that one or two cases of xerophthalmia and keratomalacia had been seen during the previous 5 or 10 years resulting from infant feeding problems. In a land of plenty the occurrence of gross vitamin deficiency disease may not be considered possible by the physician. Furthermore, any one physician, even if engaged in specialized practice, may not encounter more than one case in a lifetime and none can have extensive experience of the disease. In this way some cases may easily go undiagnosed and improperly treated.

Twins, orphans, and babies whose mothers go out to work and leave them to be fed by grandmothers or a neighbour are especially susceptible. The frequent association of infectious diseases must also have the effect of placing an additional strain on the already depleted reserves (Section A7, below). Time and again one finds that a particular child has been singled out for xerophthalmia in a home and a community where others, apparently equally exposed, are spared. The answer will usually lie in the presence of some additional adverse factor or factors.

It has been shown (Sobel, Besman, and Kramar, 1949) that infants under 1 year utilize vitamin A poorly in comparison with older children and adults.

e. The Pre-school Child (Age 1–5 Years)

It is not without reason that a division has been made at the end of the first year of life, before which the baby of a healthy and attentive mother even amid poverty may be expected to escape overt xerophthalmia. From that time onward, however, such an infant enters a danger period resulting from a combination of adverse circumstances in which the doting mother may be the unwitting means of destroying the eyesight and even the life itself of the object of her affection. What are these circumstances?

They will naturally vary from place to place and case to case, but in general they conspire to make these years of life the most hazardous of all from a nutritional point of view. It is then also that the low-protein, high-carbohydrate diet conducive to kwashiorkor takes its heaviest toll, and the circumstances are not dissimilar. It is also about this time that the mother frequently finds herself to be pregnant again. There seems to be general agreement among unsophisticated peoples that continued breast feeding during pregnancy is bad, although the reasons that are given seem to vary. The Oriyas of India believe that the milk "becomes like pus" and is therefore harmful to the suckling child, but the Chinese stop breast feeding because they believe the fetus will be harmed. A rapid and forceful weaning, onto the unsuitable adult-type diet, takes place. This constitutes the "deposed child situation" commonly seen in kwashiorkor, but also of major importance in the aetiology of xerophthalmia (McLaren, 1956). In her mistaken beliefs the Oriya mother will go to such lengths as smearing her nipples with hot chillies to make the breast objectionable to the infant. It is little wonder that this, together with the mental trauma of sudden maternal deprivation and the unpalatable food, leads to serious gastro intestinal upset which frequently tips the balance and precipitates xerophthalmia. If additional causes were needed they might be found among steadily diminishing breast output, ever increasing demands with growth, and new opportunities for infection and injury with commencing toddling. The wonder is, to those who have lived and worked with this problem, how so many escape.

A detailed analysis of 6300 cases seen in Dr Yap's hospital in Jogjakarta, Java (Fig. 40) by Oomen (1957) showed a peak incidence in both sexes in the year of life, with more than half of the total cases occurring in the 3rd and 4th years. He pointed out (Oomen, 1955) that this is nearly 2 years later than the peak for kwashiorkor and suggested that storage and the protective effect of prolonged breast feeding in the case of vitamin A may account for this.

Ultimately it is the vitamin A potentialities of the weaning diet that will be all-important at this stage. The word "potentialities" is used advisedly, for it must be remembered that carotene, and not the preformed vitamin, is the mainstay. This raises the question of the efficacy of carotene and the possibilities of failure of conversion and absorption being responsible for xerophthalmia in the presence of adequate carotene intake. Tijssen (1936), from his experiences as an itinerant ophthalmologist in Sumatra, even went so far as to say that xerophthalmia was a constitutional disease, due to "apraxia" in toddlers, quite separate from keratomalacia in breast-fed infants, a nutritional disease.

There are reasons to believe that associated deficiencies, particularly of protein and fat (Section 7, below), interfere with the metabolism of both carotene and vitamin A. That these play a relatively minor role in comparison with actual dietary deficiency is clear from the innumerable observations in parts of the world where kwashiorkor is common but quite small amounts of carotene in banana and other fruits and vegetables protect completely from xerophthalmia.

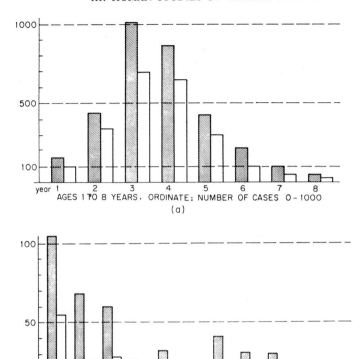

FIG. 40. Age distribution of 6300 cases of xerophthalmia in the Eye Hospital at Jogjakarta, Indonesia, from 1935 to 1954. Hatched bars are males. Note the differences in preponderance of males in low age and older groups. From Oomen (1961).

Considerable emphasis has been laid by some (e.g. Oomen, 1958) upon the occurrence of the xerophthalmia problem in close association with the consumption of a mainly rice diet. It is true that rice is devoid of carotene and that xerophthalmia in overwhelming magnitude is found largely in the rice-eating areas of Southeast Asia. Of fundamental importance and common to all parts where xerophthalmia occurs are the absence of such items as milk, eggs, and meat which provide the preformed vitamin, and at the same time the limited intake being in the form of the pro-vitamin.

In areas where there is a constantly recurring food shortage problem there may be much less xerophthalmia than where rice is plentiful. This apparent paradox is readily understood when it is realized that famine may force people to eat plants and leaves which may not otherwise be regarded by them as suitable for human consumption. This happens in Indonesia where cassava leaves, rich in carotene, are consumed under near-famine conditions (Mulock Houwer, 1956; Timmer, 1961).

Serious xerophthalmia problems exist in Central America and parts of Africa where rice is not eaten. Here, however, one also finds just as in Asia, although usually to a lesser degree, the desperate triad of population pressure, high infant mortality, and what one might term "landless poverty." That factors such as these, and others that depend upon them, and not the nature of the staple food in the diet are the primary culprits, might be illustrated by many examples. That known best to the writer, and observed by him during the 5 years he lived in India (McLaren, 1956), concerned two racial groups living in and near the Khond Hills of Orissa. Both groups, the Oriyas and the Khonds, were rice eating and both showed a similar incidence of the milder signs of vitamin A deficiency, such as night blindness, early conjunctival xerosis, and Bitot's spots, but the gross corneal destruction of keratomalacia occurred almost exclusively among Oriyas. The explanation seemed to lie in the rapid succession of pregnancies among the Oriyas and the subsequent forcible weaning of the "deposed child". The Khonds are a more primitive, aboriginal, group who rather strictly adhere to a tribal taboo on the resumption of sexual intercourse within a year or so of the birth of a child, thus having, as do some tribes in Africa, a built-in family planning system. It is interesting that the Koran states that it is a mothers' duty to devote herself fully to bringing up her child for the first two years of life. To this end, her husband should not have intercourse with her during that time. In traditional Islamic society, where most men had more than one wife, this taboo probably worked very well; today, for economic and other reasons, most have only one.

Under the pressure of the triad of factors referred to above, family life becomes disturbed and distorted and the infant and toddler are the first to suffer. As early as 1938 Donath and Gorter noted that in Indonesia most xerophthalmia is seen where the women have an occupation away from home, working on estates or in weaving mills, and the composition of the baby's menu is neglected, being left to some other adult. When one has repeatedly seen old crones left to stuff handfuls of dry rice into the mouths of hungry infants to keep them quiet one ceases to wonder that xerophthalmia is rife.

f. The School-age Child (Age 5–15 Years)
As subjects for clinical nutritional examination schoolchildren have proved to be the most convenient age group. The facility with which they may be investigated in large numbers is outweighed by the disadvantage, as far as vitamin A deficiency is concerned, that this is a relatively immune age group. Only about 10% of all patients are of this age and the majority have

mild signs. These consist of xerosis conjunctivae and Bitot's spots, the former being very difficult to diagnose in isolation and the latter not necessarily associated with vitamin A deficiency (Section 3b, above). If, for instance, this criterion had been adopted during the ICNND survey of Ethiopia the deduction would have been made that there was a serious vitamin A deficiency problem in Addis Ababa and some other parts of the country. Among a total of 6417 school children in Addis Ababa there were 157 with Bitot's spots—an incidence of 2.4%. Dark adaptation studies, conjunctival scrapings, and plasma vitamin A levels, however, failed to show any relationship of Bitot's spots to vitamin A status (Section 3b, above). It cannot be too strongly emphasized that any investigation directed toward revealing the presence of a vitamin A deficiency problem in a population must concentrate on the pre-school child. Only in this group may an appreciable number of the severe eye lesions be expected. If older groups are also examined tests for impairment of dark adaptation will be found the most revealing and reliable methods, but here again the incidence of deficient subjects will be very low.

g. The Adult

In the population at large, instances of the severer degrees of corneal damage are extremely rare. It is not uncommon for nursing mothers of children with xerophthalmia to have mild xerosis and Bitot's spots, but special circumstances of privation are necessary before permanent impairment of vision results. The only case seen by the writer was a 26-year-old Oriya woman who had given birth to a normal infant one month previously (McLaren, 1956). Both eyes showed advanced keratomalacia when first seen. Fuchs (1947) mentioned similar instances in Mysore, India of women giving birth to unaffected infants but themselves going blind from keratomalacia in the postpartum period. It is difficult to understand the pathogenesis of such cases.

Night blindness, on the other hand, is a not uncommon complaint among adults where xerophthalmia occurs in the children. There are numerous stories in this connection such as those concerning Newfoundland fishermen who had to be led from the landing stage to their sleeping quarters after a long sunny day at sea, and how seamen would bandage one eye during the day and so preserve it for use in the twilight. Platt (1958) told the story of the old ladies of a village in Teso, Uganda who have the reputation for being able to foretell when the rains are coming. They remain in the hut all day, not exposed to bright sunlight, and therefore have the ability to detect "summer lightning" in the distance, not visible to those out of doors all day.

Night blindness is a more distinct and arresting symptom than any other manifestation of vitamin A deficiency. Probably because of this and because it is an early manifestation, the occurrence of night blindness in epidemic form has been carefully noted on numerous occasions. Those affected have included troops in the field (Hicks, 1867; Ishihara, 1913), the besieged (Meyerhof, 1916), sailors on long sea voyages, jail (Buchanan, 1900) and concentration camp populations (Salus, 1957), those undergoing Lenten fasts (Blessig, 1866), and famine victims (Balletto, 1954).

Reports of seasonal night blindness in areas where the people rely almost entirely upon locally grown food are numerous (Bloch, 1917; Jess, 1921; Blegvad, 1924; Pillat, 1929; Milano, 1936; Bietti, 1940).

The development of night blindness may depend upon the availability of vegetables and fruits which may not be very rich in carotene but contain sufficient to be protective when eaten in large quantities. Thus in Guatemala (MacPhail, 1929) gangs of railway workmen received maize cakes, beans, rice, coffee, and sugar, with meat once a week. Night blindness occurred only in those labourers working on those parts of the line which did not run through banana country.

The results of the Sheffield experiment (Section 4a, above) showed that very exceptional circumstances are necessary before really marked evidence of vitamin A deficiency occurs. Even in the Far Eastern prisoner-of-war camps where other nutritional deficiencies were rife xerophthalmia was not usually encountered. Pohlman and Ritter (1952) reported that 90 prisoners were transferred from a camp on North Luzon to Manila for treatment. All were emaciated, some had severe pellagra, and all had xerophthalmia; about 10% going on to phthisis bulbi and total leucoma. In a concentration camp in central Europe night blindness was universal but keratomalacia was seen only in children (Salus, 1957).

The majority of cases described by Pillat (1929) and Sweet and K'ang (1935) in China were young adults, soldiers and apprentices living on diets devoid of vegetables and consisting mainly of rice, corn, and millet. It needs to be emphasized that such cases are quite exceptional and that some of the appearances of the eye described with such a wealth of detail by Pillat were in adults suffering from very prolonged vitamin A deficiency and therefore not to be expected in children.

7. Contributory Factors

a. Protein—Energy Malnutrition

In man, malnutrition is invariably complex and primary xerophthalmia is virtually always found against a background of protein—energy malnutrition (PEM) (Fig. 41). The highest reported rates of clinical xerophthalmia complicating PEM in hospitalized patients were about 75% some years ago in Indonesia (Oomen, 1954). The rate ranges down to almost zero in such places as Santiago (Chile), Beirut (Lebanon) and Kampala (Uganda) where PEM itself is common. In much of South and East Asia the rate is likely to be 20–40% and elsewhere usually does not exceed 5–10% (Oomen *et al.*, 1964). This speaks strongly for a primary role for dietary intake of vitamin A and only a secondary one for such factors as are mentioned below. The vitamin A status of PEM cases without eye lesions has repeatedly been found

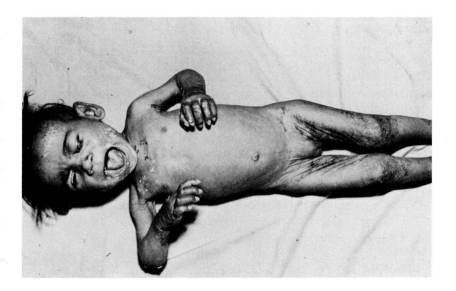

FIG. 41. Xerophthalmia accompanying kwashiorkor in a Jordanian child.

to be low as measured by plasma levels (Trowell *et al.*, 1954; Scrimshaw *et al.*, 1956; McLaren *et al.*, 1965).

Xerophthalmia occurs more frequently in kwashiorkor than in marasmus, and plasma levels are lower in the former (McLaren, 1966). RBP levels are very low in kwashiorkor but normal in marasmus (Smith *et al.*, 1973). Liver vitamin A was found to be equally low in kwashiorkor and marasmus (McLaren, 1966).

Malabsorption accompanying PEM may impair absorption of vitamin A and conversion of carotene and the common intestinal infections may do the same. Impaired synthesis of RBP may prevent release of vitamin A from the liver (Arroyave *et al.*, 1961; Smith *et al.*, 1973).

From time to time it has been suggested that keratomalacia is specifically related to protein deficiency and not to deficiency of vitamin A (Yap Kie

Tiong, 1956; Kuming and Politzer, 1967). However, evidence in experimental animals and clinical experience do not support this, although protein deficiency usually accompanies this late stage (Section IB).

The mortality in severe PEM is raised severalfold if there is accompanying xerophthalmia (McLaren et al., 1965; see Section 8a).

Skimmed milk, devoid of vitamin A unless specially fortified, is frequently used for distribution to undernourished children and initiating recovery in PEM. It has precipitated xerophthalmia under these circumstances (WHO, 1976) and milk fortified with vitamin A is increasingly being used.

b. Dietary Fat

Most tropical dietaries are low not only in certain of the vitamins and protein, but also in fat. What little fat there is tends to be from vegetable sources and high in the unsaturated fatty acids. There does not seem to be any evidence that fat is necessary for proper absorption of pre-formed vitamin A. The more important matter from a practical point of view, which has been investigated in both experimental animals and in man, is that it is necessary for utilization of dietary carotene (WHO, 1967). Roels et al. (1958b) showed that schoolboys in Ruanda Urundi absorbed carotene much more efficiently when a small quantity of fat was added to the diet.

c. Vitamin E

Animal studies have shown that deficiency of vitamin E may impair absorption and storage of vitamin A. Malnourished children frequently have lower serum tocopherol levels (McLaren et al., 1965). For these reasons 40 i.u. vitamin E is usually incorporated in the 200 000 i.u. vitamin A capsule used in treatment (Section 10) and prevention (Section 11).

d. Infections

The whole subject of the relation between nutrition and infection is a very involved one. Both of these entities are in themselves highly complex and, as might be expected, different combinations of various infections and nutritional deficiencies give different results. Many other factors such as stage of infection and degree of deficiency are of importance. As far as vitamin A is concerned the pendulum has swung between the concept of this vitamin in an all-important anti-infective role, and the view that certain infections, especially some of the exanthemata such as measles and smallpox, frequently precipitate xerophthalmia. In recent years laboratory animal studies have shown that vitamin A is an important enhancer of the immune response and that in deficiency cell-mediated immunity in particular is markedly depressed (Section IB).

Measles was first associated with xerophthalmia by Fischer (1843). This relationship is considered in detail later (Chapter 11, Section C). Many since have emphasized the role of both acute and chronic febrile illnesses (Sweet and K'ang, 1935; Oomen, 1961). Some, such as pertussis, have their main effect by causing prolonged anorexia; those causing gastrointestinal upset will impair absorption (Ramalingaswami, 1948), while even quite short periods of fever are known to lower serum vitamin A levels, through depression of RBP mitosis by the liver, although usually only temporarily. In India keratomalacia was almost universally accompanied by hookworm or giardia infestations in one study (Tiwary, 1966) and was frequently associated with tuberculosis in another (Bhattachayya and Chatterjee, 1964). Bacteriuria is more common (Brown *et al.*, 1979).

e. Sex Differences

Investigations in the experimental animal in general point toward the greater susceptibility of the male to the effects of vitamin A deficiency (Section IE). This is also true for the less severe manifestations in man, but keratomalacia in very young infants seems to behave rather differently. Oomen (1957) analysed the very extensive data of Yap, consisting of 6300 cases of all ages, and concluded that there are two quite distinct attack rates by sex for xerophthalmia. These consist of a low one for the preschool child (1.4 male:1.0 female), and much higher one after the age of 10 years or so (6.0 male:1.0 female). These conclusions are largely substantiated by the smaller series of other workers. Thus among 1511 cases of "hikam" or xerophthalmia described by Mori (1904) 862 or 57%, were boys, and in the comparable stage of deficiency in Denmark (Blegvad, 1924) 53% were males. The larger sex difference applying to the older age groups with milder deficiency is also exemplified by the 330 cases of night blindness seen by Birnbacher (1928) in Vienna after the first world war. Of these 88.5% were boys and men, with the greatest male preponderance between the ages of 10 and 30 years. In data such as these there is always the possibility that more male cases may have presented for various reasons, creating a false impression of the actual incidence of the disease in the community as a whole. This criticism would seem not to apply to Yap's data for hospital attendances for all other causes were equally distributed between the sexes.

Examination of unselected groups has shown a higher incidence of Bitot's spots in males than in females; Roels *et al.* (1958a) in Ruanda Urundi—boys 1.00%, men 0.85%, girls 0.20%, and women 0.10%; and in Ethiopia (Paton and McLaren, 1960). It must be remembered, however, that the children in the latter study showed no accompanying evidence of vitamin A deficiency and these data cannot be taken to support a male preponderance in vitamin A deficiency. Many conditions are known to occur more commonly in the male although the reasons for this are not understood.

The sex differences in the metabolism of vitamin A have been summarized by Moore (1957c) and these tend to show a greater vulnerability in the male. The writer is inclined to agree with Oomen (1961) that incidental reasons for the sex difference in man, such as readiness with which medical help may be sought, availability of carotene sources, and exposure to sunlight, are not convincing and most likely to cancel one another out.

When we turn to keratomalacia in the first year or two of life we find no evidence of a definite preponderance in males. Mori (1904) separated 116 such cases from those with "hikam," and of these 51% were boys, this proportion not differing from the sex distribution at birth. Oomen also feels from his experience in Indonesia that any sex difference there may be in the first year of life is very slight, and Tijssen (1936) from his close observation of the rural population in Sumatra contended that keratomalacia was a nutritional disease affecting the sexes equally in the first two years of life, but that xerophthalmia was a constitutional condition arising later on in boys twice as frequently as in girls. On looking over his own original data at Udayagiri the writer was surprised to find that they show a similar effect of age on sex distribution (McLaren, 1956). Of the nine cases under 3 years of age all were female except one. From 4 until 6 years the sex ratio was reversed, i.e. 18 males to seven females.

The average adult male has about 20% more vitamin A in his serum than the female (Leitner et al., 1960). At birth his level is the same as or slightly lower than that of the female (Lund and Kimble, 1943) both values being lower than in the adult. These levels correlate, nor surprisingly, with those of serum RBP (mean adult male 47 μg/ml, female 42 μg/ml and 20–30 μg/ml up to the age of 10 years). Liver vitamin A is similar in male and female accident victims (Raicha et al., 1972) and clinical differences appear to be cultural rather than biological.

f. Season

Plasma levels of vitamin A and carotene tend to fluctuate seasonally with the availability of fresh vegetables and fruit. Outbreaks of night blindness tend to occur towards the end of prolonged dry seasons.

In many parts of the world PEM has a marked seasonal incidence, with a major peak towards the end of the "summer diarrhoea" season and a minor one associated with respiratory infections in the winter (McLaren, 1966).

PEM is usually then of the marasmic type and xerophthalmia follows a similar course. Sinha and Bang (1973) carried out an extensive study of seasonal variations in rural West Bengal.

8. The Magnitude of the Problem

It is probably true to say that the enormity of the problem of infant xerophthalmia is only apparent to those who have at some time or another had to witness the hopeless procession of human tragedy through hospital wards and outpatient departments. When the cause is known, prevention and early cure are cheap and effective, and yet the flow of incurable cases is undiminished year by year, it is little to be wondered at that the attitude of the observer may become cynical when the academic achievements of Western medicine are seen to be so powerless in practice.

a. The Contribution to Young Child Mortality

It is especially in the infant that the severe eye lesions are found and it is also in this age group that the severe systemic effects may result in death. Even the advanced cases of keratomalacia in adults seen by Pillat (1929) were not usually fatal. In Denmark 24% of the affected children died (Blegvad, 1924) and in Djakarta (de Haas et al., Meulemans, 1940) the mortality was 35%. In Jordan, McLaren et al. (1965a) found that the mortality of PEM of 15% was raised to about 60% in cases with accompanying xerophthalmia, even if the lesions were only XI or XIB. In the overcrowded and poverty stricken parts of the world where xerophthalmia is common the child mortality may lie somewhere in the region of up to 500 per 1000 live births. Just what contribution vitamin A deficiency may make to this appalling wastage of young life cannot be precisely known. It probably plays its part in two ways. Firstly, there is the mortality of cases of xerophthalmia. Oomen (1961) reported a rate of 1% of all infants with overt xerophthalmia common in many parts of Indonesia and this was also the rate among Gogo babies in Central Tanganyika (McLaren, 1960). Recent figures from Indonesia (see Section 9aiii) suggest that in this country about 30 000 of the 12 million preschool children die annually with xerophthalmia. This in itself is a relatively minor contribution to the 15 million annual preschool-age deaths in developing countries estimated recently by UNICEF.

Secondly, it is clear that in those countries where 1% of all infants have the gross eye lesions, many more will be at risk and have milder clinical or subclinical deficiency. This may very well lead to susceptibility to infections and reduction of resistance but the extent of this has not been determined.

Experimental animals suffering from vitamin A deficiency frequently deteriorate rapidly in health and die before ever developing gross eye lesions. If this is any indication of what may sometimes happen in man, then there may well be an additional, albeit indefinable, role of vitamin A deficiency in infant mortality.

b. As a Cause of Blindness

The overwhelming effects of xerophthalmia are borne by the young. From what has been said it is evident that a large proportion do not survive, receiving no medical care, but a minority do, bearing the indelible marks of scarring and destruction for the rest of their days. Again referring to the series of Blegvad (1924) we find that among the 298 survivors, 27% were totally blind, 59% had greatly reduced vision (24% both eyes, 35% one eye), and only 14% had no impairment of vision. De Haas *et al.* (1940) found that in Djakarta of 152 infants a closely similar proportion (29%) became totally blind, and 18% were blind in one eye. In two blind institutions in Tanganyika the writer found that 14 and 25% of the inmates had ocular appearances suggestive of, and gave a history compatible with, a diagnosis of keratomalacia.

The blinding sequelae of vitamin A deficiency consist of varying degrees of corneal scarring—nebulae, maculae, and leucomata, together with distortion of the globe consequent upon softening of the cornea. If this structure ruptures then the lens may be extruded with vitreous, leaving a sightless shrunken remnant known as phthisis bulbi. If the cornea holds out under a rising intraocular tension then it becomes ballooned forward in a nipple-like protrusion and the sclera behind is distorted and thinned—ectasia of the cornea and anterior staphyloma.

On the basis of early data from Indonesia, the writer made an estimate that about 20 000 children became blind annually from xerophthalmia (McLaren, 1963). Later, a countrywide registration programme and epidemiological study in Jordan formed the basis for an upward revision to about 100 000 (McLaren *et al.*, 1966b; WHO, 1976). Most recently the extensive survey carried out in Indonesia (Section 9*aiii*) again raises the estimated figure to about 250 000.

c. Other Effects

Dry scaly skin, associated with xerophthalmia, was first noted by de Gouvêa (1883). Fuller accounts were subsequently given by Pillat (1932) (see Section 3*b*, above) and Frazier and Hu (1936) from China, Nicholls (1933) in Ceylon where he called it phrynoderma, or toad skin, and from East Africa (Loewenthal, 1935). The characteristic change is a heaping up of keratinized material around hair follicles with plugging of the follicle giving a "nutmeg grater" appearance and feel to the affected skin, usually the outer aspects of the upper parts of the limbs (Fig. 42). This is frequently termed perifollicular hyperkeratosis. It is rarely seem in young children. It occurred in the

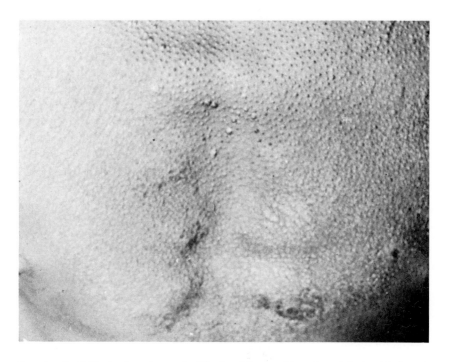

FIG. 42. Perifollicular hyperkeratosis. The heaping up of hyperkeratinized epithelium is confined to the hair follicles, which it tends to block. It is not seen in young children and is not confined to cases of vitamin A deficiency.

human deprivation studies of Hume and Krebs (1949) and Sauberlich *et al.* (1974), but also in the starvation experiment of Keys *et al.* (1950) and is not pathognomonic of vitamin A deficiency.

Haemoconcentration was reported to be a very early feature of the vitamin A-deficient rat (McLaren *et al.*, 1965b) and this has been repeatedly confirmed. More recently the paradoxical finding of anaemia has been described in human deprivation and animal experiments (Hodges *et al.*, 1978). Iron accumulates in liver and spleen and there appears to be a failure in reutilization. These authors suggest that loss of taste and smell, a recognized feature of vitamin A-deficient animals, may lead to inanition and dehydration, resulting in haemoconcentration that masks the anaemia.

9. Global Occurrence

Since *Malnutrition and the Eye* was published in 1963 a number of events have occurred which necessitate complete revision of this section. In 1962–63 WHO undertook a worldwide survey of xerophthalmia (Oomen *et al.*, 1964). Much evidence was collated, mostly based on hospital experience, and a great deal of interest in the subject was aroused, and a further compilation of data was made more recently (WHO, 1976). An important step forward in methodology was taken in the 1970s when point-prevalence surveys were undertaken in several countries, and these will be referred to under the respective countries. Survey technique was discussed by Sommer (1978). Several organizations have been responsible for initiating and fostering these studies and related activities. Prominent among these are Helen Keller International and USAID with its International Vitamin A Consultative Group (IVACG). WHO, UNICEF, the Royal Commonwealth Society for the Blind, and the Nutrition Foundation, New York, have also assisted many action programmes which frequently provide new data on the occurrence of vitamin A deficiency and xerophthalmia.

The decision has been made to retain earlier references to the occurrence of xerophthalmia in addition to the more up-to-date accounts. Mention is made wherever appropriate to changes that are thought to have occurred in more recent years. Furthermore, reports in the literature tend to be sporadic, usually unrepresentative of a country or region as a whole, and the quality of the reports varies tremendously. No doubt there are many sins of omission, as well as those of commission, in the account that follows and the overall intention is to paint a picture in outline.

A good starting point is the map that was prepared recently by the Protein Calorie Advisory Group of the UN (1976) based on a tentative list of 73 countries and territories where vitamin A deficiency is a public health problem (Fig. 43).

The map does not give any indication of the relative importance of the problem in various countries and inclusion or exclusion are subject to the limitations that have already been referred to. It is therefore useful to make a broad division of the world along the following lines. Technologically developed countries are free of the problem although some, like Japan, that

FIG. 43. The global distribution of vitamin A deficiency as a public health problem. From Protein-Calorie Advisory Group (1976).

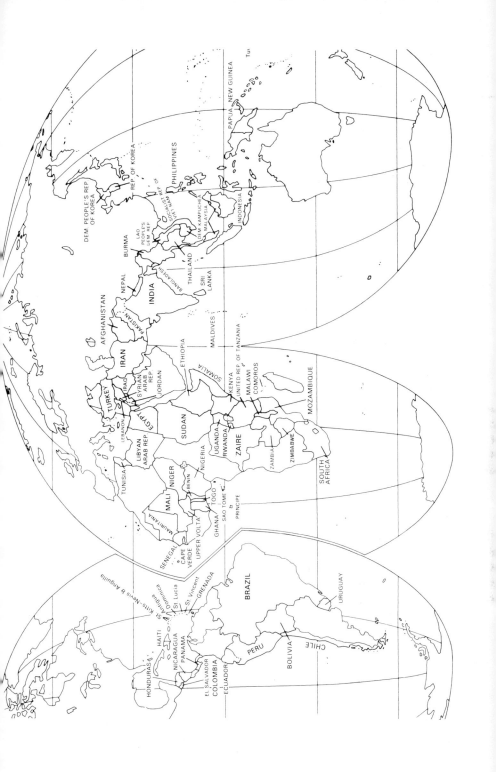

have developed rapidly and recently did have one in the not-so-distant past. Xerophthalmia reaches its highest incidence in the rice-dependent areas of south and eastern Asia, that is to say where rice is the staple, forms the bulk of every meal and young children often receive little else besides. Elsewhere in the developing world, in much of the Middle East, Africa and Central and South America, xerophthalmia is less common and its emergence or disappearance is rather closely related to changes in social and economic conditions.

a. Asia

It is undoubtedly in the over-populated and poverty-stricken countries of Asia that the heaviest toll of sight and life is taken by deficiency of vitamin A. The following accounts, while being very selective, and some of these indicative of the recent past rather than the present time, may be taken to represent the situation in all parts of these countries where living standards are low, population pressure high, and medical services quite inadequate for the needs of the people.

i. China. In the 1930s there were many reports of xerophthalmia, frequently associated with what can now be recognized as protein malnutrition. The accounts of Pillat (1929, 1930, 1931, 1939) are some of the most lucid, and reference is frequently made to his work earlier. Most of his cases were young adults, many of them soldiers in a military camp near Peiping, as were some of those of Sweet and K'ang (1935). It has to be remembered that the xerophthalmia and keratomalacia they described had developed under exceptional circumstances, and that some of the appearances are not typical of the more usual condition in the infant.

That keratomalacia was not uncommon in the Chinese infant is suggested by the following reports taken from among many. Hsu (1927) treated 10 cases, all with general dystrophy, and of the 11 infants reported by Keefer and Yang (1929) to have been fed exclusively on milk for many months, resulting in anaemia and undernutrition, three also had keratomalacia. It was stated by Gow (1934) that 2.9% of all eye cases attending the Mukden hospital in Manchuria were suffering from keratomalacia. Weech (1930) in Peiping noted oedema in five of his 13 children under the age of $3\frac{1}{2}$ years with keratomalacia, and called attention to the marked undernutrition of the entire group. There seems little doubt that these infants and also those described by Chen (1942) in Shanghai were suffering from kwashiorkor as well as keratomalacia.

In the Peoples' Republic of China enormous strides have been made in the improvement of living conditions, control of epidemic disease and provision of primary health care. WHO observers have stated that childhood malnutrition is no longer a public health problem. Recent evidence of peasant unrest suggests that this may not be true for the more remote areas. Millions of Chinese are still rice-dependent.

ii. India, Pakistan, Sri Lanka and Bangladesh. Xerophthalmia continues to be an important cause of blindness, particularly in the rice- and cassava-eating southern part of India and rice-dependent Bangladesh more than half a century after the account Wright (1922) gave of his extensive experience. Kirwan, Sen, and Bose (1943) described many cases of keratomalacia in young Bengali children who were also often emaciated, with distended abdomen, dry, brittle, and scanty hair, and with loose, dry, and darkened skin. In the neighbouring province of Orissa the writer (McLaren, 1956) described cultural practices related to the incidence of infantile keratomalacia (Section 6e, above). Large numbers of cases, frequently presenting in association with kwashiorkor, still occur in Madras (Achar, 1950; Achar and Benjamin, 1953), Poona (Khalap, 1956), Hyderabad (Chandra *et al.*, 1960), and Madhya Pradesh (Rambo, 1958). Xerophthalmia is still the most important single cause of blindness in childhood in central and southern India (WHO, 1976). In a recent report to the Royal Commonwealth Society for the Blind, Shah (1978) estimated that among the 92 million children aged 1–5 years in India 7.4 million have non-corneal and 0.22 million corneal xerophthalmia.

In 1942 it was considered (Wickremesinghe, 1942) that two thirds of the blindness in infants and young children in Sri Lanka was due to keratomalacia and in 1958 another worker (Sivasubramaniam) pronounced it the major cause of blindness in children under 5 years. A recent survey of 13 450 children (aged 6 months to 6 years) in 15 health areas has revealed a public health problem to exist in only two of these (Brink *et al.*, 1979).

In the predominantly wheat- and dairy produce-consuming north of the Indian subcontinent nutrition in general is much better than in the south and severe vitamin A deficiency is less common. Of the 200 children suffering from malnutrition studied by Manchanda and Gupta (1958) in Amritsar, Punjab only four had keratomalacia.

Individual reports refer to a massive vitamin A deficiency problem in Bangladesh. Large numbers of cases of keratomalacia are seen in hospitals in Dacca and other urban centres. Initial examination of 21 300 children for a prevention programme showed 1% XN, 31.89% XI and 0.18% XS.

iii. Southeast Asia. Although the problems of nutrition have been investigated more thoroughly in some of these countries than in others, there is reason to believe that the reports published from Indonesia, and the Philippines may largely reflect conditions throughout this whole area. Several hundred million people live in these countries and the density of population is greater than anywhere else of comparable size. Rice is the staple diet and is universally employed to supplement breast feeding. It is little wonder then that infant xerophthalmia is so common.

It has been from Indonesia in particular that a close association between keratomalacia and kwashiorkor and marasmus was early reported. The blinding results of vitamin A deficiency were recognized before the equally serious effects of protein and energy deficiency were known. That xerophthalmia was not an isolated phenomenon, affecting only the eyes, was evident to de Haas *et al.* (1940) when they commented on the presence of general dystrophy in more than 70% of their cases in the Central Hospital, Batavia (now Djakarta). A similarly high correlation between the two conditions has been noted by many others: Oomen (1953, 1954, 1955) in Macassar and Djakarta and Jogjakarta; Hoogenkamp (1956) in Kalimantan, and Darby and McLaren (1957) in several parts of Java, to mention only a few. The experience of the Chinese ophthalmologist Yap Kie Tiong in his eye hospital in the city of Jogjakarta in southern Java is perhaps unrivalled. The records of his cases, which have been analysed by Oomen (1961) and Timmer (1961), reveal as many as 11000 cases of xerophthalmia and keratomalacia seen between 1934 and 1954. Only on the island of Flores, where yellow maize is eaten in abundance (Oomen, 1958) and in sparsely populated West Irian does xerophthalmia seem to be rare.

Over a period of several years ten Doesschate (1968) made an intensive study of all cases of blindness in an eye hospital in Surabaya, East Java. Keratomalacia was the commonest cause of blindness in children. Follow-up over a 2 to 3 year period showed that more than 30% patients had died at home.

Since 1973 Helen Keller International has sponsored field projects and research on xerophthalmia in Indonesia. In a prevention pilot project a 4.7 per cent overall prevalence rate was found in Central Java (American Foundation for Overseas Blind, 1975). The Nutritional Blindness Prevention Project based in Bandung, West Java is entering its closing stages at the time of writing. It has included a countrywide survey of more than 27 000 rural and 9000 urban preschool children in more than 250 single sites in seven regions of the country. In 11 out of 23 provinces the WHO criteria for a public health problem were exceeded. Analysis of the data shows the following figures:

	Preschool	Annual incidence population at risk	Cases per year
Corneal	4/1000	12 million	48 000
Non-corneal	104/1000	12 million	1 250 000

The risk of contracting nutritional eye disease before the fifth birthday is thus 2% for corneal and 52% for non-corneal xerophthalmia. It is estimated that 60 000–80 000 preschool children in Indonesia develop corneal xerophthalmia per year of whom 50% go blind. Mortality of corneal xerophthalmia cases is 50–80%. The prevalence of corneal scars was negligible, most of whom became blind, died.

In Vietnam, Nguyen Dinh Cat (1958) reported seeing 1502 cases of keratomalacia in the north during 1951–53, but only 181 in the south during a similar period in 1955–57. With the continual unrest throughout the whole of the Indochina area since that time it is unlikely that the situation has improved.

Sporadic reports have come from Burma (Postmus, 1956; Sarin, 1957; Ko-Lay, 1968) and on a visit to Rangoon in 1972 the writer found about 20% of hospitalized children with PEM to have xerophthalmia. It is reported to be the most common cause of blindness in young children in Nepal (Prasad and Upadhaya, 1967). Vitamin A deficiency appears to be fairly widespread in Thailand (Netrasiri and Netrasiri, 1955; van Eekelen, 1956) and has been investigated at Chengmai (Smith *et al.*, 1975) and in Bangkok (Suthutvoravoot and Olson, 1974). Xerophthalmia was previously common in Hong Kong (Dansey-Browning, 1958) but is rare at the present time.

The problem of keratomalacia in Malaysia has been recognized for some time, commonly in association with kwashiorkor (Martin, 1930; Said, 1955). Field (1931) gave an early account of xerophthalmia in Perak where he found it affected 4% of the children of immigrant Tamils but less than 0.5% of Malays and was very rare in Chinese. Oomen (1960) found xerosis conjunctivae and Bitot's spots as the most common evidence of vitamin A deficiency, but even so agreed with McPherson (1956), working in Kelantan, that in some parts it may account for a large proportion of the blind. Chen (1972) reported on the importance of sociocultural factors. Williamson (Section 6d, above) described the disastrous effect the replacement of breast feeding by sweetened condensed milk had in Singapore. Loh (1967) reported a marked fall in prevalence over 10 years, and Lim (1975) stated that xerophthalmia was then non-existent.

In the Philippines keratomalacia frequently accompanies kwashiorkor (Stransky, 1950; Stransky, Dauis-Lawas, and Lawas, 1951). De Ocampo (1956) reports that xerophthalmia was still a frequent cause of blindness. In recent years xerophthalmia has been intensively studied on the island of Cebu (Solon *et al.*, 1978).

iv. Japan. The account of "hikam" by Mori (1904) was one of the first indications that infant xerophthalmia is a widespread scourge in some countries. Japanese ophthalmologists, with whom the matter was discussed in Tokyo in 1960, agreed that xerophthalmia was then only rarely seen. That the situation had radically changed, particularly since the end of the second world war, was evident from data compiled by Professor Irinoda of Hirosaki University. Studies by these workers between 1910 and 1930 showed a high incidence in the general population of xerosis, night blindness, and keratomalacia. That in many instances of vitamin A deficiency disease the eyes were permanently damaged is shown by figures Irinoda gives for the percentage of blindness due to keratomalacia according to various workers. The results of 14 such studies carried out between 1909 and 1953 showed a range of from 4.90 to 34.83%. Majima et al. (1960) reporting on the examination they made of the causes of blindness in Shizuoka blind school in 1958–59 found that 12 (six males and six females) out of 37 cases due to other than congenital conditions had been caused by keratomalacia. Japan forms the prime example of how xerophthalmia has disappeared as a by-product of economic and social advance.

b. The Middle East and North Africa

The countries of this region have a cultural unity, comprising the heart of the Moslem world and the people for the most part being Arab. Geographically north African countries, like those of the Middle East, have large arid tracts. Some are also undergoing rapid development as a result of new-found oil wealth but this has not necessarily benefited the ordinary man.

Many of these countries were visited by the writer during the survey for WHO (Oomen et al., 1964) and evidence gained at that time and subsequently for the not infrequent occurrence of xerophthalmia in Syria, Jordan (McLaren et al., 1965a; Patwardhan, 1969), Egypt (Smith et al., 1973), Sudan (Mekki el Sheikh, 1960), Upper Volta, Libya, Tunisia (Rezgallah et al., 1967), Morocco, Iraq, parts of Iran, and Afghanistan.

However, a note of warning has to be sounded. Xerophthalmia is frequently overlooked as a cause of blindness in young children, especially in countries like those of this region where communicable ophthalmia, particularly trachoma, is endemic (Jones et al., 1976).

c. Africa South of the Sahara

Traditionally it has not been considered that xerophthalmia is an important problem in this part of the continent. Certainly most of the population are protected in those parts of West and Central Africa, where red palm oil, containing about 20 000 $\mu g/100$ g of carotene, is used for cooking, but even there keratomalacia has been reported in infants too young to receive the family diet. More frequently than elsewhere an association has been noted with measles (see Chapter 11, Section C) and native medicine frequently complicates the picture.

Early reports include those of Williams (1933) from Accra, Trowell (1937) from Kampala, McKenzie (1939), Balletto (1954) and McLaren (1960) from Tanzania, Stock (1946) from northern Nigeria, Scragg and Rubidge (1960) from Durban, and Squires (1956) from Bechuanaland.

Friis-Hansen and McCullough (1962) reported low serum vitamin A levels and frequent conjunctival changes in three rural parts of Zambia. In the 1950s one of the highest rates of blindness in the world was reported from the Luapula valley of Zambia; 3235/100 000 in those under 18 years old. Much of this was attributable to a combination of vitamin A deficiency and measles (Cobb and Awdry, 1968).

Recent reports include those of McManus (1968) from Matabeleland, Rhodesia, Lechat et al. (1976) from Niger, Ben Sira et al. (1972) from Malawi, Yassur (1972) from Rwanda, Voorhoeve (1966) and Oomen (1971) from Nigeria, and Quéré et al. (1967) from the former West African Territories.

Two reports from the Republic of South Africa illustrate how the situation may vary in different parts of a country. While PEM is common in both Johannesburg and Cape Town, xerophthalmia was a frequent accompaniment in the former, 9.7 per cent in 1116 cases of kwashiorkor with 24.8% deaths (Kuming and Politzer, 1967) among the Bantu. In Cape Town among the Cape Coloured people xerophthalmia is rare (Konno et al., 1968) and the authors considered that the squash and pumpkin readily available there might be protective.

d. Europe.

There are very few accounts of endemic foci of xerophthalmia since the second world war and none within the past decade.

Frontali (1948) reported keratomalacia as a frequent complication of kwashiorkor in southern Italy. From Poland, Juzwa (1958) described 17 cases, most of the patients under 1 year of age, 10 of whom died with severe marasmus accompanying keratomalacia. Puretić et al. (1967) over 15 years collected a series of 19 cases in Jugoslavia; infants $1\frac{1}{2}$–9 months of age, most of them coming from rural areas. Keratomalacia was present in 17 and Bitot's spots and xerosis in two. Five died, four were blind in both eyes, seven in one eye, and only three recovered completely or with a nebula.

e. The Americas

Endemic xerophthalmia in the Western Hemisphere is now confined to the parts of Central and South America where living standards are low. Night blindness used to be common among the fishing communities of Newfoundland and Labrador (Aykroyd, 1930; Steven and Wald, 1941), but has greatly diminished following the fortification of margarine with vitamin A. In some parts, however, for instance the West Indies (Jelliffe, 1955) and British Guiana (Herlinger, 1950), other forms of malnutrition are common but the abundance of carotene available seems to be utilized in infant feeding and vitamin A status is generally adequate. Formerly xerophthalmia was a problem among East Indians in Trinidad and in remote districts and on mines in British Guiana (Committee on Nutrition in the Colonial Empire, 1939).

The survey carried out in the Central American countries by Autret and Béhar (1954) revealed that xerophthalmia is one of the most common complications of kwashiorkor in this area. The writer had the opportunity to travel extensively in Guatemala and in El Salvador in 1960 and saw many such cases in hospitals in both these countries. The importance of the problem appears to be related here, as elsewhere, to the density of population.

Many of the reports from South America have been available to the writer only in abstract form, and in those read in full little more than passing reference has been made to ocular manifestations. If one may safely argue from personal experience in part of Central America together with the detailed studies carried out from the Institute of Nutrition for Central America and Panama (INCAP), then in similar parts of the rest of Latin America a comparable problem may be inferred. In Mexico, Pagola (1948) found a high incidence of conjunctival xerosis and occasional corneal ulcers and Bitot's spots in kwashiorkor cases, and according to Gil (1934) keratomalacia is a prominent part of the infant malnutrition syndrome there. Other reports associating xerophthalmia with protein deficiency come from Cuba (Castellanos, 1935, 1937), Honduras (Vidal, 1938), Curaçaco (van der Sar, 1951), Rio de Janeiro in Brazil (Carvalho, 1946, 1947; Pernetta and de Martino, 1945), Caracas in Venezuela (Oropeza, 1946), and Santiago, Chile (Meneghello et al., 1949, 1950).

Rather indefinite accounts of xerophthalmia come from Peru (Huenemann et al., 1955) and Colombia (Thonnard-Neumann, 1957) and it is stated that in Uruguay both xerophthalmia and kwashiorkor are rare (Carlos Negro and Gentile Ramos, 1957).

Most of the South American countries do not report a major xerophthalmia problem despite quite low intakes and blood levels of vitamin A. The north-eastern part of Brazil has long been considered to be an exception, especially in the sugar cane area. Numerous cases of xerophthalmia have been reported by hospitals in this area.

Vitamin A status in the Central American countries has been extensively surveyed by the Institute of Nutrition of Central America and Panama (INCAP). In 1965–67 very low vitamin A levels were found, particularly in the rural areas, and these findings were supported by a high prevalence of low serum vitamin A values. However, clinical signs indicative or suggestive of the deficiency were not encountered on a significant scale. In April 1973, a biannual mass distribution of vitamin A capsules began in El Salvador in conjunction with a countrywide vaccination campaign and a study was carried out from September 1973 to December 1974 consisting of a nationwide prevalence survey of vitamin A-related pathological occular signs among preschool children and a retrospective chart review of hospitalized keratomalacia patients Sommer *et al.* (1975a,b). The prevalence survey, which covered 9508 children, did not reveal any cases of active corneal involvement, but five children with Bitot's spots, and three with healed corneal lesions thought to have been due to vitamin A deficiency were found. On this basis it was estimated that in the whole country (total population, 5.5 million) there are about 43 new surviving cases of X3A+3B per year, about 1 in 3 of which is likely to progress to blindness. A point prevalence survey in Haiti (Toureau *et al.*, 1976) revealed few active lesions. XS in children 0–6 years was 8.1/1000 in the north, but only 1.2/1000 in the south.

f. Australasia

Despite the primitive conditions under which nomadic hunting aborigines live in the interior of Australia nutritional eye disease does not occur, according to Mann (1959). In Papua xerophthalmia is not a problem (Dr R. F. R. Scragg, personal communication), but in Fiji it has been reported in young children (Thomson, 1949) and is occasionally associated with kwashiorkor (Manson-Bahr, 1951). Night blindness and other eye conditions due to vitamin A deficiency were described as frequent in the Solomon Islands (Committee on Nutrition in the Colonial Empire, 1939). Neave (1968) reported two fatal cases of keratomalacia among 106 children hospitalized with PEM.

10. Treatment

The physician who finds himself with the responsibility of treating cases of xerophthalmia will probably be subjected to a wide range of emotional feelings. On the one hand he will feel gratified with the dramatic response made by even quite advanced cases of xerosis corneae, and frequently even when there is residual scarring a useful degree of vision will have been preserved. All the difference will be made to the future of the child if some vision can be saved in even one eye. Nevertheless, there will be occasions, and these will be disconcertingly numerous, where the disease is especially common, when one glance at the screwed-up soggy eyelids and the underlying disorganized globes will be sufficient to tell him that all is already lost. Such cases usually are also severely generally undernourished and in the existing circumstances of neglect and poverty it is providential for family and sufferer alike that death is the rule.

Once subclinical and biochemical changes have been superseded by structural changes the process, especially in very young children, may proceed with alarming rapidity and it is essential that treatment be initiated forthwith. Unfortunately the decision to seek medical care in the first place is in the hands of the mother. Delay of a day or two at this stage, in the vain hope that things will improve, or worse still recourse to an indigenous medicine man as ignorant as herself but with an armamentarium containing some positively harmful applications, may prove decisive.

If there is any degree of corneal haziness there is the possibility of vision being permanently damaged and there is no reason to withhold a full course of treatment even if the conjunctiva alone is affected. There is no precise upper limit on the dose and as is mentioned later (Section IVB, below) the symptoms of hypervitaminosis A induced by a single dose are readily reversible. The relatively few instances reported have been usually with very large doses, with one exception in individuals without manifest xerophthalmia, and the symptoms which have never left any residual effects may have resulted from some idiosyncrasy. Occasional instances of apparent mild hypervitaminotic reaction have been encountered in massive dose preventive programmes (Section 11). These facts should not deter one from giving fully adequate treatment for established xerophthalmia.

Treatment consists of a capsule of vitamin A palmitate in oil (200 000 i.u., or about 66 000 μg) daily for 2 days and repeated on discharge. The dose is halved for infants under 1 year and for pregnant women. Oily vitamin A is not absorbed from the site of injection if given intramuscularly. If oral administration is not advisable because of severe vomiting, diarrhoea or other reasons water-dispersable injection in the above dosage must be given. Despite repeated representations oil injections are still on the market and largely account for the reported unresponsiveness of xerophthalmia to vitamin A. Vitamin A in tablet form rapidly deteriorates and should not be used. Cod or shark liver oil may be used for maintenance, 1 ounce providing about 10 000 μg. Halibut liver oil is about 50 times more potent.

The practice of putting cod liver oil drops into the eye as the only means of therapy cannot be deprecated too strongly. Records of response to this method and also by the administration of vitamin A to the lactating mother for treatment, through the milk, of her child's xerophthalmia, do not justify these practices. In a large clinical trial Sommer et al. (1980) found 200 000 i.u. oral oil to be as effective as 100 000 i.u. intramuscular water-dispersible vitamin A in the treatment of severe xerophthalmia. From recent studies in both the experimental animal (Pirie, 1977) and human patients (Sommer and Emran, 1978) topical application of retinoic acid 0.1% in oil has been shown to enhance the healing of corneal lesions and may form a useful adjunct to systemic treatment.

Useful vision may be restored by penetrating keratoplasty (Singh Gurbak and Malik, 1973), and in Malawi Ben Sira *et al.* (1972) were able to restore the anterior chamber permanently in 48 out of 50 cases of active keratomalacia by a "covering graft."

11. Prevention

When I was writing *Malnutrition and the Eye* in the early 1960s there had been no systematic attempt to combat the problem of xerophthalmia, even in those few countries like India and Indonesia where it was recognized to be a problem. Government and international agencies alike showed very little interest in the subject.

What has happened in the intervening 20 years gives much cause for gratification although much remains to be done. One of the most important factors in contributing towards control has undoubtedly been the enormous intensification of work in the field leading to a much better understanding and more widespread recognition of the existence of the problem of xerophthalmia. This means that doctors, nurses and even parents have learned to recognize the earlier stages, resulting in more effective treatment of established disease rather than prevention.

a. Nutrition Education

In the context of prevention I believe it is fundamental to recognize that xerophthalmia has the unusual characteristic of usually being a disease of "poverty in the midst of plenty". Where it is a serious problem there is no lack of provitamin A, in the form of dark-green leafy vegetables. The proper use of these cheap and readily available sources must be the cornerstone of any public health approach. A recent monograph (Oomen and Grubben, 1977) constitutes a useful, practical guide. Where xerophthalmia complicates PEM, nutrition rehabilitation centres should include in their programme the use of locally available, carotene-rich food and education of the mothers in their use. In Madurai, south India, Venkataswamy *et al.* (1976) have shown that such a centre is as effective as, and much less expensive than, hospital-based facilities.

Other approaches that have been adopted are based on the assumption that in communities at risk health and nutrition education measures cannot provide a quick answer in the existing circumstances and in view of the enormous toll on sight and life.

b. Periodic Massive Dose Programmes

The basis of the periodic massive dose programme is the 200 000 i.u. vitamin A capsule, available in many countries now from UNICEF, twice or three times a year, usually to children between the ages of 6 months and 5 years. Only half the capsule is used for those under 1 year. Several studies have shown that such a programme is safe and effective in lowering the prevalence of eye symptoms and maintaining plasma vitamin A levels (e.g. Vijayaraghavan et al., 1975; Tarwotjo et al., 1975). Programmes have been carried out in a number of countries including India, Bangladesh, Sri Lanka, Indonesia, Philippines, El Salvador and Haiti. Many millions of children have been covered annually by the programmes and the benefit, although difficult to measure, must be considerable. The problems in practice are also not inconsiderable. The programme has to be maintained indefinitely, so long as the underlying conditions persist. The cost is something like US$ 100 000 annually per million children covered, even in a country like India where health personnel in the rural areas are relatively numerous and well organized. Those children at risk to severe blinding xerophthalmia are the most inaccessible (Sommer et al., 1975b).

c. Fortification

Wheat flour is routinely fortified with vitamin A and other nutrients in some technologically developed countries. The first vitamin A fortification programme to combat vitamin A deficiency and xerophthalmia was undertaken by the Institute of Nutrition for Central America and Panama, using sugar as the medium. This is now being carried out in several of the countries of the area and being evaluated (Aguilar et al., 1977). The three types of intervention strategy described here are being evaluated in Cebu, Philippines with monosodium glutamate being the medium for fortification (Solon et al., 1978).

B. Secondary Vitamin A Deficiency

Secondary or endogenous nutritional deficiency arises in the presence of an adequate diet. It results from a failure at one or more stages in the proper utilization of nutrients within the body. Disorders of digestion, absorption, transport, storage, cellular metabolism, elimination or basic requirements may be responsible (McLaren, 1976).

In the case of vitamin A several of the possible mechanisms may be implicated. Adams *et al.* (1960) reported vitamin A deficiency following gastrectomy in five patients. Four had night blindness and the fifth perifollicular hyperkeratosis. All had very low fasting levels of vitamin in plasma (4–10 μg/100 ml; normal 20–50 μg/100 ml), and impaired vitamin A absorption tests. Jejunal biopsies were normal. Night blindness responded to vitamin A therapy in three patients, the fourth was not tested, and there was no definite improvement in the skin changes of the fifth.

Failure in the transport of vitamin A occurs in abetalipoproteinaemia (Chapter 8, Section IIIB). One instance in which disturbed cellular metabolism may have been responsible has been reported (Mullins, 1960). Keratomalacia failing to respond to treatment associated with adrenal hypoplasia occurred in a mentally defective black infant. McLaren and Zekian (1971) reported what appears to be a unique case of vitamin A deficiency in a 9-year-old Lebanese girl, due to failure of enzymic cleavage of β-carotene. Conjunctival xerosis, Bitot's spots and impaired dark adaptation were present. Plasma vitamin A was only 4 μg/100 ml, but total circulating carotenoids were high, the majority being β-carotene. Large oral doses of β-carotene in oil failed to raise the vitamin A level in this patient but did so in three other malnourished children. There was rapid response to vitamin A of the plasma level and the clinical signs. The dietary history revealed almost sole reliance on vegetable sources for the vitamin. This defect would clearly only manifest itself when preformed vitamin A is excluded from the diet.

A metabolic defect in mongolism has been postulated (Griffiths and Behrman, 1967) on the finding of a high incidence of impaired dark adaptation, but as this is a subjective test and the subjects were mentally defective, these results cannot be accepted.

Malabsorption states have frequently been reported to result in vitamin A deficiency. Impaired visual function in chronic pancreatitis has usually been attributed to vitamin A deficiency, but Toskes *et al.* (1977) have recently provided evidence for zinc deficiency as a cause (Chapter 5, Section IIC). Another recent report (Vahlquist *et al.*, 1978) described impaired dark adaptation and lowered plasma RBP in patients suffering from various intestinal diseases. Vitamin A therapy brought about a return to normal. In another series (Russell *et al.*, 1973) vitamin A was effective only in some.

Cystic fibrosis (mucoviscidosis) appears to occupy a rather special position. Ullerich and Witte (1961) described a 6-month-old infant with bilateral xerophthalmia and keratomalacia in one eye. The goblet cells are normal (Holm and Kessing, 1975). Petersen *et al.* (1968) reported night blindness and xerophthalmia in a 16-year-old girl, responding to vitamin A therapy. Bruce *et al.* (1960) described venous engorgement and oedema of the disc with haemorrhages and cystic changes at the macula which they regarded as characteristic. There was no evidence of vitamin A deficiency. Lietman *et al.* (1964) and Wong and Collins (1965) reported in addition to the retinal changes optic neuritis leading to atrophy. They attributed the latter to prolonged chloramphenicol therapy.

There are many accounts in the early literature of night blindness and xerosis of the conjunctiva associated with chronic liver disease (Moore, 1957d). A typical series was described by Patek and Haig (1939) 19 out of 24 having impaired dark adaptation, although none complained of night blindness. Most were malnourished, with weight loss, peripheral neuritis, glossitis, pellagrous dermatosis and lustreless conjunctivae. Scrapings from the conjunctiva in several patients showed keratinization of the epithelium and at postmortem three cases had typical keratinizing metaplasia of the pancreatic ducts. The impairment of dark adaptation responded to vitamin A.

In two patients with chronic alcoholism, goblet cells were absent on conjunctival biopsy and the eyes were dry with keratotic conjunctivae, despite normal tear volumes. Vitamin A therapy restored goblet cells to the conjunctivae (Sullivan *et al.*, 1973).

Bronte-Stewart and Foulds (1972) reported dyschromatopsia in two patients with cirrhosis, and a return to normal cone function with vitamin A. Sandberg *et al.* (1977) reported two patients with impaired rod and cone function which responded to vitamin A. In the study of Vahlquist *et al.* (1978) mentioned above, there were also patients with diseases of the liver. In these there was no response of dark adaptation or plasma RBP to vitamin A therapy. Response occurred, however, in the series of Russell *et al.* (1978).

The role of zinc is discussed later (Chapter 5, Section IIC; Chapter 10, Section IIA2).

IV. Human Studies of Hypervitaminosis A

In recent years this subject has rightly received a great deal of attention. Today, while on the one hand the classical deficiency diseases have been abolished from the more advanced countries, although continuing almost unchecked in the greater part of the world, on the other the dangers of excessive intake of nutrients are becoming apparent. Hypervitaminosis A is but one of these.

The problem of vitamin A toxicity has two main aspects. The first of these is the damage to the embryo resulting in congenital malformations (Chapter 9, Section IIB). There is no evidence at present that this may happen in man, as it does in animals, although precautions against such a possible occurrence should be taken. There is no doubt, however, about the harmful effects that a prolonged and excessive intake of vitamin A may have on both children and adults. This second aspect of vitamin A intoxication is important not only in connection with the way it may arise from an abuse of vitamin preparations, but also concerning the safety of therapeutic regimes for correction of actual clinical deficiency. The second of these matters is discussed above (Section IIIA*10*). The manifestations of hypervitaminosis A may best be considered separately as they occur in acute and chronic poisoning.

A. Acute Hypervitaminosis A

A number of instances recorded in adults has arisen from the ingestion by arctic explorers of polar bear or bearded seal liver. The concentration of vitamin A is so high in these, approximately $5000 \mu g/g$, that millions of units have probably been consumed at a single meal. Children have usually become affected through the injudicious therapeutic use of a single large dose of vitamin A amounting to many thousand micrograms.

In both age groups the main symptoms are nervous due to a sudden and marked rise in cerebrospinal fluid (CSF) pressure. Papilloedema has been observed in some cases and some adults have complained of visual disturbances including diplopia and lights before the eyes. Marie and Sée (1951, 1954) noticed that vomiting and bulging of the anterior fontanelle occurred in three infants aged under 1 year within 24 hours of the ingestion of 350 000 i.u. vitamin A. Recovery was rapid.

It is not known how the rise in CSF pressure is produced. In experimental animals hydrocephalus has resulted in the offspring of mothers with either hyper- or hypovitaminosis A (Chapter 9, Section IA). The rise in CSF pressure in young and adult animals on vitamin A-deficient diets is well established (Section IC). It has been reported that avitaminosis A can cause hydrocephalus in infants (Section III&*c*, above) although this is a most unusual manifestation.

Nearly all the children in whom hypervitaminosis A was produced were being treated for skin or other complaints in which there was some evidence of a mild deficiency of the vitamin. The case reported by Ehrengut (1955) differs from these in that the condition developed in an artificially fed $4\frac{1}{2}$ month old infant with severe keratomalacia. In the course of 2 days 187 000 i.u. vitamin A were given. After a further 2 days the child became febrile, and developed opisthotonus, bulging of the anterior fontanelle associated with somnolence, raised CSF pressure, petechiae, and rhinitis. Immediate improvement followed cessation of the vitamin therapy, but relapse followed a further 44 000 i.u. 2 days later. When the vitamin was again given after a further 17 days in small doses the keratomalacia healed.

This unusual case is instructive for it does indicate the possibility of producing alarming, albeit benign, symptoms with vitamin A therapy even in young subjects in whom all stores of the vitamin are totally depleted and signs of deficiency are present. The amounts given to this child are by no means excessive in keratomalacia and the writer and many other workers in the tropics have given as much for several days without ever having observed untoward effects. It seems that the manifestation of acute intoxication results from direct toxic effects on certain tissues, and is not dependent upon saturation of liver stores (Brëslau, 1957). This child may have had some defect that prevented liver storage and caused the circulation to be flooded with the vitamin. Just how much vitamin A is necessary to bring about the optimum cure of xerophthalmia and just how much may be given without causing side effects has never been decided (Section IIIA*10*).

B. Chronic Hypervitaminosis A

This was first described in a 3-year-old child (Josephs, 1944) and since then many well-documented cases, mostly in infants and young children, have been put on record. The onset is insidious and follows on a period of many weeks or months during which the daily ingestion of vitamin A has been in the region of 100 000 i.u. (33 000 μg). The clinical features vary considerably but in children tend to consist of various skin changes, hepatomegaly, and painful swellings of bones and joints. Hepatomegaly and bone involvement are less prominent in adults and the haemorrhagic phenomena, so common in animals, rarely occur in humans.

The ocular features include papilloedema, extraocular muscle paralyses, diplopia, and occasionally exophthalmos (Oliver and Havener, 1958). The case reported by Turtz and Turtz (1960) had—in addition to diplopia, poor visual acuity, and early papilloedema—discrete superficial haemorrhages throughout the retinae of both eyes. This 17-year-old boy had been taking 200 000 i.u. vitamin A daily for the previous 18 months for the treatment of acne.

Morrice *et al.* (1970) and Mikkelsen *et al.* (1974) report several cases in which papilloedema and other eye signs were accompanied by symptoms of raised intracranial pressure, simulating brain tumour, "pseudotumour cerebri".

C. Hypercarotenosis

Mention should be made of the effects of accumulation of excessive amounts of carotenoids in the body. Hypercarotenaemia (plasma carotenoids greater than 300 mg/100 ml) leads to the staining of tissues, especially the palms of the hands and soles of the feet, due to secretion of pigment in the sebum. The condition may arise by excessive ingestion, as in West Africa and elsewhere where red palm oil, a rich source, is used in cooking, or excessive drinking of carrot juice (Abrahamson and Abrahamson, 1962).

It is also seen in diabetes mellitus, myxoedema, and anorexia nervosa occasionally, probably due to a defect in conversion of carotene to vitamin A. Hypervitaminosis never results and the abnormal pigment disappears when consumption ceases.

Giorgio *et al.* (1964) reported the case of a 42-year-old white male in whom pseudo Kayser-Fleischer rings of the cornea were found to be due to carotenoid deposition in arci senili.

Chapter 3

Vitamins of the B Complex

While other vitamins have been given a special letter to identify them and have been regarded as quite separate and unrelated substances, those grouped together under the letter B have been treated in this way for a very definite reason. A B vitamin has been defined as an organic substance which acts catalytically in all living cells and which is essential for the nutrition of higher animals. Until 1926 it was generally believed that "vitamin B" was a single entity, but in that year it was shown to consist of two factors differing in their reactions to changes of temperature. The thermolabile factor was shown to have the ability to cure the symptoms of beriberi, while the quite separate thermostable factor had growth-promoting properties. The thermolabile factor proved to be a single vitamin, thiamine, but the heat stable factor turned out to be a complex with several members.

Just as the existence of thiamine had been demonstrated by feeding experiments on birds and human beings suffering from deficiency disease so were four other members of this complex shown to exist. Thus, Goldberger's studies on pellagra in the southern United States and his experiments on humans and dogs pointed the way to the discovery of the biological importance of nicotinic acid. Riboflavin was shown to be a vitamin necessary for the growth of rats, pyridoxine as a factor that cured dermatitis in rats, and pantothenic acid as being curative of a dermatitis in chicks. It was pantothenic acid that formed the link between the group of vitamins of the B complex and what was known as the "bios" complex. It has been observed many years before that certain yeasts failed to develop on a medium of purified constituents but that they grew satisfactorily when a yeast extract was added. It was concluded that these organisms required a factor for their growth derived from living cells and this was called "bios". It was later shown that this was not a single substance and various components were shown to be identical with thiamine, riboflavin, nicotinic acid, and pyridoxine. Thus the vitamin B complex and the bios complex were seen to have much in common, if not being actually identical. One member of the bios complex not then identified with any member of the vitamin B complex was a substance to which the name of pantothenic acid had been given. Concentrates prepared from liver showed chemical properties similar to those of the filtrate factor that cured dermatitis in chicks. An interchange of specimens by the workers concerned showed that pantothenic acid cured the dermatitis in chicks and the filtrate factor stimulated the growth of yeast. Shortly afterward the identity of the two substances was established by degradation and synthesis.

This new development was followed up with important results. Biotin, another member of the bios complex with biological activity in extremely high dilution, was found to relieve the symptoms produced in animals by deficiency of what was then called vitamin H. In almost exactly the same way it was found that a factor termed vitamin Bc, essential for the chick, was identical with folic acid, a growth factor of certain bacteria. In this case there are several closely related substances exhibiting similar biological properties, as it were a folic acid complex within the vitamin B complex. Similarly both p-aminobenzoic acid and inositol were shown to be not only essential growth factors for many bacteria but also vitamins for certain animal species.

There are several substances of doubtful status as members of the vitamin B complex but these need not be considered here as a deficiency of them is not known to cause any ocular lesions. The latest firmly established member of the complex is vitamin B_{12} or cobalamin. This is the extrinsic factor of Castle, the anti-pernicious anemia factor in liver, as well as being the essential growth factor for *Lactobacillus lactis* found in refined liver extracts.

Because of the close association in nature of members of the B vitamin complex and the multiple deficiency states produced particularly in the earlier work, it has seemed best to deal with the vitamins as a group, considering together their various ocular manifestations.

I. Animal Studies

A. The Ocular Glands and the Lids

1. "Spectacle Eye"

The first account in which the eye was implicated in deficiency of vitamins of the B complex seems to be the short note by Goldberger and Lillie (1926) on the state of albino rats fed on the heat-stable fraction of yeast. They mentioned "ophthalmia" as one of the clinical features but gave no further details. Shortly afterward a similar account was published by the English workers Chick and Roscoe (1927). A more detailed description of the ocular signs was given by Sherman and Sandels (1931) who noted in rats deficient in riboflavin, then known as vitamin G, a denudation of the eyelids identical with that already described in vitamin A-deficient rats (see Chapter 2, Section IB). This was named by these workers "spectacle eye" on account of the spectacle-like ring of bare skin immediately surrounding the eyes, part of a generalized dermatitis. It was subsequently shown by György and Eckardt (1940) that deficiency of pyridoxine could also produce this change in the rat. Spectacle eye is not confined to the rat: Irinoda and Mikami (1958) described it in rabbits as well as rats suffering from pyridoxine deficiency. In both these animals the palpebral margin was congested and moist and in some cases resembled a true blepharitis angularis. Histologically the lids showed hyperkeratosis of the skin of the eyelids with oedema and dilatation of blood vessels. In the subcutaneous tissue there was infiltration of lymphocytes, plasma cells, and monocytes. The purpose of this study was to investigate the role of pyridoxine deficiency in the angular blepharoconjunctivitis of man associated usually with infection by *Haemophilus duplex* (Morax-Axenfeld bacillus). When this organism was inoculated into the conjunctival sac of pyridoxine-deficient animals it tended to survive longer than in the case of controls. From these results and from other work carried out in man (see Section IIA5) the authors concluded that deficiency of pyridoxine plays a primary part in this clinical condition, and infection with *H. duplex* has only a secondary significance. From the same laboratory blepharoconjunctivitis has been reported in pantothenic acid-deficient rats (Tomizawa, 1959) and more severe destructive changes in the lids in biotin deficiency (Ichinohe, 1960) identical with the desquamation, thinning, and atrophy found elsewhere in the skin, in addition to the blepharo-dermatitis of "spectacle eye" (Irinoda and Ichinohe, 1961). Sekino (1960) noted marginal blepharitis in the folic acid-deficient rat.

2. Porphyrin Incrustation

All animals possessing a third eyelid have a large gland of Harder situated in the orbit posterior to the eyeball. McElroy *et al.* (1941) demonstrated that the pigment responsible for the so-called "blood-caked whiskers" secretion seen in rats in a number of deficiency states is coproporphyrin. Among these deficiency states are included those involving pantothenic acid (Oleson *et al.*, 1939), riboflavin (Bessey and Wolbach, 1939), nicotinic acid (Krehl, 1949), biotin (Ichinohe, 1960), vitamin B_{12} (Takahashi, 1958), essential fatty acids (see Chapter 8, Section IC), water depletion (Figge and Atkinson, 1941) (see Chapter 1, Section IB2), and protein deficiency (McLaren, 1959) (see Chapter 6, Section IB). In the writer's experience the porphyrin incrustation does not always take precisely the same form. The term "blood-caked whiskers" has the unfortunate implication that the material is blood, which it is not. It describes the main feature of one form of porphyrin incrustation which affects not only the whiskers but also the snout and the paws to some extent by transfer. The eyelids are not involved. Deficiency of vitamins of the B complex produces this appearance. In deficiency of vitamin A and protein the secretion is strictly limited to the lids and the end of the snout. In one vitamin A-deficient rat the writer found that the posterior surface of the upper central incisor teeth showed the characteristic fluorescence around the ends of the nasolacrimal ducts which run through these teeth.

It was shown by Collins et al. (1953) that the porphyrin incrustation resulting from deficiency of vitamins of the B complex was enhanced by an accompanying high relative humidity. Animals kept at 90% relative humidity developed this staining within a period of 1 to 3 weeks while those maintained below 50% relative humidity showed hardly any. The most marked effect was in rats on diets deficient in riboflavin, pantothenic acid, or pyridoxine and also subjected to the stress of a high relative humidity. In view of the reported beneficial effects of certain flavonoid compounds in a variety of pathological conditions in which capillary fragility and permeability were interfered with, these workers (Schreiber and Elvehjem, 1954) decided to see what effect the flavonols rutin, quercetin, and quercitrin had on porphyrin incrustation. From their experiments it was evident that these flavonoid compounds essentially prevented the discharge of pigment in vitamin-deficient animals and in those on a restricted water regime maintained at 90% relative humidity. They suggest that under conditions of stress, exemplified by a high relative humidity in these experiments, the rat may have special requirements for flavonoid compounds.

The ocular glands in the vitamin B-deficient animal have not received much attention. It was Philpot and Pirie (1943) who made the interesting suggestion that the corneal epithelium might obtain some of its riboflavin from the eye secretions as a result of their discovery that the concentration of this vitamin was higher in the lacrimal and Meibomian glands of the ox than in any other tissue of the eye. In addition to the porphyrin secretion already referred to, Bessey and Wolbach (1939) also found that the Harderian gland of the rat showed dense infiltration of darkly staining lymphocytes which replaced the glandular tissue. According to Salmon and Engel (1940) the Harderian gland shows some sloughing and haemorrhages into the lumen of the ducts in pantothenic acid deficiency.

In an attempt to reproduce in the experimental animal the syndrome of infantile malnutrition as observed in the South African Bantu, Gilbert and Gillman (1944) fed albino rats for 2 years on a diet consisting of maize pap and fermented milk. After 15 months the majority of the animals had developed porphyrin incrustation of the whiskers and around the eyes and snout. The aetiology of these changes was not ascertained but lack of the B vitamins and protein may well have been involved. The same group (Gillman *et al.*, 1947) subsequently showed that the extraorbital lacrimal glands of these animals were microscopically extensively mottled with yellow areas alternating with white. Histologically there was hypertrophy of nuclei, metaplasia of the gland cells, cystic dilatation of the ducts, and marked accumulation of fat. Both the appearance of porphyrin secretion and the severity of the changes in the glands were much more pronounced in the male than in the female. This marked sexual dimorphism of the exorbital gland of the albino rat was also noted in respect of changes due to the ageing process by Walker (1958). Surprisingly this dimorphism was not present in Norwegian grey rats.

B. The Conjunctiva and the Cornea

The bulbar conjunctiva and cornea may conveniently be considered together as they are examined at the same time and their metabolism is closely related. In the rat, the species which has been most frequently used for experimental study of ocular signs of B complex deficiency, the conjunctiva is nothing more than an inconspicuous narrow ring of tissue, and attention has been concentrated on the cornea.

1. Riboflavin

Sherman and Sandels (1931) reported vascularization of the cornea in rats suffering from vitamin "G" deficiency. Histological sections of the eyes of these animals showed a slight keratitis, infiltration with a few polymorphonuclears, and some newly formed blood channels. In the same year, Day *et al.* (1931) noted that most of their riboflavin-deficient rats with cataract also had superficial corneal vascularization. Several years later a more thorough study was made by Bessey and Wolbach (1939) and comparison was made with results obtained much earlier (Wolbach and Howe, 1925) in vitamin A deficiency. Apart from the accompanying keratinization of corneal and conjunctival epithelia in vitamin A deficiency there was very little difference noted. They fed 300 rats on a synthetic diet in which casein and cornstarch were freed from riboflavin by extraction and refluxing with alcohol. In every instance after the 4th week of the deficiency, microscopic examination or India ink injections produced evidence of corneal vascularization. From the 5th to the 7th week the palpebral fissures became narrowed and the eye receded, the lids being rather swollen. The corneae became slightly dull as if finely sanded and after the 7th to the 10th week one or both corneae might become turbid and white. By the 10th or 11th week blood vessels extended inward for more than one third of the diameter of the cornea. Venous connections were even more abundant than arterial and the conclusion was drawn that simultaneous growth from arterial and venous sources took place. The invading capillaries at first lay just beneath the corneal epithelium but later others came to lie deep in the substantia propria. Only in very advanced stages of deficiency were vessels seen deeper than the junction of the middle and lower third of the stroma. The capillaries lay between the lamellae of the stroma and as the deficiency advanced, so the endothelial cells became more prominent and the mitotic figures more numerous in the capillary walls. Leucocytes, mostly polymorphs, accumulated beneath the epithelium especially near the centre of the cornea and appeared to be invading the epithelium. The stromal collagen became replaced by a lightly staining non-fibrillary material and the fibrils appeared to have swollen and fused. In the epithelium there was remarkably little change in the deeper layers but the superficial cells became separated and vesicles sometimes formed between the superficial and deep layers. Recovery took place rapidly. Moderate corneal turbidity cleared in 12 hours after 60 μg riboflavin by mouth, and after 2 weeks of 20 μg daily blood vessels were no longer visible by slit lamp. Five μg of riboflavin daily was found to be an adequate protective dose against vascularization. In a further comparative study of the corneal vascularization in vitamin A and riboflavin deficiency (see also Chapter 2, Section IB), Bowles *et al.* (1946) described initial changes of conjunctival oedema and congestion followed about a week later by congestion of limbic vessels. Soon after this, capillary "sprouts" of the terminal loop type were seen to extentd a short distance into the cornea. This was followed a few days later by intense oedema and opacification of the cornea which slowly subsided, leaving the cornea extensively vascularized usually with vessels of the terminal loop type.

Professor Irinoda and his colleagues at Hirosaki University in Japan carried out much experimental work in connection with the effects of a deficiency of various members of the vitamin B complex on the eye, and this will be described in subsequent pages. The writer has had the privilege of being entertained by Professor Irinoda and his colleague Dr Mikami in Tokyo and of seeing their work. These studies have been prompted by the occurrence of a disease in the Aomori perfecture known locally as "shibi-gattchaki", apparently due to deficiency of vitamins of the B complex and in which eye lesions are a prominent feature. The clinical aspects of this work are described in Section IIA4.

In the rabbit, Irinoda (1955) produced corneal vascularization in 3 animals and diffuse corneal opacity in 5 out of a total of 26 rabbits. Histologically he found vacuole formation in the cells of the superficial layers of the corneal epithelium and subepithelial cellular infiltration and vessel formation. In an electron microscopic study (Takahashi, 1959) the cells of the corneal epithelium showed degeneration and swelling of the mitochondria and vacuole-like swelling of the cytoplasm in the early stages of deficiency, with partial breakdown of the nucleus in the later stages.

It was suggested by Johnson and Eckardt (1940) that vascularization due to riboflavin deficiency was hastened by exposure to sunlight, due to destruction of the vitamin. Lowry and Bessey (1945) could not confirm this, and suggested that this was probably because riboflavin is in a bound form in the cornea. In excised ox eyes Philpot and Pirie (1943) showed that the dinucleotide of riboflavin in the epithelium is stable. Almost nothing is known about the nature of the biochemical lesion in the cornea resulting from deficiency of riboflavin apart from the observation of Lee and Hart (1944) (see also Chapter 2, Section IB) that the oxygen uptake of the epithelium is diminished.

Subsequently similar changes have been reported in other species. In the dog, Street et al. (1941) described corneal opacities with the appearance of a deep punctate keratitis but did not mention vascularization. However, Potter et al. (1942) found that in their riboflavin-deficient dogs eye signs appeared in 4 to 9 weeks and consisted of a purulent discharge, followed in a few days by vascularization, and later by opacities. Both of these groups of workers mention that the nictitating membrane was pulled forward and the eyeball rotated dorsally in a peculiar manner. In the pig (Patek, et al., 1941) changes in the corneal epithelial cells occur but in the absence of vascularization. This was confirmed by Wintrobe et al. (1944), who examined two pigs which lived for 91 and 135 days on a diet deficient in riboflavin. In mice (Lippincott and Morris, 1942), cats (Gershoff et al., 1959), and monkeys (Waisman, 1944) corneal changes were absent. The chinook salmon (Halver, 1957) in riboflavin deficiency is photophobic and develops corneal vascularization. The baby pig (Miller et al., 1954), in addition to developing a heavy sebaceous exudate about the eye, showed an interesting histological change in the corneal epithelium although, as in the adult animal, there was no vascularization. This consisted of a ballooning of the columnar cells of the basal layer very similar to the appearance of these cells in the epithelium of rats fed a diet of cassava by the writer (see Fig. 83). It may have been that these latter changes were in part due to a deficiency of riboflavin rather than of protein.

2. *Other B Vitamins*

Deficiency of vitamins of the B complex other than riboflavin as far as is known plays a much smaller role in pathology for the cornea. Bowles *et al.* (1949) reported corneal vascularization in rats deficient in either pyridoxine or pantothenic acid. More severe lesions consisting of keratitis, corneal ulceration, and abscess formation were described by Musini (1954) in the pyridoxine-deficient rat, and Irinoda and Mikami (1958) noted vascularization in their rabbits. Tomizawa (1959) investigated the ocular changes in albino and in hooded rats. Corneal vascularization and opacity were present in both strains and actual ulceration occurred in the hooded strain in pantothenic acid deficiency.

Van Bijsterveld (1976) inoculated the conjunctiva of pyridoxine deficient and control guinea pigs with three strains of *Moraxella* organisms. In the deficient group there was decreased tear flow and the organisms survived longer. Lysozyme concentrations in tear fluid were similar in both groups.

Minimal changes, consisting of slight vascularization, increase of pigment at the limbus, and what the authors called "separation and movement" at the basal cell layer of the conjunctiva were seen by Irinoda and Yamada (1956) in rabbits deficient in nicotinic acid. Agarwal and Datt (1954) claimed enhanced healing with diminished scarring of corneal incisions in normal rabbits dosed with micotinic acid (see also Section IIA6).

Ichinohe (1960) in an investigation of acute and chronic biotin deficiency in albino and hooded rats reported superficial diffuse keratitis, corneal opacity with vascularization, and ulceration in a few animals chronically deficient.

Claims have been made for a role for vitamin B_{12} in experimental corneal wound healing (Menna and Rosati, 1953) and regeneration of corneal nerves (Martini, 1955), but in the study undertaken by Takahashi (1958) on the ocular manifestations of vitamin B_{12} deficiency in the rat the cornea appears to have escaped and the main lesions were in the retina. Sekino (1960) described thinning of the corneal epithelium with nuclear degeneration and diminished glycogen and nucleic acid in folic acid deficiency.

The work of Gilbert and Gillman (1944) in the rat in relation to the role of a diet of corn pap and fermented milk in producing malnutrition in South African Bantu children has already been mentioned (Section A2 above). In addition to porphyrin incrustation and lacrimal gland changes they described vascularization of the cornea under the slit lamp microscope with vacuolation of the epithelium and scarring. The diet was probably especially low in protein and vitamins of the B complex but it is not possible to relate any specific deficiency to these eye changes.

C. The Lens

1. Riboflavin

In 1928 it was mentioned by Salmon *et al.* in an account of the effects of a diet deficient in certain members of the vitamin B complex in the rat that an occasional feature was cataract. This is the first report of a nutritional deficiency leading to cataract which has since been substantiated although it will be recalled that von Szily earlier claimed that vitamin A deficiency could do so, but this has never been confirmed. Shortly afterwards Day *et al.* (1931) found that 94% of their rats on a riboflavin-deficient diet developed cataract in from 60 to 87 days. Day and his colleagues subsequently reported that such a diet also produced a similarly high percentage of lens opacities in wild rats (Langston and Day, 1933), mice (Langston *et al.*, 1933), and chicks (Day *et al.*, 1934). This work has been confirmed many times but other investigators have never been able to obtain the very high incidence of cataract reported by Day. It seems unlikely that species or strain differences could account for this in view of the uniformly high incidence in the animals studied by Day. It is more likely that differences in the composition of the experimental diets were responsible. By the substitution of egg albumin for casein, Day *et al.* (1934) completely prevented the development of cataract in both rats and chicks. Supplementation of the diet with cystine also appeared to decrease the incidence. It was later shown (Day and Darby, 1936) that the rate of growth of the animal was an important factor. In those rats that gained less than 10 g body weight weekly 63% developed cataract but among those gaining 60 g or more not one showed lens changes. From the work of Baum *et al.* (1942) it appeared that cataract occurred more consistently when there was a trace of riboflavin in the diet than when the diet was completely riboflavin-free. Relatively minor dietary changes resulted in marked differences in the incidence of damage to the lens. The many differences and discrepancies in all this work have never been satisfactorily resolved but recent work suggests that factors other than riboflavin may have played a part. Hasegawa and Yagi (1975) failed to produce typical cataract, and on electron microscopic examination there was only swelling and degeneration of mitochondria and vacuolation of the cytosol in epithelial cells. Srivastava and Beutler (1972) reported a higher incidence of cataract in rats fed a high galactose diet when they were also deficient in riboflavin. They found that deficient animals, as was to be expected, had reduced activity in the lens of glutathione reductase, but normal levels of reduced glutathione, total thiol and protein thiol seemed to rule out thiol deficiency as a factor. Polyols, such as galactitol and sorbitol, have been shown to accumulate in the lens in sugar cataracts (Chapter 7,

Section I), and it is suspected that they produce osmotic and permeability changes in the lens capsule and thus contribute to opacification. Srivastava and Beutler (1972) suggest that as NADPH is a cofactor for glutathione reductase as well as for aldose reductase, and since the latter enzyme catalyses the reduction of galactose to galactitol, riboflavin deficiency might facilitate galactitol formation by increasing the availability of NADPH for the aldose reductase reaction. Recent human studies on this subject are discussed later (Chapter 11, Section B).

Cataract has also been observed to occur as a feature of riboflavin deficiency in certain other animal species. It is possible that Day (1934) also induced

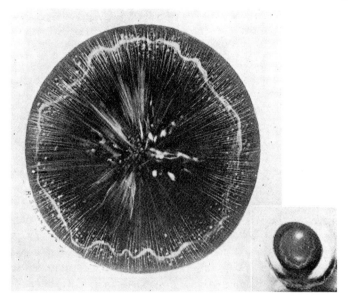

FIG. 44. Cataract in riboflavin deficiency in a pig (slit lamp composite drawing). Insert: Photograph of the same eye showing the equatorial opacities. From Wintrobe *et al.* (1944)

cataract in the monkey in this way but the published data are not adequate for independent evaluation of this point. Lippincott and Morris (1942) noted, in passing, that cataract occurred infrequently in their riboflavin-deficient mice. Although no corneal changes were seen by Wintrobe *et al.* (1944) in their pigs they did develop cataract (Fig. 44). In the baby pig, Miller *et al.* (1954) found that cataract was present at about 35 days of age in animals started on the riboflavin-deficient diet when 72 hours old. The opacities were situated just posterior to the equator of the lens. The affected lens fibres were swollen and separated and the epithelial cells were also swollen, forming what were termed vesicular cells. The study of riboflavin deficiency in the chinook salmon by Halver (1957) mentions "cloudy lens" in addition to photophobia and corneal vascularization (see above, Section B*1*). The latest account of experimental cataract due to riboflavin deficiency would seem to be that of Gershoff *et al*. (1959) in the cat. In this species there was no corneal change but cataracts developed with some frequency in those animals suffering from chronic deficiency of riboflavin and receiving a high fat diet. The cataracts were bilateral in five cats. Some were nuclear and some subcapsular thus differing somewhat from the riboflavin-deficiency cataracts in other species which have tended to be only cortical. In two cases the capsule was loosened and a material giving the Liebermann–Burchard reaction for unesterified cholesterol was present under the capsule. Tryptophan metabolism is disturbed in riboflavin deficiency (Mason, 1953) and this may play a part in cataract formation (Chapter 6, Section ID).

2. Other B Vitamins

As in the case of the cornea, so for the lens, most of the changes have been with a deficiency of riboflavin and there are few accounts of work with the rest of the B group vitamins. Most of these are concerned with the effect of maternal dietary deficiency on the embryo and are therefore considered in Chapter 9. A passing reference was made to the development of cataract in some of the rats fed a choline-deficient diet in a study of the effect of subcutaneous injections of serotonin creatinine sulphate by McDonald *et al*. (1958). Whether the lens damage was due to the choline deficiency or accentuated by the high calorie, high fat diet is not clear. That it was solely due to the choline deficiency is unlikely, for numerous accounts of the effects of such a deficiency in the rat have not previously included cataract, although other ocular lesions are known to occur (see below, Section IG). It is possible that the state in rats attributed to a diet poor in methyl groups, one of the features of which was reported to be cataract (Cristini, 1950), was really choline deficiency although lack of methionine may also have played a part.

Inositol is usually grouped among the B vitamins. Chemically it is *meso*-cyclohexanehexanol and is similar in structure to "gammexane", the insecticide which may act as an anti-metabolite. It is possible that, unlike other vitamins of the B complex, it is not a prosthetic group of an essential enzyme system but that it is an essential component of living tissue. Deficiency of inositol produces alopecia and loss of weight in mice and rats but deficiency symptoms in man have not been described. It was detected in the lens by Krause and Weekers (1938) and was shown by van Heyningen (1957) to be present in that tissue in concentrations almost higher than anywhere else in the body. The mere presence of inositol and other organic compounds in high concentration in the lens does not necessarily mean that they enter into the metabolic processes of that tissue. It does, however, invite enquiry as to why they should be there, but at present there is no answer to this question.

D. The Retina

Riboflavin has been detected in the retina of many species. Pirie (1943) found only small quantities in the mammalian retina and this was nearly all bound as riboflavin-adenine-dinucleotide which is light-stable. Clear evidence that riboflavin acts as a photosensitizer in the mammalian retina is lacking. The tapetum lucidum is a structure lying behind the light-sensitive cells of the retina in such a way that any light not absorbed during its first passage through these cells is reflected back again and has a second opportunity to be absorbed. Man and the higher apes do not have a tapetum but many lower animals do, including the lemur *Galage crassicaudatus*, and in this species Pirie (1959) found this structure to be made up of crystals of riboflavin. It is suggested that riboflavin may increase the light stimulus in two ways, by acting as a reflector and by its property of fluorescence.

Once again it is Japanese workers who have given descriptions of the retinal changes in vitamin B complex deficiency. In the riboflavin-deficient rabbit (Irinoda and Sato, 1954) most of the animals showed evidence of degenerative changes in the retinal ganglion cells indicated by chromatolysis and chromatophilia of Nissl's bodies and vacuole formation in the cytoplasm. Similar changes were found in rabbits deficient in nicotinic acid (Irinoda and Yamada, 1956), together with a movement of the pigment of the pigment epithelium into the visual cell layer. In the rat deficient in pantothenic acid (Tomizawa, 1959) the visual cell and outer nuclear layers degenerated, the changes being especially marked in pregnant animals, and there was a thinning of pigment granules in the choroid. Degenerative changes were slight in the ganglion cell layer of a few rats deficient in pyridoxine (Mikami, 1956). Some of the most marked ocular lesions occurred in the retina and choroid of rats deficient in vitamin B_{12} (Takahashi, 1958). These consisted of dilatation of the retinal veins and pallor of the fundus. Histologically there was an oedematous swelling and atrophy of the retina, dilatation of the choroidal vessels, and thickening of the choroidal tissues.

Koyanagi et al. (1966) found that in the riboflavin-deficient rat the ratio of amplitude of b-wave: a-wave of the ERG decreased after 6 weeks and returned to normal after 4 weeks on a normal diet.

In folic acid deficiency dilatation of retinal vessels and haemorrhages were reported (Sekino, 1960). Exudative haemorrhages were associated with the retinal veins in choline deficiency (Konta, 1960).

E. The Optic Nerves and Pathways

One of the earliest studies undertaken of nutritional disease in animals was the classical work of Dr C. Eijkman, a Dutchman employed in his country's colonial service in Java, in 1897. Eijkman became interested in beriberi, a disease extremely common in that country then and in many other parts of the tropics. Hitherto it had been attributed to a bacterial infection. He noticed that hens in the prison yard in Batavia, now Djakarta, had a weakness of the legs similar to the paralysis of beriberi from which the prisoners were suffering. Eijkman made a further, and all-important, observation; he noticed that the hens recovered when their diet was inadvertently changed from polished rice, similar to that consumed by the prisoners, to unmilled rice. This suggested to him that beriberi was connected with diet rather than infection. Experimentally, Eijkman then showed that he could induce paralysis in hens by feeding them on polished rice and that this could be cured by adding rice polishings to the diet. His fellow worker, Grijns, later demonstrated that beans also prevented paralysis in birds and that extracts of rice polishings or beans were curative of the disease in both birds and beriberi patients. It was many years later that the active principle, thiamine, was shown to be one of the vitamins of the B complex.

The effects of deprivation of thiamine on the nervous system have been studied extensively, but in most of this work the eyes and optic tracts have received little attention. There are considerable difficulties inherent in this particular kind of experimental work. Different species vary very much in the ease with which they develop neurological signs in thiamine deficiency. It is necessary for the experiments to be prolonged, for it has been shown repeatedly that acute deficiency results in no histological changes in the nerves. That some of the changes may be due to accompanying inanition, as a result of the marked depression of appetite that is characteristic of thiamine deficiency, also has to be borne in mind. To safeguard against this problem entails pair-feeding of control animals over a long period.

It does seem clear, however, that a chronic deficiency of thiamine produces degenerative changes in the peripheral nerves of the rat (Prickett *et al*. 1939; Rodger, 1953; North and Sinclair, 1956) although only after a considerable period of marked deficiency. Degenerative lesions are readily induced in the pigeon, of course, and these have been studied thoroughly by Swank and

Prados (1942). Wintrobe *et al.* (1944), on the other hand, found no nervous system changes in the pig. Intermittent periods of acute thiamine deficiency superimposed upon chronic deficiency and pantothenic acid deficiency did not produce any changes in the rat (North and Sinclair, 1957) and it has been the general finding that acute deficiency has little or no effect. The exception to this was the work of Swank and Prados (1942) in which acute thiamine deficiency did produce in the pigeon damage to the central terminations of optic fibres and the secondary optic centres. These changes were also present in their chronically deficient birds, together with lesions in the oculomotor and trochlear nerves and their nuclei.

A more thorough study of the optic pathways was made by Rodger (1953) in the rat. He found that about half of his animals suffering from chronic thiamine deficiency showed changes in the optic nerves, the lateral geniculate bodies, and the dorsal nuclei (Fig. 45). The retina was unaffected. He went on to show (Rodger, 1954) that in a chronic deficiency of both thiamine and riboflavin the rats lived longer than those that had been deficient in thiamine alone and that all showed degenerative changes in the optic tract. North and Sinclair (1957) criticized this and other earlier work that had claimed to show degenerative changes based upon examination of the material by the Marchi method or examination of the nerves under polarized light. They are of the opinion that these changes were the result of inanition, for they were also present in their control material. They advocated the use of other methods, such as staining with osmium tetroxide and Sudan black, for these methods gave normal results with myelin and the axis cylinders in their material from both experimental and control animals.

In man there occurs a condition of the central nervous system usually known as Wernicke's encephalopathy, the manifestations of which are considered to be largely due to deficiency of thiamine (see Section IIB2). The main clinical features include disturbances of consciousness, vomiting, nystagmus, and paresis of the ocular muscles. Haemorrhagic lesions of the mammillary bodies in the midbrain occur in man and have also been found in pigeons deficient in thiamine (Alexander, 1940). In the rat, Prickett (1934) observed foci of congestion, haemorrhage, and degeneration in the pons, medulla, and cerebellum. In the monkey, Rinehart *et al.* (1949) reported areas of degeneration in the corpus striatum, globus pallidus, substantia nigra, mammillary bodies, corpora quadrigemina, cerebellar cortex, and nuclei of the 3rd, 6th, 8th, and 10th cranial nerves.

Thiamine deficiency may result from the ingestion of certain animal and plant tissues containing the enzyme thiaminase that destroys the vitamin. Chastek paralysis occurs in foxes fed on raw fish on fox ranches, and a factor in fern pasture fed to horses and cattle may have a similar effect (Chapter 10, Section I). Thiaminase may also produce deficiency symptoms in chicks, cats, and pigeons. In all these animals certain of the features closely resemble the Wernicke's encephalopathy-like syndrome produced experimentally in animals fed on a thiamine-deficient diet.

The effects of vitamin B_{12} deficiency on the optic nerve have mainly been studied in relation to the aetiology of nutritional retrobulbar neuropathy in

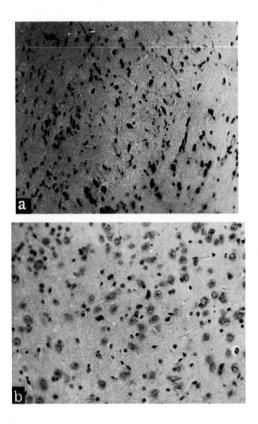

FIG. 45. (a) Sclerosis and hyperchromatism of visual neurones in chronic thiamine deficiency. (Giemsa. ×175.) (b) Unaffected visual neurones of dorsal nucleus in paired control animal. (Giemsa. ×175.) From Rodger (1954).

man (Section B1). The possible role of cyanide, from tobacco smoke, in this group of conditions has also been investigated experimentally.

Van Bogaert (1927) described the spontaneous development of funicular spinal disease in monkeys that were caged. Orang-utans are particularly susceptible. The optic nerve is markedly affected. He attributed the changes to the vegetarian diet fed, and the animals were found to respond to liver extract. Hind (1970) studied a group of rhesus monkeys kept on a vegetarian diet for more than 2 years. Demyelination of the optic nerve occurred, notably in the region of the papillo-macular bundle. The lesions were usually bilateral and affected the entire course of the bundle. Control animals fed a vitamin B_{12}-enriched diet showed no degeneration of the myelin sheath. Contrary to the findings of Wilson and Langman (1966) in man (Section B*1e*) there was a rise in levels of cyanide and thiocyanate. (Agamanolis *et al.* (1976) maintained a group of monkeys on a vitamin B_{12} deficient diet. After

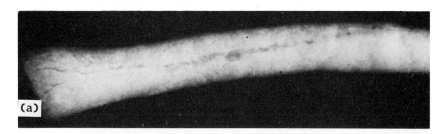

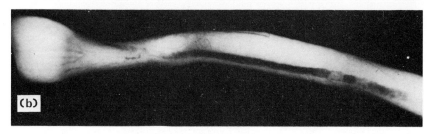

FIG. 46. Degeneration of rat optic nerves in experimental cyanide intoxication. (a) Normal (control) rat optic nerve. (b) Optic nerve of intoxicated rat. Note focal constriction of nerve corresponding to immediate retrobulbar portion. From Lessell (1971).

5 years the blood and marrow pictures were normal. Over periods of 33 to 45 months five monkeys developed gross visual impairment with lesions similar to those of human nutritional retrobulbar neuropathy, and cord lesions. A control animal receiving vitamin B_{12} remained normal throughout.

Injection of large doses of cyanide, producing coma and death in about 1 hour, resulted in bilateral, focal demyelination in the region of the optic nerve in about 20% of rats under study (Lessell, 1971). The corpus callosum was affected in 70% (Figs. 46, 47). This acute intoxication clearly differs from the human situation. Hydroxocobalamin in large doses has been shown experimentally to protect against otherwise fatal doses of cyanide by a reversible conversion to cyanocobalamin (Boxer and Rickards, 1952). Smith and Duckett (1965) confirmed this and found cyanocobalamin ineffective.

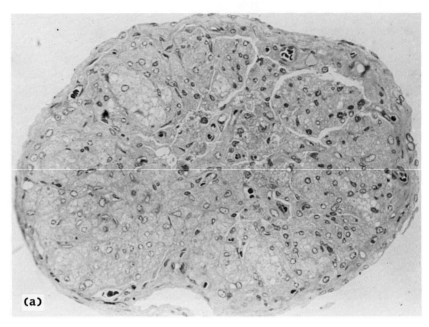

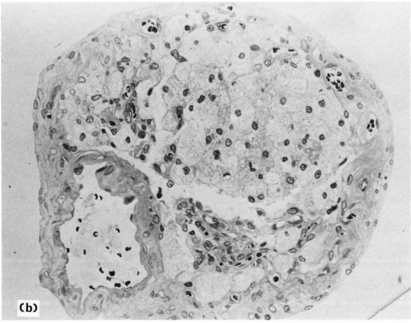

FIG. 47. (a) Cross-section of optic nerve of intoxicated rat. Nerve is vacuolated and glial cells appear pyknotic (toluidine blue). (b) Cross-section of optic nerves of intoxicated rats with severe necrotic lesions. Cells present are pyknotic macroglia and macrophages (toluidine blue). From Lessell (1971).

F. The Uveal Tract

In choline deficiency mucoid degeneration and thickening and proliferation of endothelial cells occur in the iris, ciliary body and choroid, resulting in haemorrhages (Konta, 1960). The uveal vessels are dilated in folic acid deficiency (Sekino, 1960).

G. The Vitreous Body

Choline is a lipotropic factor, preventing the excessive deposition of fat in the liver. In some species haemorrhagic degeneration of the kidneys results from choline deficiency and this may lead to hypertension. Griffith and Wade (1939) noted that in their choline-deficient rats, in which the kidneys were most severely affected, intraocular haemorrhages also occurred. This lesion was studied more fully by Bellows and Chinn (1943), who found that the most frequent occurrence was a column of blood in Cloquet's canal. This is a structure within which runs the hyaloid artery, the blood supply of the lens during fetal life. In the rat this whole system is absorbed and disappears just after birth. These workers also noted that no eye changes occurred in young puppies. This species difference was explained by the work of Burns and Hartroft (1949), who showed that the haemorrhages arose by the process of diapedesis from the hyaloid arterial system which had to be patent at the time of the deficiency for this to occur. In the dog, as in man, the hyaloid system had closed before birth and the intraocular haemorrhages did not take place. Nor do they in the mature rat for the same reason. In the young rat, however, with the system still open at birth, they do occur. It was also noted that the most severe kidney damage occurred in the weanling rat and this might also be related to the ease of diapedesis of cells.

II. Human Studies

A. The Anterior Segment

1. Corneal Vascularization

Invasion of the clear corneal substance by capillary vessels from the limbus has been observed in some animal species, notably the rat, dog, and rabbit, as a result of riboflavin deficiency, but not in others Section IB2). The evidence as to whether or not this may occur in man, and if it does, how frequent it may be, is conflicting. Although a deficiency of several of the other vitamins of the B complex has resulted in corneal vascularization in experimental animals, in man the only vitamin of this group implicated so far is riboflavin.

The first description of human hyporiboflavinosis in patients fed on an experimental diet low in riboflavin mentioned inflammation of the lips, fissures at the corners of the mouth, and glossitis, but made no reference to the eyes (Sebrell and Butler, 1938). Spies, Vilter, and Ashe (1939) in their nutrition clinic in Birmingham, Alabama noted that about 70% of their patients had ocular symptoms which appeared to respond to riboflavin. These consisted of conjunctivitis, especially affecting the lower lid, lacrimation, burning eyes, and failing vision.

Corneal vascularization was mentioned for the first time in a preliminary report (Kruse *et al.*, 1940) and shortly afterward in a full account (Sydenstricker *et al.*, 1940) of work in which Sebrell had now joined Sydenstricker's group in Georgia. The study was made on 47 patients, of whom 16 were hospitalized for nutritional disease (11 with pellagra), 13 were outpatients (three of these were pellagrins in whom signs of hyporiboflavinosis developed during treatment with nicotinic acid), and 18 were well nourished institutional employees—all but two of whom complained of cheilosis or visual disturbances such as photophobia, dimness of vision, or eye strain not relieved by correction of refractive errors. The institutional employees were physicians, nurses, and technicians.

In these 47 subjects the following ocular signs were observed: circumcorneal injection (45), actual vascularization of the cornea (37), superficial nebulae (18), superficial punctate keratitis (2), interstitial nebulae (6), and posterior punctate keratitis (4). In addition certain other signs were noted which were not regarded as being causally associated with the nutritional deficiency. They were frank iritis (4), pigment accumulation in the anterior iris (19), striking mydriasis (4), and cataract in elderly subjects (6).

The changes in the anterior segment cleared up with riboflavin therapy. It is not possible for the reader of the original account to gain a very clear picture of precisely how the eyes of these patients looked. Only one case is illustrated and then only the whole face is shown and the pictures reproduced poorly. There seems to have been marked exudation around the lids and exfoliation of most of the face in this case (No. 8). After "5–15 mg of riboflavin" (presumably daily) for 4 days there was no change. After 10 days the eyes were much improved and there was a relapse after cessation of therapy for 9 days, which was again cured on the 11th day of resumed treatment.

Following upon the publication of these reports nutrition surveys were carried out by workers who jumped to the conclusion that circumcorneal injection and corneal vascularization were pathognomonic of riboflavin deficiency. Two important points were not appreciated at that time and even today misinterpretation sometimes occurs. The work of Scott (1944), Ferguson (1944), Gregory (1943), and many others has shown conclusively that vascularization of the cornea of the type observed in riboflavin-deficient subjects is not in any way specific and may occur in many other states. It is important to recognize that the vascularization found in true riboflavin deficiency occurs equally in all quadrants of the cornea and is not localized to any one part, as for instance that due to trachoma, which starts invariably in the upper limbus. Secondly, it was not long before ophthalmologists began to point out that the limbic plexus is a capillary bed which is liable to great physiological variation. The filling up of previously constricted and empty limbic vessels has frequently been mistaken for vascularization. It is only when the clear corneal substance becomes actually invaded by new vessel formation that corneal vascularization may be said to be present. The pericorneal limbus is in two layers, the superficial conjunctival part and the deep episcleral. Deep ciliary congestion is always a serious sign indicating uveal disease but superficial circumcorneal injection can be transiently produced by vigorously rubbing the eye for a moment and may also result from numerous other kinds of local irritation. It is quite normal for vessels to occupy the whole width of the limbus and there is not necessarily an avascular zone between the plexus and the corneo-scleral junction.

Despite the errors in observation and interpretation that followed the reports from the southern United States there seems little reason to doubt that deficiency of riboflavin was partly responsible for at least the corneal changes in those patients. Several years later, reporting on ocular disturbances in riboflavin deficiency, Spies et al. (1945) had this to say on the uncertainties of this subject.

> We freely admit that we do not know what specific ocular symptoms and lesions are caused by riboflavin deficiency. It is to be admitted freely that the picture described is not one which is pathognomonic of riboflavin deficiency or one that can be immediately and specifically differentiated from superficial inflammation of the eye from numerous other causes.

The economic and social conditions that resulted from and followed the depression in the early 1930s caused many of the people in the southern United States to subsist on a diet of corn bread, "fat back"—the fat of the pig—and some beans. This particular kind of diet does not seem to have an exact counterpart in any other part of the world. With increased prosperity, movement of the black population away from plantations in the South, and recognition of the effects of deficiency of members of the B complex of vitamins, such cases are no longer seen.

There appear to be very few well documented cases of corneal vascularization responding to riboflavin from other areas despite the widespread deficiency of this vitamin in most tropical dietaries. The single case reported by Mann (1945) is one of these few (Fig. 48). The writer has had the opportunity in many countries to examine the eyes of subjects of all ages living on a diet deficient in the B vitamins and has been struck by the lack of evidence of eye lesions, apart from occasional photophobia and circumcorneal injection which might well have a different cause. (McLaren, 1960a).

Prominent among the features of deficiency of the vitamin B complex are the involvement of skin, mucous membranes, and nervous system. Most

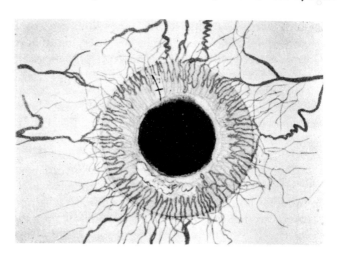

FIG. 48. Corneal vascularization in riboflavin deficiency. From Mann (1945).

accounts have come from different parts of the tropics or from prisoner-of-war camps during the Second World War. One remarkable fact is the virtual absence of any account of true vascularization of the cornea as part of a symptom-complex responsive to therapy with B group vitamins. Many reports fail to mention the eye, but quite a number specifically state that the cornea was clear. Thus corneal vascularization did not accompany the nutritional amblyopia reported so frequently among the inmates of Japanese prisoner-of-war camps (Ridley, 1945; Dansey-Browning and Rich, 1946; Smith and Woodruff, 1951; Pohlman and Ritter, 1952) nor was it a feature of the "corneal epithelial dystrophy" in these same patients to be discussed below (Section IIA2) (Shapland, 1946; Smith and Woodruff, 1951). Similarly vascularization of the cornea has not been a feature of proven or suspect vitamin B complex deficiency states in the West Indies (Métivier, 1941; Cruickshank, 1956; Degazon, 1956), or West Africa (Moore, 1930; Money, 1959; Rodger, 1959) where these appear to be peculiarly common.

Further support for the idea that corneal vascularization is not a constant, or even prominent, feature of riboflavin deficiency disease in man comes from several human experimental studies. Gordon and Vail (1950) carried out a carefully controlled study of mental patients kept on a diet severely restricted in riboflavin for as long as 15 months. None showed any change in the limbal blood vessels or any corneal vascularization. In another study Horwitt *et al*. (1949) noted no corneal vascularization, no change in tear flow or corneal sensitivity and no diminution of visual acuity, although the posterior segment was affected (Section IIB5). Negative results have also been obtained by Boehrer *et al*. (1943) and Hills *et al*. (1951) in human volunteers over shorter periods.

It would seem safe then to conclude that corneal vascularization is by no means one of the more frequent manifestations of riboflavin deficiency in man, and furthermore that when invasion of the cornea by capillaries is observed it should not be attributed to nutritional deficiency until other causes have been eliminated.

2. Corneal Epithelial Dystrophy

This name was given to a condition observed by Métivier (1941) in Trinidad and attributed by him to vitamin B deficiency. According to Duke-Elder (1946) two Japanese workers, Miyashita (1923) and Takada (1934) had given prior accounts of superficial keratitis in vitamin B deficiency. Métivier collected 192 cases in which there was a greyish-white disturbance of the epithelium, made up of fine dots running typically in a double line transversely across the cornea at the level of the lower part of the pupillary area. Sometimes the double line was incomplete, often there were prolongations of it above and below, and occasionally the whole corneal surface was covered with greyish-white spots (Fig. 49). Other ocular symptoms were photophobia, lacrimation, circumcorneal injection, diminution of visual acuity, and increased pallor of the temporal half of the optic disc. Other symptoms suggestive of a deficiency of the B complex included burning feet, cheilosis, and sore tongue. It was claimed that the corneal dystrophy cleared up after 2 weeks on riboflavin 5 mg daily, but took 5 to 12 weeks when foods rich in the B complex were given. Aykroyd and Verma (1942) described 13 cases of a similar condition of superficial keratitis associated with fissured tongue and angular stomatitis with response to riboflavin.

It was Burgess (1946) who drew attention to the close similarity between the condition described by Métivier and that which occurred in large numbers of prisoners of war treated in the Australian General Hospital at Changi in Singapore (Smith and Woodruff, 1951). Changi was the largest military prisoner-of-war camp in the Far East. Burgess was himself interned in Singapore and at the time Nutrition Officer, Malaya Command. Reference will be made again below (Section B1*b*) to the combined account of the wartime experience of Smith in Hong Kong and Woodruff in Singapore in connection with the related subject of nutritional amblyopia, but at this

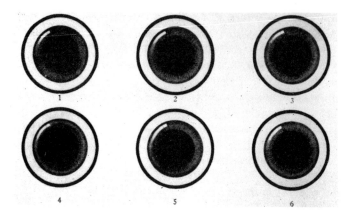

FIG. 49. Corneal epithelial dystrophy. From Métivier (1941).

point their very full description of what they refer to as "corneal degeneration" or "superficial keratitis" provides the main source of information about this condition in Japanese prisoner-of-war camps.

During the period June 1942 to January 1944, 711 cases were seen in the military hospital at Changi. Although hundreds of cases of nutritional amblyopia occurred in both Singapore and Hong Kong and the disease was described as essentially similar in the two camps, responding to B vitamin therapy, especially riboflavin, as did the corneal disease, the corneal condition was seen only at Changi. In view of the similarity of dietary conditions and occurrence of deficiency syndromes in the two camps it is difficult to understand why no cases of corneal epithelial dystrophy were reported from Hong Kong or from most of the other camps in the Far East. The authors suggest that minor degrees may have been missed in Hong Kong because there was no slit lamp available there, but they also state that only a few patients were examined in this way at Changi because the instrument was not very satisfactory. That the condition was not nutritional in origin does not seem to have been considered.

The description of the eye lesions corresponds very well with that of Métivier. There was usually slight circumcorneal injection with quite marked conjunctivitis and blepharitis in some cases. Strong focal illumination of the cornea revealed many minute superficial, punctate, greyish patches, usually staining with fluorescein. Sometimes the patches were scattered diffusely over the whole cornea, in other cases they were confined to the more exposed part, and in 3% of the total were arranged in the linear fashion similar to that described by Métivier. Corneal sensation was never impaired, and vascularization of the cornea did not occur.

In support of a nutritional aetiology for the condition was the association with nutritional amblyopia, nearly half of the cases with corneal lesions having definite central scotomata, and 34% of the amblyopia cases also having corneal involvement. The main peak of incidence coincided with that for nutritional amblyopia. Local treatment consisting of covering the eye, and the instillation of paraffin or drops of zinc sulphate or quinine sulphate appeared to have only a temporary effect on the corneal lesions. Antibiotics were not available.

Under prison camp conditions it was possible to carry out only a limited therapeutic trial. Of ten patients with amblyopia, five also had corneal degeneration with staining of the cornea with fluorescein. On a diet containing about five times the normal requirements of riboflavin, but with approximately adequate amounts of other vitamins, all these cases were cured within 3 weeks.

One other account may be considered before passing on to try to evaluate the significance of this lesion. During four years Nañagas (1953) in the Philippines encountered 44 cases, mostly in young adults, in whom the main symptoms were "foggy" vision and dazzle, often accompanied by a peripheral polyneuropathy and angular stomatitis. The corneal lesions were confined to the epithelium and consisted of grey punctate dots, situated in the pupillary area. In only one case was there vascularization, and in another there was xerosis of the conjunctiva. The lesions did not always show a definite pattern, but sometimes they did, in one case consisting of dots arranged in two transverse bands precisely as described by Métivier, although Nañagas makes no reference to his work. The optic nerves appear to have been occasionally involved; eight patients had central or paracentral scotomata.

Nañagas drew attention to a previous report from the Philippines (de Ocampo, 1941) in which vitamin A deficiency was held responsible. His cases did not respond to vitamin A but good results were obtained with whole B complex. He also expressed the opinion that the three cases of corneal lesion occurring in beriberi patients described by Ayuyao (1933) may have had the same aetiology.

What then, is the evidence for and against a nutritional aetiology for corneal epithelial dystrophy? Perhaps the strongest point in favour is the frequent association with nutritional amblyopia, and the orogenital and burning feet syndromes, about the aetiology of which all are agreed to the extent that they are nutritional, although there are differences of opinion as to what B vitamins are primarily involved (Section B*hii*). Granted that there is such an association this does not mean that it is a causal one. Those who have reported the condition agree that vitamin B complex therapy is effective, and in particular riboflavin. Apparent response to vitamins of a host of conditions has led to innumerable errors in the past, and there has not been a truly critical evaluation made yet in the case of this corneal condition.

The contention of Smith and Woodruff (1951) that corneal vascularization does not occur in this condition until later on and that other workers who have described vascularization only in riboflavin deficiency have missed the epithelial changes is open to criticism. The corneal vascularization produced in experimental animals and seen in man in riboflavin deficiency has always preceded opacity formation and keratitis.

It is now apparent that there is a multiplicity of viral infections of the eye, some of which have a worldwide distribution and occur in epidemic form. Of these, epidemic keratoconjunctivitis is known to have originated in the Orient from whence it was transferred via the Hawaiian Islands to the United States in 1941 (Thygeson, 1957). The disease characteristically has an acute phase of several weeks' duration with preauricular and sometimes submaxillary adenopathy. A conjunctivitis with scanty exudate is followed in from 7 to 10 days by a corneal phase in which subepithelial opacities develop, sometimes preceded by minor epithelial changes. These opacities may persist for many months before they finally disappear spontaneously. It is now generally accepted that epidemic keratoconjunctivitis is caused by type 8 Adenovirus of many strains.

The suggestion is therefore made that corneal epithelial dystrophy is nothing more than epidemic keratoconjunctivitis, possibly conditioned and modified by a deficiency of vitamins of the B complex. This might account for the frequent breaking down of the epithelium over the sub-epithelial opacities and consequent staining with fluorescein. The absence of vascularization in both these conditions is a point in favour of their identity. Some support for this hypothesis has come from work in Japan (Shinozuka, 1959) where it has been found that patients with corneal involvement in epidemic keratoconjunctivitis have lower blood riboflavin levels than patients without keratitis and lower than those of controls. It is also claimed that riboflavin therapy benefits the corneal condition.

3. *Pellagra*

It is not certain that nicotinic acid deficiency itself is ever responsible for eye lesions in man. However, as has already been pointed out, pellagra is a multiple deficiency disease and in addition to lack of nicotinic acid, other B vitamins are also likely to be on the low side in the diet. The eyes are not commonly affected in pellagra; several reports have mentioned amblyopia (Section IIB*1hii* below) but this and the occasional instance of anterior segment involvement (shibi-gatchaki, see below, and Djacos, 1949) would seem to be due to lack of one of the B vitamins other than nicotinic acid, most likely riboflavin.

In Chapter 1, Section II reference was made to the description by Djacos of "superficial polymorphous keratopathy" in patients with starvation oedema in Athens. Apparently at the same time pellagra in an acute form assumed epidemic proportions. Relatively few developed eye trouble and the report was based on 41 cases. These eye lesions accompanying pellagra, and attributed by Djacos to deficiency of riboflavin, are quite different from those he saw in cases of hunger oedema and they are treated by him as separate entities.

The bulbar conjunctiva was injected and oedematous, with linear erosions in the temporal part of the interpalpebral fissure. A corneal dystrophy was seen in some cases, being of two types, superficial and deep. In the superficial type the slit lamp revealed many small epithelial erosions staining with fluorescein, usually concentrated in the lower half of the cornea. The deeper form consisted of several ovoid opacities situated in the deep part of the stroma, usually placed in semicircular fashion with the concavity of the semicircle upward. Vascularization of the cornea was seen frequently. Three types of opacity were described in the lens: minute punctate opacities distributed evenly over both anterior and posterior surfaces; larger irregularly shaped opacities, possibly formed by confluence of the punctate form; and tongue-like opacities extending from the superficial cortex toward the nucleus.

There was no diminution of visual acuity, fundus change, or evidence of retrobulbar neuritis. Djacos suggested that the anterior segment changes were due to acute riboflavin deficiency and that the posterior segment lesions occurred only in prolonged deficiency.

From India, where vitamin B complex deficiency is widespread, brownish pigmentation of the corneal substance, corneal nerves and the lens, visible with the slit lamp, have been reported by Mathur *et al.* (1968). Venkataswamy (1967) described blepharoconjunctivitis and epithelial keratitis.

4. *Shibi-gatchaki*

This disease was first reported by Masuda and Aoyama (1951) from the Tsugaru district of Aomori prefecture of Japan. The name they gave to the condition is made up of two words, *shibi* meaning "roughness", and *gatchaki* meaning "itching of the anal and genital regions". These refer to two of the main features of the syndrome, the roughness of the skin, as in pellagra, and the scrotal or vulval dermatitis of hyporiboflavinosis. Large numbers of cases were seen annually among the rural population of the district, the highest incidence being in the springtime at the end of the hard winter when the paddy fields had been covered with snow since November. Most of the land was given over to rice cultivation and apple orchards and the people had insufficient land to grow kitchen garden produce. Their diet consisted mainly of highly polished rice, with a small amount of green vegetables and an occasional dish of fish or meat. All ages were affected. The stress of pregnancy often precipitated the disease, and some of the cases in infants also had evidence of kwashiorkor.

The ocular lesions were a prominent feature of the condition and have been described by Irinoda and Sato (1954). They include many of the symptoms described already from other parts of the world in vitamin B complex deficiency, such as dim vision and photophobia, angular blepharoconjunctivitis, conjunctival hyperaemia, superficial diffuse keratitis, and temporal pallor of the optic disc. Nodule formation on the iris, and retinal changes such as silver-greyish patches and brownish pigmentation are of more doubtful significance. Riboflavin blood levels and urinary excretion after a loading dose were very low in these cases, and similar results were obtained for nicotinic acid. The histological changes in the conjunctiva consisted of vacuole formation and hyperkeratinization of the epithelial layer with neovascularization and cellular infiltration in the anterior portion of the cornea. The best response occurred with riboflavin.

There seems little doubt that shibi-gatchaki was due to deficiency of vitamins of the B complex with the features of pellagra and of riboflavin deficiency predominating. Professor Irinoda showed the writer colour transparencies of the clinical signs and discussed with him the aetiology and prevention of the condition. With economic advance in the region the condition has disappeared in recent years.

5. *Angular Blepharoconjunctivitis*

It is the form of blepharitis located at the outer canthi that is of special interest to the nutritionist. Fissuring and sogginess in this situation are frequently associated with identical changes at the angles of the mouth in subjects with other evidence of vitamin B complex deficiency (Fig. 50). When there is conjunctivitis accompanying the blepharitis there is frequently infection with the Morax-Axenfeld bacillus (*Haemophilus duplex*).

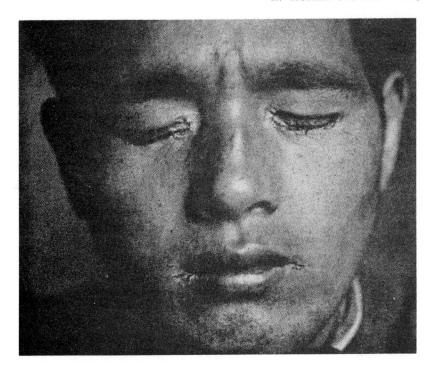

FIG. 50. Angular blepharo-conjunctivitis and angular stomatitis in riboflavin deficiency. From Bicknell and Prescott (1953). "The Vitamins in Medicine", 3rd ed. Heinemann, London.

Views differ as to whether this condition is infectious in nature or whether it is primarily a deficiency state. Verma (1944) claimed that riboflavin in doses of 3 to 5 mg daily, although sometimes 40 mg daily was needed, cured the conjunctivitis, blepharitis, and stomatitis of cases in India, including disappearance of the Morax-Axenfeld bacillus infection. Among 97 prisoners in Nanking 23 were found to have evidence of riboflavin deficiency and three of these had angular blepharitis responding to riboflavin (Chen Tzu-Ta, 1948). Angular blepharoconjunctivitis was also a feature of shibi-gatchaki, and Irinoda and Mikami (1958) claimed that it is due to pyridoxine deficiency. They produced similar lesions in deficient rabbits (Section IA1). It would seem from the reports of several Japanese workers that H. duplex may be present in the eye without causing any symptoms (Yasuda and Goto, 1940; Mitsui and Hinokuma, 1950). Response of angular blepharitis to pyridoxine therapy was claimed by Hinokuma and Yamashita (1950) and Asahiuga and Goto (1943). Irinoda and Mikami (1958) found a significantly higher excretion of pyridoxine in the urine of patients with blepharoconjunctivitis than of controls, irrespective of whether they had *H. duplex* infection or not.

Vilter and his associates at Cincinnati (Mueller and Vilter, 1950; Vilter *et al.*, 1953) induced changes in human subjects by feeding them on a diet low in vitamins of the B complex together with doses of the pyridoxine anti-metabolite deoxypyridoxine. Glossitis, stomatitis, and seborrhoeic dermatitis around the eyes, nose, and mouth failed to respond to riboflavin, nicotinic acid, or thiamine but cleared up within 3 days after administering pyridoxine. Two subjects in the earlier experiment and three in the later had scaling at the outer canthus and conjunctivitis. These results are suggestive, although by no means conclusive, of pyridoxine deficiency being the cause of at least some cases of angular blepharoconjunctivitis. Here, as in other conditions apparently related to deficiency of B complex vitamins, different vitamins may conceivably be implicated in the same process.

6. Miscellaneous Conditions

The rather vexed question of eye involvement in beriberi will be considered mainly in the discussion of the posterior segment (Section IIB*1hii*, below) because amblyopia is by far the most important aspect of this subject. There is considerable evidence that, along with paralysis of other muscles in this disease, there may also be paralysis of the external ocular muscles, particularly those served by the abducens nerve, and less frequently there may be ptosis and paralysis of accommodation (Bietti, 1940). It is uncertain whether the diminished sensitivity of the cornea frequently mentioned as an ocular sign of beriberi is really part of the disease or whether it is due to an associated deficiency of vitamin A. Thiamine has been claimed (Sysi, 1946) to increase the amplitude of accommodation of non-deficient subjects.

In subjects with corneal ulcers and not deficient in nicotinic acid Agarwal and Datt (1954) observed a beneficial effect on the time the ulcers took to heal and the ultimate scar formation as a result of therapy with nicotinic acid. This was more marked when the vitamin was given subconjunctivally than when it was given intramuscularly. Similar results were obtained in the rabbit (Section IB2).

B. The Posterior Segment

1. Nutritional Retrobulbar Neuropathy

This term is employed here to cover a group of conditions that have many clinical features in common, but in which the aetiologic factors differ widely, and which present many puzzling features. Nutritional factors, either primary or secondary, play an important part in production of the lesion, common to all, but various other precipitating factors have also to be considered.

In deciding how to approach a subject as diverse and complex as this, considerable difficulties are encountered. It seemed desirable to treat together those aspects that are common to all the conditions. These include the early accounts of amblyopia associated with undernutrition or heavy tobacco and/or alcohol consumption, and also the clinical features and the pathology. Thereafter this form of amblyopia arising under very different circumstances has been dealt with separately. On occasion the amblyopia is only part of a more generalized ocular involvement, and reference should also be made to other parts of this chapter, especially those relating to thiamine and niacin (Sections B2 and B3). Heavy reliance has been placed on recent reviews by Dreyfus (1976), Kunze and Leitenmaier (1976) and Foulds and Pettigrew (1977).

a. Early Accounts

The earliest known reference to what may have been this condition is found in Aristotle's *Ethica Nicomurchia*, published in 350 B.C. (cited by Esser, 1928), in which impaired vision was associated with alcoholism.

Failure of vision in the absence of any gross external eye disease has long been associated with what we can now recognize as beriberi and pellagra. Perhaps the first account was that of Jacobus Bontius in 1645 among the rice-eating inhabitants of Amboina and the Moluccan Islands (Indonesia). In Chapter XVI of De Medicina Indorum he wrote:

The inhabitants of these islands impute it [blindness] to eating hot rice, and that such is really the cause of it, seems to be confirmed by experience . . . our sailors are prohibited from eating hot rice under a certain penalty . . . which blindness, however, is not perpetual, but often ceases on a change of air, or better diet. . . . But the grand specific in this disorder, and a medicine of which I have often experienced the virtues, is the liver of the fish Lamia, eaten crude with salt. . . . Upon the whole, though the blindness is often transitory, yet if neglected and an improper diet persisted in, with an unseasonable use of arrack, it often degenerates into a total deprivation of sight, of which everywhere here we meet with instances.

Bontius also speaks of the optic nerves being affected but there is no mention of night blindness or corneal change, and there seems little doubt that the condition described is nutritional amblyopia and not xerophthalmia.

Boerhaave (1749) described a patient with disturbed vision associated with excessive wine consumption; abstinence was reported to have brought about prompt and complete recovery. Numerous accounts of amblyopia associated with chronic alcoholism and smoking referred to the possibility of poor nutrition as a factor, and advocated dietary measures in addition to abstinence from alcohol and tobacco (Sichel, 1837, 1865; Horner, 1878: Förster, 1880; Sachs, 1889; Deschweinitz, 1896).

Many of the older writers on pellagra, especially those working in Italy, made reference to visual disturbances in this disease and although their accounts are incomplete they are very suggestive of nutritional amblyopia. Cajetani Strambio in his classical account "De Pellagra" of the disease in Milan (1789) was probably the first when he refers to "crepuscular amblyopia", diplopia, and failing vision.

Many of the early accounts of pellagra include references to visual defects. Calderini (1847) stated that 48% of men and 72% of women with pellagra complained of visual disturbances, and one of his patients had contraction of the visual fields. Lombroso (1892) referred to two cases with optic atrophy, and Guita (1884) and Rampoldi (1885) reported retinal changes. Ottolenghi (1890) described a variety of abnormalities of the retina and optic nerve in most of his 36 cases of pellagra. Bietti (1901) found frequent loss of visual acuity, but in 55 cases there were no defects in the visual fields. Pallor of the disc and blurring of the margins were seen in about 10% of his cases; in the remainder the fundus was normal. Sections of the optic nerves and retinae at postmortem showed no changes.

The role of tobacco dates from 1817 with the work of Beer. Hirschberg (1879) in his historic account linked tobacco and alcohol, and the term tobacco–alcohol amblyopia has been in common usage ever since.

b. Clinical Features

With only few exceptions, to be mentioned later, the ocular syndrome has presented a remarkably uniform picture. This has been true for descriptions coming from prisoner-of-war camps or of sporadic cases or endemic foci of the disease in malnourished population groups. Tobacco–alcohol amblyopia appears to be essentially a deficiency and not a toxic amblyopia (Section IIB*1d*), identical in every clinical and pathological feature with nutritional amblyopia. The rather rare complication of optic neuropathy in pernicious anaemia has the same symptomatology (Section B*1i*) and can only be differentiated by the accompanying haematological findings. The main complaint is blurring of vision for both near and distant objects, frequently accompanied by photophobia and aching behind the eyeball made worse by strong light.

The onset of impairment of central vision is usually gradual. In the prisoner-of-war camps the first symptoms did not appear until the patients had been consuming the deficient diet for a matter of some months, usually from about 6 months to a year. There is slow and chronically progressive decline in vision and together with the loss of visual acuity initially there is already a central scotoma for red and green. With the progression of the amblyopia within the red scotoma there is additionally relative or absolute scotoma for white, the scotoma having a centrocoecal localization in the temporal region of the middle of the visual field. This also explains clinically the finding described as the "temporal letter sign", consisting in the fact that the patient has more difficulty in recognizing the temporally arranged letters, on the sight-testing chart, than the nasal. The acquired loss of red/green colour discrimination may be detected using Ishihara pseudoiso-chromatic plates; or more reliably by the use of the Farnsworth-Munsell 100-hue test, when an elevated score and a characteristic polarity are found (Chisholm et al., 1970). The remainder of the visual fields is usually normal although there may occasionally be slight general peripheral contraction. All the conditions mentioned above differ from the true toxic amblyopias in that the area of field involved is confined to that served by the papillo-macular bundle, while much larger areas are affected by the latter.

One of the most precise accounts of the nature of the visual field defects has been given by Durran (1946) of fellow prisoners of war in Hong Kong. In his cases the field defects were central, and did not closely resemble those of tobacco amblyopia in shape or nuclei but were mostly roughly circular. The severer ones showed a central nucleus for a 10 mm white object at 1 metre extending to 2 or 3 degrees from the fixation point, with roughly concentric zones for 5 mm and 1 mm, or there might be no field for 1 mm. In others the defect might be only a relative one for red, and during the course of recovery a scotoma for white might regress to a relative scotoma for red. A few of the severer cases showed some peripheral contraction by the confrontation test; no perimeter was available. Those with dense scotomata frequently had a concentric depression of the 1 mm isoptre to within the blind spot, and in some cases the 5 mm isoptre was also depressed.

The visual acuity loss is usually of the same order in both eyes and varies with the intensity and size of the central scotoma. It rarely falls below 6/60 and it is doubtful if complete blindness ever occurs in an uncomplicated case. Among 4000 recently released prisoners from Japanese camps Denny-Brown (1947) found 185 cases with residual disability from nutritional amblyopia but no case of complete blindness.

Most authors agree that there is frequently an increase in the normal pallor of the temporal side of the optic disc, although it is difficult to decide whether some cases are pathological. The more marked degrees of pallor, going on to optic atrophy, are usually found in cases of long standing with major visual loss.

Retinal haemorrhages have been seen in a few cases and it may be that they have the same aetiology as those in Wernicke's encephalopathy (Section IIB2, below). Some degree of recovery is the rule, its extent probably depending upon the severity of the amblyopia and the time it has existed before therapy is instituted. Clarke and Sircus (1952) were able to follow up patients with nutritional neuropathy who were seen by one of them (Clarke and Sneddon, 1946) 6 years previously when they were newly released from Japanese prison camps in Hong Kong. At that time a well-balanced diet and massive doses of vitamins failed to bring about any improvement in the neurological signs including amblyopia. Of the 26 cases found to have loss of visual acuity on the first examination, 15 were judged to be severe and 11 mild. Six years later 14 of the severe cases were unchanged and one was worse. In the mild group six were unchanged, two had fully recovered, one had improved, and two were worse. Where examination was possible no change was found in scotomata, appearance of the optic disc and evidence of macular degeneration. This and other experience of the long-term prognosis show that cases that are of severe degree before treatment begins almost invariably fail to improve and that the results in the milder cases are very variable, making the prognosis for any case extremely guarded.

Certain other visual disturbances have been reported in prisoners of war, not necessarily associated with nutritional amblyopia in the same individual, and for which there was no real evidence that they were caused by malnutrition. Asthenopia, fatigue of the eye muscles with blurring, diplopia, and headache after short periods of concentration were extremely common and often associated with, and possibly due in part to, what appeared to be the premature onset of presbyopia (Chapter 11, Section A). Sudden temporary, complete loss of vision in one eye was reported in 11 men by Smith and Woodruff (1951). It appeared to be due to vasomotor spasm associated with extreme hypotension. The development and progression of myopia was noted by some observers and will be considered with other evidence relating refractive errors to malnutrition (Chapter 11, Section A).

Harrington (1962) appears to be alone in claiming that the visual field defect in alcohol amblyopia can be differentiated from that due to tobacco. He stated that in the former the scotoma is small, central, with steep margins; in the latter centrocaecal with sloping margins.

c. Pathology

The papillomacular bundles are fibre tracts which connect the macular ganglion cells of the retina with the lateral geniculate ganglia. Common to the various forms of nutritional retrobulbar neuropathy described here is a bilaterally symmetrical loss of myelinated fibres in those bundles occupying the central parts of the optic nerve, chiasm and tract.

In the retina there is a pronounced loss of ganglion cells in the macula extending within a radius of 1–2 mm from the fovea centralis. Peripherally the ganglion cell layer remains intact. Demyelination of the papillomacular bundle appears to begin in the retro-orbital parts of the optic nerve (Victor and Dreyfus, 1965) (Fig. 51). It tends to spread in a centrifugal and axial

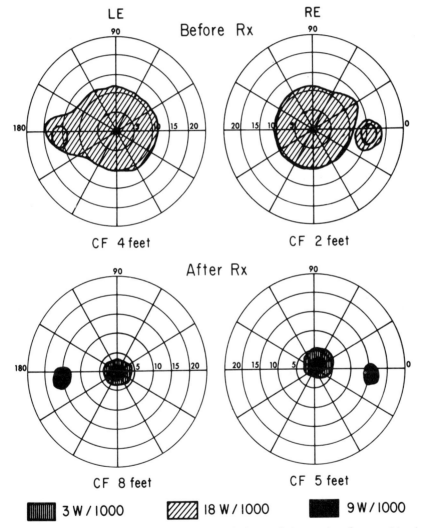

FIG. 51. Visual defect in alcohol amblyopia, before and 2 months after nutritional replenishment. From Dreyfus (1976).

fashion. In the lateral geniculate ganglion transsynaptic degeneration results in zonal loss of small nerve cells in the most dorsal layers of this multilayered structure. The optic radiations and the calcarine cortex remain normal (Figs. 52–55) (Victor *et al.*, 1960). In advanced disease it has been observed that

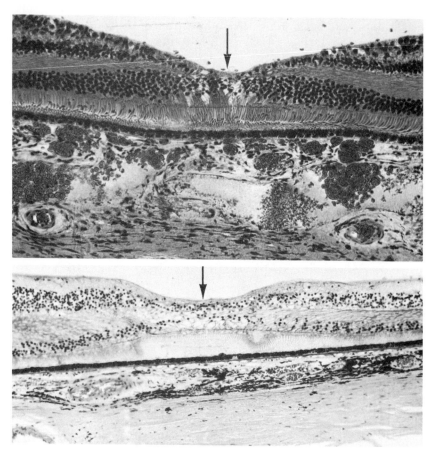

FIG. 52. Sections of the retina in alcohol amblyopia: sections through the macular region. Above: Normal control. Below: Alcohol amblyopia. Note severe loss of ganglion cells. The arrow points to the fovea. From Dreyfus (1976).

collagenous tissue, fibroblasts and glial cells replace medullated fibres and axis cylinders in the zones of maximal demyelination.

Dreyfus (1976) observes that the primary site of the pathological process has not been firmly established, but suggests that it is most likely to be the retro-orbital and centrally located myelinated fibres of the optic nerve, as found by many early workers (Samelsohn, 1882; Uthoff, 1886; Sachs, 1889;

Scott, 1918; Kagoshima, 1918; Krylov, 1932). This was also the experience
of later workers with amblyopia in prisoners of war (Fisher, 1955) (Fig. 56)
and in chronic alcoholism (Victor and Dreyfus, 1965). The eventual
centrifugal spread, as described above, appears to lead to secondary degenera-

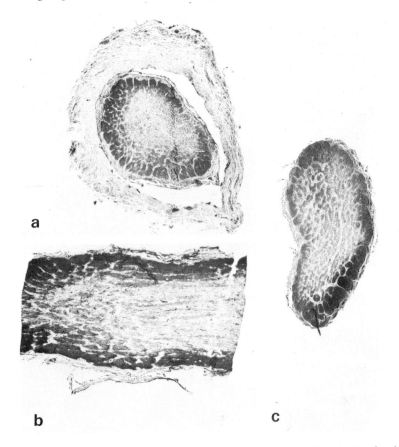

a

b   c

FIG. 53. Retrobulbar parts of the optic nerve in alcohol amblyopia (a) Cross-section showing
extensive destruction of medullated fibres in the centre of the nerve. (b) Longitudinal section
at the same level as in (a). (c) Cross-section through the optic nerve anterior to the chiasm.
Extensive destruction in the area of the papillomacular bundle is evident (Spielmayer stain for
myelin).

tion of retinal ganglion cells within the maculae. This would explain why the
retinal ganglion cells have been found normal in some reports (Sachs, 1889;
Deschweinitz, 1896), while in others loss of these cells has been prominent
(Samelsohn, 1882; Birch-Hirschfeld, 1902; Rönne, 1910).

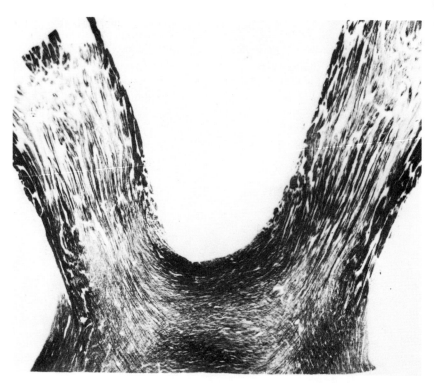

FIG. 54. Optic nerves and chiasm in alcohol amblyopia; horizontal sections of the chiasm and proximal portions of the optic nerves. Pallor of myelin staining is noted to decussate in the middle third of the chiasm. From Dreyfus (1976).

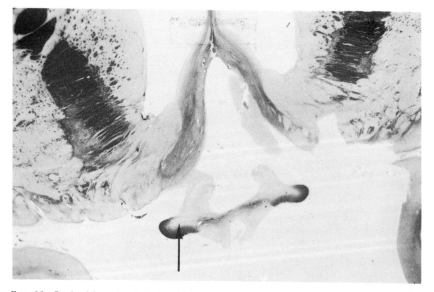

FIG. 55. Optic chiasm in alcohol amblyopia: coronal section of the brain at the level of the posterior part of the optic chiasm. The arrow points to the zone of demyelination. From Dreyfus (1976).

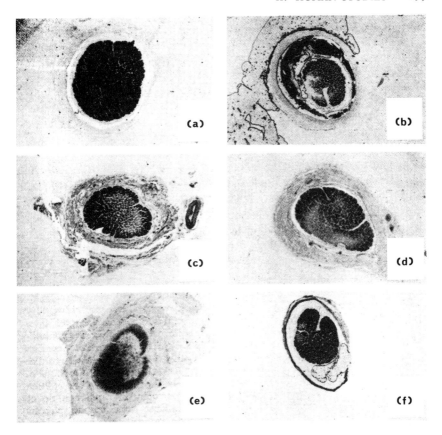

FIG. 56. Degeneration of nerve fibres in the region of the papillomacular bundle in nutritional amblyopia. From Fisher (1955).

d. Tobacco-related Retrobulbar Neuropathy

There is general agreement that tobacco consumption alone cannot explain the incidence. Only a very minute proportion of all tobacco smokers contract the disease. Cigars and cigarettes, especially the latter, are only rarely causally associated, the smoking of strong tobacco in pipes being the typical finding. The reason for the great preponderance of pipe smokers is not known. It has been suggested that one factor may be that the increase in the proportion of pipe smokers that occurs in middle and old age, together with the known decrease in serum vitamin B_{12} level with age, make the development of amblyopia more likely in aged pipe smokers. It may also be that pipe smoking, unlike that of cigarettes, does not cause stimulation of gastric juice secretion and serum vitamin B_{12} levels may not be thus raised

(Heaton, 1960). Tobacco chewing or snuff taking have on rare occasions been implicated, but then these habits are relatively uncommon. It is well authenticated that the use of tobacco alone may cause amblyopia. although it is more common for it to be associated with alcohol intake. It has been shown that the amount of tobacco consumed by those who develop amblyopia varies enormously, although the usual history obtained is of heavy smoking over a period of years.

In an extensive review Silvette *et al.* (1960) showed that during the past 100 years there has been a steady decline in the number of publications on tobacco amblyopia, despite the equally steady increase in tobacco consumption. If it can be assumed that the degree to which a disease is reported reflects to some extent the true incidence of that disease, then any number of factors may be at work, of which improved general health and nutrition are probably among the more important.

Potts (1973) stated that the incidence of the condition appears to have decreased considerably over the past 50 years in the United States, but to a lesser extent in the United Kingdom. According to the data compiled by Lee (1975), in that period in the United States cigarette consumption (per head of the population over 15 years of age) increased sixfold, but pipe tobacco consumption dropped tenfold. The corresponding figures for the United Kingdom are a threefold rise for cigarettes and threefold fall for pipe tobacco. In 1920 pipe tobacco consumption in the United States was twice per head what it was in the United Kingdom. It has now dropped to two-thirds.

e. Cyanide and Vitamin B_{12} Deficiency

Wokes (1958) suggested that cyanide, known to be in high concentration in tobacco smoke, was the toxic factor in tobacco amblyopia. Heaton *et al.* (1958) reported significant lowering of plasma vitamin B_{12} and good response to parenteral vitamin B_{12} therapy. In this study 13 patients with classical centrocaecal scotomata had markedly depressed plasma vitamin B_{12} levels (15–350 pg/ml). Five of these patients had additional neurological involvement and one had pernicious anaemia. All showed ocular improvement with vitamin B_{12}, even if they continued smoking. Pipe smoking has been shown to impair absorption of vitamin B_{12} (Foulds *et al.*, 1969; Watson-Williams *et al.*, 1969). Smith (1961) postulated that cyanide might result in the conversion of hydroxocobalamin to cyanocobalamin. Support is lent to the idea of a toxic role for the cyanide radical by the demonstration of the greater effectiveness of hydroxocobalamin in the treatment of tobacco amblyopia than cyanocobalamin (Chisholm *et al.*, 1967). Response to cyanocobalamin reported by some workers is not incompatible with this finding, as ampoules of cyanocobalamin contain varying amounts of hydroxocobalamin (Smith, 1961).

The major metabolite of cyanide, of high concentration in tobacco smoke, is the non-toxic thiocyanate. Conjugation requires sulphur and is controlled by the enzyme rhodanese (E.C.2811) and by mercaptopyruvate sulphur transferase (E.C.2812). Normal smokers have higher thiocyanate levels in body fluids than do non-smokers, and these levels parallel closely tobacco consumption. Despite the fact that patients with tobacco amblyopia tend to smoke more heavily than non-amblyopic smokers they have lower thiocyanate levels, suggesting reduced ability to detoxify cyanide (Foulds *et al.*, 1968a; Pettigrew and Fell, 1972).

Foulds and Pettigrew (1977) have presented evidence of a defect in the metabolism of sulphur, necessary for the detoxication of cyanide, in patients with tobacco amblyopia. They have lower than normal levels of reduced glutathione in erythrocytes (Pettigrew *et al.*, 1972), which return to normal, despite continued smoking, with dietary supplements of cystine or parenteral inorganic sulphur; and improved vision is accompanied by increased plasma and urinary levels of thiocyanate (Phillips *et al.*, 1970).

Hydroxocobalamin therapy, even in the absence of demonstrable vitamin B_{12} deficiency, may result in improved vision and return towards normal of the indicators of restored sulphur metabolism noted above. It is postulated that vitamin B_{12} deficiency might lead to a deficiency of a sulphur donor, necessary for the conversion of cyanide to thiocyanate, by its known role as methylcobalamin in the transmethylation of homocysteine to methionine referred to earlier (Foulds and Pettigrew, 1977).

f. Other B Group Vitamins

Providing optic atrophy has not occurred, improvement in vision may be expected by preventing further consumption of tobacco or alcohol. Attention to the diet, with special emphasis on vitamins of the B complex, gives greater improvement and is further evidence for the role of nutrition in the aetiology of the condition. Furthermore, some workers have been able to obtain just as good results by dietary means in the presence of an unaltered consumption of tobacco and alcohol as when these were prohibited. Carroll (1944) was the first to demonstrate this. He treated patients on a variety of dietary regimes, at the same time allowing them to continue the use of tobacco and/or alcohol as before. The recovery in these patients was at least as good as those treated similarly but deprived of tobacco and alcohol. Thiamine alone gave good results, but there was some evidence that there was more complete restoration of vision if the whole B complex was given (Carroll, 1966).

Other B-group vitamins, such as pyridoxine and folic acid, are also involved in the metabolism of sulphur, and this might explain the improvement noted in some patients with B complex therapy, but not with vitamin B_{12} alone. Philipsen and Hommes (1970) reported response to pyridoxine in three patients who had abnormal tryptophan load tests. Foulds and Pettigrew (1977) also reviewed experimental evidence for the impairment of choline synthesis from ethanolamine in the presence of impaired conversion of cyanide to thiocyanate. Choline is a precursor in the production of myelin.

g. Retrobulbar Neuropathy in Chronic Alcoholism

This syndrome afflicts a relatively small proportion of all chronic alcoholic patients, probably no more than 1 in 200 of those hospitalized (Victor *et al.*, 1960). Other neurological disorders related to vitamin deficiency, such as the Wernicke-Korsakoff syndrome (Section B2), or polyneuropathy, usually due to vitamin B complex deficiency, are often present.

Patients have usually been drinking excessively and steadily over many years. Wasting of tissues is usually evident and systemic signs of nutritional deficiencies are common. Amblyopia is most frequently seen in the fourth and fifth decades of life, and men and women are equally affected, suggesting that heavy pipe smoking with possible cyanide intoxication is probably not important in this group (but see Section B*d*).

In the early stages response to vitamin B complex therapy and good diet is usually prompt and complete. Thiamine appears to give especially good results in these patients (Carroll, 1944, 1966), even if alcohol consumption is not curtailed.

h. Retrobulbar Neuropathy in Undernourished Communities

i. Global Occurrence As in the case of xerophthalmia, so now for nutritional amblyopia it does seem to be worth-while to attempt to map out the known distribution throughout the world of this condition. The same difficulties over incomplete reporting, inadequate knowledge of the literature, and alterations with time are also inherent here. Of even more importance in the production of nutritional amblyopia than of night blindness and xerophthalmia has been the wilful man-induced malnutrition of the prison camp. In this way the number of reports and volume of case material from Southeast Asia in particular has been much greater than it would otherwise have been. Nevertheless it would seem that wartime conditions only served to show up certain basic inadequacies in the Oriental diet, for the neuropathies and other signs associated with deficiency of vitamins of the B complex were not in evidence in camps in Europe. With these limitations borne in mind this account may be taken to form a basis for appraisal of the present-day situation.

West Indies. Some of the earliest accounts came from here and it remains today one of the most important endemic foci of the condition. In 1888 and again in 1897 Strachan reported a malady affecting 510 patients seen at the Kingston Public Hospital in Jamaica which he regarded as being due to malaria but in which he noted many features suggestive of beriberi. In addition to dim vision the symptomatology included burning pains in the palms and soles; numbness and cramps in the hands and feet; hyperaemia and desquamation of the palms and soles; branny desquamation at the margins of the eyelids, lips, and nostrils, and excoriation at the corners of the mouth, the prepuce, anus, and vulva; hyperaemia of the conjunctiva and of the mucous membrane of the mouth with loss of surface epithelium of the tongue. There was marked emaciation and some cases died. Scott in 1918 reported from Jamaica an acute outbreak of what he called "central neuritis" occurring among adult native labourers, male and female, on sugar estates during the cutting of the cane crop, and which ceased when the operation was over. The onset was very acute and there were 50 to 100 new cases every day. Invariably the first symptom was conjunctivitis with swelling, redness, and abrasions of the lids with marked photophobia. This was followed by a stomatitis with fissures at the angle of the lips. The tongue was usually not sore. Two weeks later either diarrhoea occurred, sometimes leading to death, or constipation with various nervous symptoms developed. These consisted of "burning in the toes and soles of the feet", numbness and tingling in the legs with incoordination and ataxia but no loss of power or sensation. The upper limbs were sometimes similarly affected and in some cases there was diminution of visual and auditory acuity. Ophthalmoscopic and visual field examinations were not reported. The usual diet of these people consisted of yam, breadfruit, cocoa, peas, beans, cornmeal, and salt fish, but during the harvesting the workers lived almost entirely on the sugar cane. The symptoms are very suggestive of vitamin B complex deficiency, although Scott thought the disease might be due to an ingested toxin.

Jamaica was again the scene of an outbreak of retrobulbar neuritis in 74 children living in the town of Kingston during a period of food shortage that followed a hurricane disaster (Whitbourne, 1947). Some of the children also had nutritional oedema, perlèche, and glossitis. Carroll (1947) was able to demonstrate central scotomata in many cases. There was good response to brewer's yeast. Two previous outbreaks in Jamaican children were reported by Clark (1935–36) and Dickenson (1935–36).

Polyneuropathy of obscure aetiology is still a major health problem on the island of Jamaica. In 1956 Cruickshank described 100 cases of a "neuropathic syndrome of uncertain origin" in which amblyopia was a prominent feature. In 1961 he reported that he had seen more than 300 cases during the previous 8 years with adequate records on 210 patients. The incidence of the various clinical features is given in Table IV, where it will be seen that 27% had retrobulbar neuropathy. In the Eye Department of the

Kingston Public Hospital, Degazon (1956) gave an account of what he called "tropical amblyopia" in 298 cases in the period 1948–55. There was little evidence of malnutrition and he attributed the beneficial effect of vitamin B complex therapy in early cases to a vasodilator rather than nutritional effect of these substances.

Less is known about the position on other islands in the Caribbean area but the evidence we have would suggest that nutritional amblyopia is also a problem there. In 1929 Sharples described the burning feet syndrome in Hindu Bengalis in British Guiana, stating that it was not seen in the rest of the population. Other symptoms included a complaint of "darkness of the eyes" and anaesthesia of the dorsum of the feet but no paresis or wasting. Women between the ages of 17 and 40 were most commonly affected. The diet consisted of polished rice and some meat. Symptoms subsided with improvement in the diet. A report coming 30 years later from the same area (Murray and Asregadoo, 1959) stated that optic atrophy is found only in the black population who are usually free from other signs of vitamin B complex deficiency, and that the East Indians often have these other signs but not optic atrophy. Retrobulbar neuropathy was accompanied by angular stomatitis and glossitis, however, in the condition reported in British Guiana schoolchildren by Browne (1939). These children lived in rural areas where rice was the staple and recovery of vision usually occurred with improvement of the diet. A similar ocular condition was seen in women 6 or 12 months after parturition in which there was temporal pallor of the discs, central scotomata with normal peripheral fields. This he attributed, however, to the taking of black pepper and ginger teas during the puerperium.

In addition to what he termed "corneal epithelial dystrophy" (Section A2, above) Metivier (1941) in Trinidad found many of these patients also had amblyopia and skin and mucous membrane lesions responding to riboflavin and foods rich in the B complex. Children as well as adults were also affected by the amblyopia reported from Barbados (St John, 1936) which was sometimes accompanied by the facial lesions of riboflavin deficiency. Children seem to be much more commonly affected by nutritional amblyopia in the West Indies and also in West Africa than in other parts of the world.

The condition has been reported among the West Indian community in Britain (Crews, 1963; Owen, 1966). Of the 22 patients studied by Crews, 15 had deterioration of vision before immigration. Carroll (1971) described bilateral, central or centrocaecal scotomata and temporal pallor of the optic discs in 22 Jamaican immigrants to the United States. Two also had bilateral nerve deafness. The changes remained unaltered over many years.

Africa. The earliest account of pellagra from Africa was given by Stannus (1912, 1913), who described an outbreak among the inmates of the Central Prison at Zomba in Nyasaland. Numerous subsequent reports, summarized

TABLE IV. *Incidence of Neurological Signs of Multiple Neuropathy Syndrome in Jamaica[a]*

	No. of cases[b]	Percentage
Mode of onset		
Sudden	36	17
Gradual	174	83
Symptoms include:		
Pain in back	74	35
Bladder dysfunction	107	51
Neurological findings		
(1) Motor. Exaggerated reflexes and increased tone (the majority with extensor plantar reflexes)	197	94
(2) Muscle wasting. Selective wasting of hand, calf, and peroneal muscles, occasionally of shoulder-girdle muscles, and two cases of laryngeal palsy presumably from nuclear damage	24	11
(3) Sensory loss. Posterior columns	134	64
(4) Optic nerve. Retrobulbar neuropathy	57	27
(5) Eighth nerve deafness	49	23

[a] From Cruickshank (1961).
[b] Total of 210 patients.

later by Stannus (1936), came from many other parts of the African continent. Nearly all these were of outbreaks of pellagra-like disease in prisoners and little attention was paid to the eyes, prominence being given rather to the skin changes, the sore tongue and lips, the burning feet, diarrhoea, and mental changes.

The first description of an outbreak of vitamin B complex deficiency disease in the general population would seem to be that of Bradley (1929) from the Seychelles islands in the Indian Ocean. The condition seems to have been one familiar to the people, for they had given it the name "décoquée", no doubt from the appearance of the skin. The symptoms included soreness of the angles of the mouth, redness of the eyelids, erythematous rash of the genitalia, and sometimes impairment of vision and hearing. Inhabitants of the islands receiving a good diet did not suffer from the disease and those that went to the mainland improved.

In 1934 Moore described a condition affecting African boarding school children in Nigeria. He saw about 300 cases in 5 years. While 12% of the boys who were boarders and poorly fed were affected, no cases occurred among children who lived at home or among the girls who were taught cooking. Some cases were also seen among the poorer casual labourers who lived on cassava, dried fish, oil, suet, and pepper. First, the tongue and mouth became sore with aphthous lips and this was followed by a dry scaly itching condition of the scrotum. Finally the vision became dim with loss of central acuity but with peripheral fields unaffected. In advanced cases there was pallor of the temporal halves of the optic discs.

The diet of these schoolboys consisted of one cabin biscuit and cassava soup (gari) with only 3 ounces of meat a week. During the holidays the condition improved and treatment of early cases with Marmite, oleum morrhuae, iron, and "tombo"—a fermented palm sap—gave good results. Moore (1937, 1939, 1940) carried out extensive trials later and found autoclaved Marmite just as effective as the ordinary preparation. A closely similar condition in Sierra Leone had been ascribed by Wright (1928, 1930) to a combined deficiency of vitamins A and B. In this, soreness of the mouth, eyes, anus, scrotum, and vulva was associated with a variety of nervous symptoms including impaired vision, due apparently, however, to corneal and not optic nerve disease. Dawson et al. (1948) described five cases of optic atrophy associated with contraction of the visual fields in African troops, natives of the Gold Coast, but stationed for from 1 to 3 years in Sierra Leone where they had lived mainly on a rice diet. Those less severely affected responded well to thiamine. One case had in addition a generalized polyneuritis, but none had skin or mucous membrane changes. The evidence here points to a beriberi-like condition rather than the hyporiboflavinosis generally accompanying amblyopia in these African accounts. Spillane (1947) saw more than 100 cases of a neurological syndrome in German prisoners of war in the camp in the Suez Canal zone and others in that area, occurring a few each month between August 1943 and January 1945. More than half of those affected complained of failing vision and had central scotomata and pallor of the optic discs. In this they resembled their captured British foes in Japanese hands rather than those on the continent of Europe, for despite apparently similar conditions of privation these latter did not develop this disease of the nervous system.

Money (1958, 1959) described an endemic focus of a related nutritional neuropathy in the Epe district of southern Nigeria. Between October 1954 and October 1956 he saw 100 cases of severe ataxic neuropathy in and around Ibadan. Of these, 87% complained of transient or persistent blurring of vision, but this never amounted to blindness. Perimetry was carried out on ten inpatients, the fields being normal in five, paracentral scotomata being present in two, and generalized contraction of the peripheral fields in three. In 92 patients the fundi were clearly visible and showed no abnormality in 52, pallor of the temporal halves of the discs in 27, acute optic neuropathy in five, and primary optic atrophy in eight. The author rightly points out that a simple nutritional aetiology does not fit all the facts in these cases and this is borne out as far as the ocular manifestations are concerned by their lack of uniformity. In general there was quite good response in early cases of most neurological symptoms including vision to vitamins of the B complex.

Knuettgen (1956) reported a similar neuropathy with visual failure from Liberia. Money, whose experience in Nigeria has been referred to above, later reported (Money, 1961) three cases of what he calls "obscure funicular myelopathy" seen during 12 months in Kampala, Uganda in East Africa, where such conditions are rare. One of these was of mixed spastic and ataxic type with poor visual acuity. Considerable improvement occurred with vitamin B_{12} therapy. During 4 years in Tanganyika (Tanzania) the present writer saw only three cases in which amblyopia appeared to be nutritional in origin, all responding to vitamin B_{12} (McLaren, 1960b).

Monekosso and Ashby (1963), the former being the same worker as Money referred to above, divided 74 patients with mucocutaneous signs of vitamin B complex deficiency into three groups. Nineteen were apparently healthy schoolchildren with either the entire disc swollen or pink, or pathological temporal pallor. Twenty-four patients aged 11 to 20 years were referred to hospital with amblyopia and similar fundus changes. Thirty-one patients, aged 18 to 64 years were admitted to hospital primarily for ataxia, but several had also optic atrophy.

Osuntokun et al. (1968) reported the lowering of plasma sulphur amino acids, normal or high vitamin B_{12} levels, and raised plasma thiocyanate levels in nine Nigerian patients with ataxic neuropathy. They attributed the condition to cyanide ingestion as a result of incompletely prepared cassava, known to contain cyanide. In 360 patients with polyneuropathy Osuntokun and Osuntokun (1971) found eye signs and symptoms in more than 80%, amounting to total blindness in some cases. This report differs from others in that central or centrocaecal scotoma was uncommon, and 84% of those with eye changes had contraction of the peripheral fields.

Quéré et al. (1967) reported 115 patients with the usual features in Senegal.

Asia. Many of the accounts of nutritional amblyopia in the population at large and nearly all the experience of the disease among prisoners of war has come from Southeast Asia.

Japan. Early Japanese accounts of the disease "kakke", the local name for beriberi, consistently included references to ocular manifestations, namely retrobulbar neuritis, paralyses of ocular muscles, and decreased sensitivity of the cornea and conjunctiva. The whole controversial subject of beriberi and nutritional amblyopia is dealt with in Section B1*hii*, below, and the other two features were mentioned above (Section A6). Dietary conditions have greatly improved in Japan in more recent years and frank malnutrition is now rare. In the Aomori prefecture the disease shibi-gatchaki, to which reference has already been made (Section A4, above), has ceased to be a public health problem. It was essentially due to deficiency of riboflavin and nicotinic acid. Retrobulbar neuritis occurred in about 10% of cases.

Malaya. The condition described by Landor and Pallister (1935) among a high proportion of the inmates of the prison at Johore Bahru had the usual skin and mucous membrane lesions attributable to hyporiboflavinosis. Among the associated nervous symptoms was diminution of visual acuity, to 6/60 in some cases, with poorly sustained reaction of the pupils to light. Xerophthalmia and night blindness were not seen. Similar outbreaks occurred in the Kuala Lumpur prison, the Mental Hospital at Singapore, and among the boys of the Singapore Reformatory. Some cases were also seen in poorer members of the outside population. In 50 early cases dramatic cure was obtained with 15 g of Marmite daily for one month, and of these 20 relapsed within a month of ceasing to take it. The authors believed the condition to be due to riboflavin deficiency. In an account of the diseases of a primitive tribe, the Murats, living in the interior of North Borneo, Clarke (1951) mentioned that the local Chinese and the sea-going natives very commonly suffered from beriberi, optic neuritis, burning feet, magenta tongue, and angular stomatitis but that the Murats living in their own villages were unaffected.

India and Ceylon. Most accounts of pellagra or beriberi from the subcontinent have not included references to ocular symptomatology. Again in the inmates of a jail, Nicholls (1933, 1934) from Ceylon described the skin, mucous membrane, and nervous system changes. Many of these patients went blind with keratomalacia and undoubtedly the grosser damage due to vitamin A deficiency would obscure any finer degrees of visual loss due to vitamin B complex deficiency. Of 34 patients with pellagra, beriberi or polyneuritis, 20 had evidence of retrobulbar neuropathy (Raman and Abbu, 1941). There was constriction of the peripheral fields but scotomata were not demonstrated. In Madras, Verma (1942) saw several hundred cases yearly of nutritional amblyopia. Scotomata were rarely demonstrated, corneal epithelial dystrophy was common (Section A4, above), and in early cases considerable improvement was obtained with a combination of shark liver oil and yeast.

Wadia *et al.* (1972) investigated optic neuropathy of uncertain aetiology over a $2\frac{1}{2}$-year period in Bombay. Only 20 patients were found, of whom only one had typical centrocaecal scotomata and he was a non-smoker. Six patients smoked but none a pipe. Vitamin B_{12} and thiocyanate levels were within normal limits in all cases.

Philippines. Spillane (1947) summarized the experience of a number of authors among prisoners of war, dimness of vision occurring in all camps, its nutritional nature being recognized in several. Of special interest was the description by Musselman (1945, 1946) in Cabanatuan of a neurological syndrome resembling myasthenia gravis with tiring of the eyes, diplopia, and ptosis. About 30% of 500 men at one camp were affected. It was most pronounced in men who regularly ate large quantities of dried fish, symptoms subsiding when fish was omitted from the diet and recurring when it was resupplied. Thiamine was curative and it is more than likely that this condition was an acute thiamine deficiency due to thiaminase in fish (see also Section IE, Chapter 10, Section ID).

De Ocampo *et al.* (1947) described an epidemic of nutrition amblyopia that followed the food shortage during the Japanese occupation of the islands. They found absolute central and centrocaecal scotomata and relative scotomata, especially to red, and enlarged blind spots, in some cases merging with the central scotomata. In eight of Nañagas's 44 patients with corneal changes he also found scotomata (Section A2, above).

Indonesia. Many cases of "camp eyes" occurred among the European internees on Java during the Japanese occupation. During the general food shortage afterward many more instances were seen in the local population (Sie Boen Lian, 1947).

Far Eastern prisoner-of-war camps. From the military and civilian internment camps all over the Japanese-occupied area of the Far East came, during the years immediately succeeding the 1939–45 war, report upon report of the nutritional diseases suffered by the inmates. The writer had hoped at one time to be able to summarize here this unique experience of the ocular manifestations of malnutrition. This has turned out to be impossible for two main reasons. Firstly the personnel available in most camps were not competent to make a detailed eye examination, and the few eye specialists who were there were hampered in their studies by lack of proper facilities. That work of such high calibre and great scientific value was ever carried out under such difficult conditions is a great tribute to the workers concerned who were themselves inevitably patients as well as observers. Secondly it is not possible to separate and sort out the data of a number of reports coming from the same camps and written by different workers, usually with varying special interests.

There was a remarkable uniformity about the nutritional disease observed in all the prison camps in the Far East and this applied to the eye lesions as much as it did to the other conditions. When there were conspicuous discrepancies these have been mentioned and commented upon. Individual accounts have been quoted as occasion arises but in particular those of Smith and Woodruff (1951) from Singapore and Hong Kong, which also supplied most of the data for what we know of corneal epithelial dystrophy in prisoners (Section A2, above), of Denny-Brown (1947), Clarke and Sircus

(1952) for the residual defects, and of King and Passmore (1955) for the disease in American prisoners of war in Korea, have been drawn upon throughout.

In general, the amblyopia in what must amount in all to several thousand cases in camps all over the East, in Singapore, Thailand, Java, Philippines, Hong Kong, and Korea, did not differ materially from that previously described in free living peoples in many parts of the world. On the other hand, the corneal lesions did not occur in most camps and the significance of this has already been discussed (Section A2, above). The 15 cases of Wilkinson and King (1944) are atypical in several respects. All except two showed a sluggish pupillary reaction to light and poor maintenance of contraction not reported by others. The authors were unable to demonstrate scotomata in any, but in all but two they found concentric or quadrantic contraction of the fields. The best results were claimed for nicotinic acid, not found helpful by other investigators.

At Changi military hospital, Singapore, Woodruff saw 1153 cases of nutritional amblyopia in the course of 17 months. About 34% of these also had the corneal condition, but in Hong Kong Dean Smith found amblyopia alone in 174 out of 1507 males and 196 of 986 females. Figure 57 has been constructed from data obtained in the civilian camp, Singapore. It will be seen that amblyopia, the burning feet syndrome, and the orogenital syndrome all developed a high incidence in the earlier half of 1943 and fell away sharply in August of that year when there was a marked improvement in the diet. This then included 2 oz nuts and pulses, 1 oz rice polishings, a fair supply of eggs, 3–5 oz meat daily, and an increase in vegetables, especially leafy ones. It is also noteworthy that the peak incidence occurred when there were no cases of beriberi and before pellagra had appeared. The fact that in Hong Kong more than 30 patients receiving daily injections of thiamine for beriberi or painful feet actually developed amblyopia while under treatment is very suggestive evidence against a thiamine deficiency aetiology for these cases. It would seem that a temporary excess of thiamine might have precipitated an imbalance of the B vitamins with a relative deficiency of riboflavin or some other member of the group.

The best experimental investigation into the aetiology of nutritional amblyopia was that carried out in the Selarang area of the prisoners-of-war camp in Singapore, designed by M. F. A. Woodruff and assisted by the ophthalmologist R. G. Orr, and the nutrition officer R. C. Burgess (Smith and Woodruff, 1951). Preliminary work showed that smoking, malaria, and taking of quinine could be ruled out as aetiological factors among their

FIG. 57. Monthly incidence of (a) pellagra, (b) orogenital syndrome, and (c) burning feet and nutritional amblyopia in the civilian camp, Singapore. From Smith and Woodruff (1951).

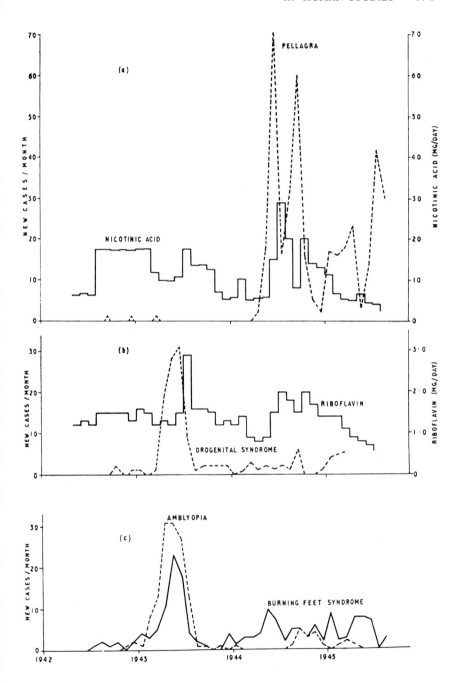

patients. Calcium, phosphorus, and nicotinic acid were not of value but Marmite gave slight improvement in all cases who received it. Other preparations high in protein, fat, and vitamin A failed to benefit the condition, but riboflavin, of which very little was available, gave promising results. A diet was devised which was better in every respect than that received by prisoners in Changi, who acted as controls, but was most markedly better as far as riboflavin was concerned. Ten relatively early cases with paracentral scotomata and visual acuity ranging from 6/9 to 6/60 in the worse eye were chosen to receive the experimental diet. The diet was continued for 4 weeks and leaf extract for a further 3 weeks. During this period the visual acuity of all cases showed a marked improvement and all eventually recovered fully.

The most recent of these accounts concerns American prisoners of war in Korea (King and Passmore, 1955) (Fig. 58a and b). The onset of visual loss was usually after about 6 or 12 months. In their 22 cases the signs of beriberi were more frequent than in prisoners without amblyopia. Only two cases showed further improvement on rehabilitation. After rehabilitation, changes were noted in the ERG that are difficult to interpret. The x-wave was reduced in amplitude and sensitivity. This was also so upon dark adaptation, the b-wave amplitude being appreciably reduced. These workers suggested that there was a disturbance of the function of rods and cones and that the optic atrophy was of the ascending type.

Western Hemisphere Mainland. In contrast to the situation on the islands of the Caribbean area the writer is aware of very few reports of nutritional amblyopia from the mainland. It is true that this may be in part due to lack of opportunity to cull much of the literature, particularly that written in Spanish. Visits to Central and South America failed however to bring this to his notice. Furthermore, writers from the West Indies and North America with better access make no such reference.

Mendoza González (1941) described seven cases of "optic neuritis" out of a large number of pellagra patients in Mexico. The reviewer states that this type of neuritis has not been previously described. Three patients were alcohol addicts however. The visual field defects were very variable, two having central defects, and two had reduced temporal fields. The pellagra was cured with a good diet and nicotinic acid, but the visual symptoms only responded to thiamine.

There have been several reports of nutritional amblyopia from the United States (Calhoun, 1918; Levine, 1934; Fine and Lachman, 1937) accompanied by some of the signs of beriberi and pellagra, but alcoholism has been

FIG. 58. (a) Central visual fields in three cases of nutritional amblyopia. (b) Electroretinographic response in the same three cases as (a). From King and Passmore (1955).

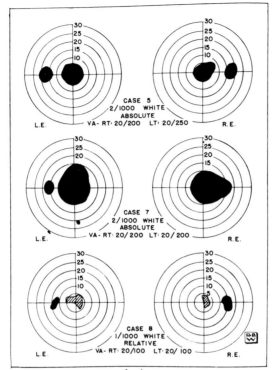

(a)

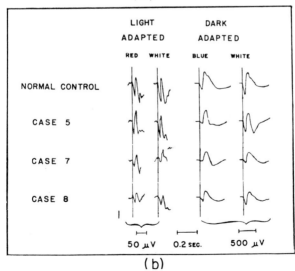

(b)

a complicating factor in many. It is of considerable interest that, during the years between the two world wars when pellagra and the associated signs of riboflavin deficiency were being so intensively investigated in the southern parts of the United States, retrobulbar neuropathy was not mentioned as part of the symptomatology. Moore (1958) in correspondence on the subject stated that in 1940 he discussed this very point with V. P. Sydenstricker, one of the leading American investigators in this field, who informed him that they had found no evidence of optic nerve involvement in their cases. In view of the ready response of the corneal, mucous membrane, and skin lesions to riboflavin therapy this must be taken as a piece of evidence against the involvement of this vitamin in nutritional amblyopia.

Europe. Nutritional amblyopia was not a feature of the effects of privation suffered by prisoners of war and civilians alike in the internment camps of Europe during the second world war (Edge, 1945; Leyton, 1946; Spillane, 1947; Medical Research Council, 1951; Helweg-Larsen *et al.,* 1952). On the other hand, during the civil war in Spain (1936–39) Jiménez Garcia (1940) observed among the civil population of Madrid 336 cases of glossitis, burning feet, and gastric disturbance. Later symptoms included dimness of vision with diplopia and scotomata. The condition responded to brewer's yeast but single members of the vitamin B complex were not very effective. The most complete account available is that in the monograph of Grande and Peraita (1941) in which details are given of nutritional neuropathies observed in more than 3000 patients. Visual disturbances were one of the most common complaints, occurring in 16.3% of all cases. They consisted of dimness of vision, with central or paracentral scotomata and varying degrees of optic atrophy. Best results were obtained with brewer's yeast—vitamins A, C, D, thiamine, and riboflavin being ineffective.

ii. The Problem of Aetiology It might be as well to make clear at the outset that the writer does not have any fixed ideas about the precise aetiology of nutritional amblyopia, beyond its being a true nutritional deficiency disease and almost certainly involving the vitamins of the B complex. It is conceivable that other factors such as heavy work, solar radiation, emotional strain, and toxins may play some additional part but the evidence for this, reviewed by Leigh (1948), is not convincing. There would seem to be three ways in which the difficulties and discrepancies that exist at present might be resolved. It is possible that deficiency of a single vitamin is responsible for the optic nerve lesion and perhaps for other manifestations also. Such a role has been suggested for vitamin B_{12}, not yet discovered when most of the work reviewed here was undertaken. It might, however, prove to be a vitamin, probably of the B complex type, still unidentified at the present time. Another possibility is that deficiency of different but closely related vitamins might have similar, although not perhaps identical, effects. If this were so, it might explain the discrepancies, although few, in the accounts of the features of amblyopia. The varieties of clinical picture are perhaps most numerous in the involvement of the peripheral nervous system (Cruickshank, 1961). A final possibility, and one which the writer tends to favour most, is that the overall balance of the B vitamins is all-important. Human dietaries deficient in vitamins of the B complex will in general tend to be deficient in all members of that complex, but there is bound to be wide variation met in practice of combination of individual deficiencies. Just what effects such combined deficiencies might have in man is quite unknown.

The intention here is merely to present the evidence, as it appears to the writer, for and against the various views that have been from time to time expressed, and to allow the reader to judge for himself.

Thiamine. Deficiency of this vitamin and an association with beriberi have been for long considered in an aetiological relationship to nutritional amblyopia. This is chiefly because of the known importance of thiamine in the metabolism of nervous tissue and the frequent mention of amblyopia as part of the beriberi syndrome in the early reports of the disease from Japan.

Unfortunately nearly all these Japanese accounts are virtually unobtainable now. What is said here is based upon the account of that literature given by Elliot (1920) in the chapter in his book written in collaboration with Miyashita, and upon discussion of the subject with ophthalmologists in Japan. There has always been some doubt as to whether the disease known as "kakke" in Japan was the same as beriberi. The frequent observation of impairment of dark adaptation and of conjunctival xerosis suggests that there was accompanying vitamin A deficiency, although these features were not separated by the Japanese authors from "kakke" itself. It is possible that there were other associated deficiencies, not recognizable at that time, and the amblyopia might have been due to these. In any case amblyopia appears to have been a rather infrequent feature of "kakke". No data concerning the incidence are given by Elliot but the Japanese authors he quotes all reported only a few cases, the largest series being only 10 in number. In a series of 217 cases of retrobulbar neuritis 6.4% were considered by Ishida (1918) to be due to beriberi. According to Miyashita, in the early stages of the condition the scotoma is small and connected to the blind spot by a narrow bridge giving it what he calls its most characteristic pestle-shaped form. Most of the early Japanese workers stressed the increased liability of women during pregnancy and lactation to develop amblyopia in association with beriberi. There is even a Japanese proverb that advises lactating women not to sew with a needle as it is a strain on the eyes at such times. Hyperemesis gravidarum may sometimes arise as a result of acute thiamine deficiency and is known to be one of the rarer causes of Wernicke's encephalopathy (Section

B2, below). Retrobulbar neuropathy has been reported as a complication (Ironside, 1938–39). The condition described by Japanese writers would appear to be different however. Of later writers, Kagawa (1938) has laid special emphasis on this association in female cases. He has thoroughly reviewed the Japanese literature on the relationship between retrobulbar neuropathy and beriberi and described his own experience in 200 cases seen in Tokyo from 1927 to 1930. He divided his patients into three groups; the largest number (123 cases) had amblyopia associated with mild beriberi, 61 cases were in lactating women, and in the remaining 16 cases amblyopia was associated with ataxia. It is remarkable that none of his cases had indisputable evidence of beriberi. In the first group the only complaint was loss of vision, and absence of the ankle jerks in about half was the only additional clinical finding. Kagawa states that this condition is known in Japan as "latent", "unripe", or "prepared condition of beriberi" but the description he gives hardly warrants such a diagnosis and one is left wondering whether it may not have been that, in a country where florid beriberi had been so rampant, a host of minor nervous disorders was ascribed to this disease. The general symptoms were also vague in the second group of cases in which amblyopia occurred in lactating women. Much more definite were the gross ataxia, disappearance of postural sensibility, and loss of power seen in the remaining small group of 16 cases. Four of these patients had glossitis and angular stomatitis and in two there was persistent tinnitus and bilateral nerve deafness. These symptoms are quite unlike those of beriberi but closely resemble the nutritional neuropathies in prisoners of war in Far Eastern camps. It is largely on the basis of Kagawa's work, and of his own extensive experience as consultant in neurology to India Command and Allied Land Forces, Southeast Asia, after the war that Denny-Brown (1947) has attacked the association of nutritional amblyopia with beriberi. According to Kagawa beriberi amblyopia is an early lesion, with truly central scotomata, closely similar to the scotomata of alcohol, tobacco, and lead poisoning. The intensity of the amblyopia did not correspond with other symptoms; it was not at the same time of the year; nor was it found in the most severe beriberi cases. Although many instances were in lactating women none of the suckled children developed infantile beriberi. All these points Denny-Brown feels militate against the condition having been one due to thiamine deficiency. Kagawa's description and Denny-Brown's appraisal of the Japanese work certainly raise serious doubts as to the validity of the supposed relationship of beriberi to nutritional amblyopia.

Most of the experience in the prison camps during the second world war also suggests no aetiological relationship with thiamine deficiency. Generally speaking, this vitamin was not effective when given even in quite large doses. In Hong Kong amblyopia commenced in more than 30 patients when they were receiving daily injections of thiamine for beriberi or painful feet (Section B*1h*, above). While many patients with amblyopia gave a history of having had beriberi these conditions did not usually coincide. There was, however, frequently a striking correspondence in time between the onset of amblyopia and of the burning feet and orogenital syndromes.

The good results obtained by Carroll (1944) with thiamine in the treatment of tobacco–alcohol amblyopia in the presence of unabated smoking and drinking have been referred to (Section B*1g*). More complete restoration of vision was obtained if the whole B complex was given.

Experimental work has shown that the optic nerves of the rat are damaged in thiamine deficiency and that these changes are enhanced by a coincident deficiency of riboflavin (Section IE).

Riboflavin. The evidence for riboflavin deficiency as the cause of nutritional amblyopia has already been presented in the accounts that have been given of the disease. It would seem from the results of therapy and the coincidence of amblyopia with other lesions responding to riboflavin that there is more support for deficiency of this than of any other single vitamin as the cause of amblyopia. Most workers agree, however, that whole B complex therapy is better than that limited to a single vitamin, whatever that vitamin be.

Nicotinic Acid. Both Bietti (1901) and Whaley (1909) described a yellowish reflex from the retina in pellagra. Cataract formation has been associated with pellagra by many writers (Chapter 11, Section B) but there is no real evidence that such a relationship is causal.

Calhoun (1918) carried out full field examinations on 13 patients with pellagra and found that all showed constriction of the peripheral fields, while in addition nine had central scotomata and one a paracentral scotoma. Riad (1929) also reported constriction of the field with asthenopia, diplopia, optic neuritis, and reduction of visual acuity in Egyptian pellagrins. Others have recorded central scotomata without alterations in the peripheral field (Jaensch, 1930; Krylov, 1932; Levine, 1934; Fine and Lachman, 1937).

In essence the visual findings in association with pellagra, as with beriberi and hyporiboflavinosis, have all tended to be very similar in nature. The degree of accuracy of observation has varied considerably, making a close comparison impossible, but the impression has been gained that contraction of the peripheral fields may possibly be more frequent in association with pellagra than with the other conditions.

Vitamin B$_{12}$. This vitamin was isolated in crystalline form from liver concentrates in 1948 and subsequently shown to be the anti-pernicious anaemia factor. It was therefore unfortunately not available for trial in nutritional amblyopia when all the tragic wealth of human material was present in the Japanese prison camps. It has been shown that vitamin B$_{12}$

deficiency is quite common in vegans, strict vegetarians who take neither eggs nor milk, and it occasionally arises after total gastrectomy and as part of the malabsorption syndrome. Detailed consideration of the role of vitamin B_{12} is given elsewhere (Sections B1e above, and B1i and j and B6, below).

i. Retrobulbar Neuropathy in Pernicious Anaemia
The nervous system is frequently involved in this disease and in about 5 % of patients there is evidence of optic neuropathy, sometimes antedating all other manifestations including haematologic changes (Cohen, 1936; Leishman, 1952; Hamilton *et al.*, 1959).

Decreased visual acuity is accompanied by central or paracentral scotoma, in one or both eyes. Extraocular muscle palsies are of rare occurrence. Heaton (1960) suggested that tobacco may be a precipitating factor in pernicious anaemia cases. More than half of the tobacco amblyopia cases studied by Leishman (1952) had a histamine-fat achlorhydria. About one-seventh of the 89 cases seen by Heaton *et al.* (1958) had pernicious anaemia. About half of the reported cases of pernicious anaemia amblyopia have been smokers, with an overwhelming majority of males. There is a female preponderance of 3 to 1 in all cases of pernicious anaemia, and it may be that the greater tendency of males to smoke, with pipe smoking being virtually confined to the male sex, accounts for this reversal of sex incidence. The presence of some other factor such as smoking, in addition to vitamin B_{12} deficiency, would seem to be indicated by the rarity of amblyopia in pernicious anaemia, sprue, and nutritional macrocytic anaemia (Adams and Hift, 1961).

Early treatment with vitamin B_{12} returns visual function to normal (Ellis and Hamilton, 1959; Hamilton *et al.*, 1959). In four patients in whom tobacco was aetiologically involved, cyanocobalamin returned the blood picture to normal, but visual improvement occurred only with hydroxocobalamin (Foulds *et al.*, 1969) (see Section B*e*). Treatment with folic acid alone has led to deterioration of the optic neuropathy, as of other nervous system changes in pernicious anaemia (Ross *et al.*, 1948).

j. Other Vitamin B_{12} Deficiency States
Infestation with the fish tapeworm, *Diphyllobothrium latum,* is known to induce a deficiency of vitamin B_{12} by interfering with its absorption from the terminal ileum. Björkenheim (1966) studied 102 consecutive carriers of the tapeworm in Helsinki. Forty had subnormal levels of serum vitamin B_{12}. Four of these subjects had centrocaecal scotomata and optic neuropathy, but none had megaloblastic anaemia, although one patient also had involvement of the cord. The eye signs were cured with expulsion of the worm and vitamin B_{12} therapy.

Resection of the terminal ileum may result in deficiency. Stambolian and

Behrens (1977) reported such a case in a 17-year-old boy who developed bilateral centrocaecal scotomata. Folic acid therapy was being given at the time and they suggest that this may have precipitated the eye changes.

k. Leber's Hereditary Optic Atrophy

The familial incidence, abrupt onset and the denser, usually permanent scotoma in this disease constitute important differences from the other optic neuropathies described here. The visual field findings differ from the other retrobulbar neuropathies in that a relative centrocaecal scotoma progresses to a large, centrocaecal scotoma which breaks through to the periphery, usually upwards or inwards (Rönne, 1910).

Smoking is not aetiologically involved, but in patients who do smoke serum thiocyanate has been found to be lowered and comparable to those values found in tobacco amblyopia (Section B*e*). Therapy with hydroxocobalamin or oral cystine is reported to cause a rise in serum thiocyanate, and in previously low levels of erythrocyte glutathione and urinary excretion (Foulds and Pettigrew, 1977). There is, however, no accompanying improvement in the disease (Foulds *et al.*, 1968b). It has been postulated that there may be an hereditary enzymic defect resulting in failure to detoxify cyanide. Nikoskelainen *et al.* (1977) treated five affected members of a family in the very early stages with prednisone and hydroxocobalamin, but failed to halt the progression of visual impairment.

l. Low Carbohydrate Diet Optic Neuropathy

The widespread use of diets for the treatment of obesity that may be deficient in vitamins as well as energy has to be pointed out. Recently Hoyt and Bilson (1977) reported two cases of thiamine-responsive optic neuropathy resulting from prolonged restriction.

2. The Wernicke-Korsakoff Syndrome (Cerebral Beriberi; Acute Superior Haemorrhagic Polioencephalitis)

There seems to be general agreement that this syndrome results from an acute deficiency of thiamine which may arise in several ways. Besides the condition caused by an acute lack of dietary thiamine and of which the main accounts have come from prisoner-of-war camps, this disease is an important manifestation of the beriberi syndrome associated with alcoholism (Victor *et al.*, 1971), and isolated cases have been reported complicating hyperemesis gravidarum, pyloric stenosis, and other types of severe, recurrent vomiting. In these circumstances the precipitation of encephalopathy by the administration of large amounts of glucose without thiamine is well known.

The symptomatology depends to some extent on the acuteness of deprivation and it has to be remembered that the signs of encephalopathy usually develop as the result of the superimposition of an acute thiamine lack on the background of chronic deficiency. Denny-Brown (1958) has described the symptoms in the order of acuteness of deprivation. The most acute are mental confusion leading to coma, and if these are accompanied by bilateral 6th nerve weakness, then Wernicke's syndrome is present. If the deprivation is less, the 6th nerve weakness becomes merely nystagmus on looking to either side, and if less still then aphonia and mental confusion may be the first or perhaps only symptoms. The 6th nerve weakness is the symptom most easily relieved by thiamine, the mental confusion being difficult to reverse. He regards Korsakoff's psychosis as a milder degree of the confusional state of Wernicke's syndrome, often appearing as this tends to subside.

The largest series of cases in which the aetiology was dietary deficiency was reported from Changi prisoner-of-war camp, Singapore (de Wardener and Lennox, 1947), these patients also being part of the larger study of deficiency diseases made by Smith and Woodruff (1951). These authors provide strong evidence for the view that this syndrome is due solely to acute thiamine deficiency. This consists of: the coincidence of the condition with a period when the thiamine: non-fat-calorie ratio was lowest; occurrence together with other forms of beriberi when no other deficiency diseases were prevalent; the coexistence of other manifestations of beriberi in 41 of these cases; and the rapidity and completeness of recovery following parenteral injections of thiamine, even in the very small doses, up to 9 mg, that were available.

In this series 31 patients recovered and 21 died. The recovery was complete in 29, and, of these, 25 received intramuscular thiamine, the others recovering on Marmite or tablets alone. Of the 25 men who were given injections, 20 are known to have improved dramatically within 48 hours, notes were inadequate on four; and one improved only slightly. Of the 25 cases recovering on thiamine, 11 had been receiving Marmite or tablets before but without effect, probably because of the severe diarrhoea that most of these patients were suffering from. Among the 21 fatal cases there were only 11 who received thiamine injections and, of these, only two died of uncomplicated Wernicke's encephalopathy.

Ocular symptoms and signs (Table V) were prominent among the clinical features of these cases. Nystagmus was the earliest of all signs and was of considerable value in diagnosis, being invariably present and only being obliterated by ophthalmoplegia in the terminal stages. The fundus was examined in only a few instances but showed small flame-shaped haemorrhages in one and early papilloedema in two cases.

TABLE V. *Ocular Signs in Wernicke's Encephalopathy in Prisoners of War*[a]

	No. of cases	Percentage
Nystagmus	52	100
External rectus fatigue and paralysis	14	26
Complete disconjugate wandering	4	8
Loss of visual acuity	2	4
Papilloedema	2	4
Pupil abnormalities	2	4
Ptosis	1	2
Complete ophthalmoplegia	1	2
Retinal haemorrhages	1	2

[a] From de Wardener and Lennox (1947).

A classic description of Wernicke's disease and Korsakoff's psychosis associated with chronic alcoholism is given in the monograph by Victor *et al.* (1971). Over nearly 20 years they studied in Boston 245 clinical cases, most with lengthy follow-up, and 82 with postmortem examinations.

In 175 patients it was possible to obtain an adequate dietary history: 84% had evidence of undernutrition as judged by gross dietary inadequacy or loss of at least 20 lb weight in the year preceding illness. In 163 patients the presenting complaint was recorded and, of these, 40% were ocular ("staring", "cross-eyed", etc.). In 86 cases the initial manifestations included ophthalmoplegia in 42%. In only nine of 232 patients carefully examined were ocular abnormalities of some kind absent. Table VI gives details of these findings. Analyses of nystagmus and of conjugate gaze palsies found are given in Tables VII and VIII.

Retinal abnormalities were confined to small haemorrhages in six cases. Bilateral central or centrocaecal scotomata were an associated finding in six patients. Papilloedema or other abnormalities of the optic disc were not seen. Bilateral ptosis occurred in six patients and a questionable unilateral ptosis in two others.

In this series the ratio of men to women was 1.7:1.0, considerably less than the 4:1 ratio for alcoholism in general, and 7:1 for particular complications of alcoholism such as "rum fits".

The major pathological changes occurred symmetrically in the paraventricular parts of nuclei of the thalamus, the mammillary bodies, periaqueductal region, floor of the fourth ventricle, and the anterior lobe of the cerebellum. Microscopically they consisted of vacuolation and looseness of tissue and destruction of parenchymal elements, where there was marked increase of pleomorphic histocytes and astrocytes. Myelinated fibres appeared to be more affected than nerve cells. Blood vessels were prominent in early

TABLE VI. *Incidence of ocular abnormalities in 232 cases of the Wernicke-Korsakoff syndrome*[a]

Sign	No. of cases		Percentage	
Nystagmus		198 (65)[b]	85	
Lateral rectus palsy, bilateral		125 (7)	54	
Complete	38 (5)			16
Partial	87 (2)			38
Conjugate gaze palsy		102 (6)	44	
Pupillary abnormality		43	19	
Retinal haemorrhages		6	3	
Ptosis		8	3	
Bilateral	6			3
Unilateral	2			<1
Central or caecocentral scotomata		6	3	
No ocular abnormality		9	4	

[a] From Victor *et al.* (1971).
[b] Figures in parentheses indicate the number in which this was the only ocular abnormality.

TABLE VII. *Analysis of nystagmus in 198 cases of the Wernicke-Korsakoff syndrome*[a]

Sign	No. of cases		Percentage
Horizontal nystagmus		192	97
Horizontal alone	87 (42)[b]		
Horizontal + vertical	100 (20)		
Horizontal + rotary	2		
Horiz. + vert. + rotary	3 (3)		
Vertical nystagmus		109	55
On upward gaze	88		
Upward + downward gaze	18		
Downward alone	3		
Rotary nystagmus		5	3
Vertical nystagmus alone		6	3
On upward gaze	5		
On downward gaze	1		
On upward + downward	0		

[a] From Victor *et al.* (1971).
[b] Figures in parentheses indicate number of cases in which this sign was the only ocular abnormality.

TABLE VII. *Analysis of conjugate gaze palsies in 102 cases of the Wernicke-Korsakoff syndrome*[a]

Sign	No. of cases		Percentage
Horizontal gaze palsy		88	86
Horizontal alone	49 (4)[b]		
Horizontal + vertical	39		
Vertical gaze palsy		48	47
Upward	34		
Upward + downward	14		
Downward	0		
Vertical gaze palsy alone		9	9
Upward	8		
Upward + downward	1		
Complete ophthalmoplegia		3 (2)	3
Internuclear ophthalmoplegia		2	2

[a] From Victor *et al.* (1971).

[b] Figures in parentheses indicate the number of cases in which this sign was the only ocular abnormality.

lesions, but the "classical" petechial haemorrhages occurred in only 20% of cases and many appeared to be agonal in nature (Figs. 59, 60 and 61).

The ocular muscle and gaze palsies are attributable to lesions of the 6th and 3rd nerve nuclei and adjacent tegmentum, and the nystagmus to lesions in the region of the vestibular nuclei. The lack of significant destruction of nerve cells was consistent with response of these signs to thiamine alone within a few hours, clearing completely in a few days or several weeks at the most.

3. Nicotinic Acid Deficiency

An encephalopathy was first described by Jolliffe (1939; Jolliffe *et al.*, 1940) and Cleckley *et al.* (1939) in America. It may or may not be accompanied by pellagra and polyneuritis, having a high mortality in the untreated but responding dramatically to nicotinic acid. The clinical features closely resemble those of Wernicke's encephalopathy and the oculomotor disturbances vary from bilateral nystagmus to complete ophthalmoplegia.

Mathur (1969) studied the macular area in 61 patients with pellagra in Udaipur, India. More than half showed vascularization and hyperaemia, and in about a third there was loss of the yellow reflex and hyperpigmentation

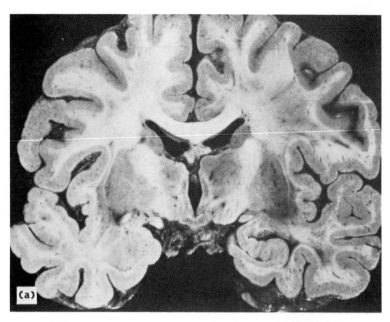

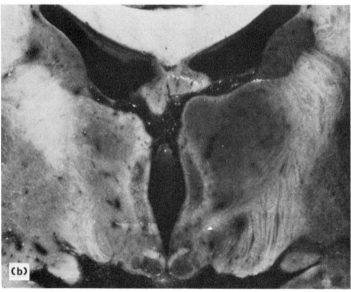

that resembled a burn. There was little improvement after cure of the pellagrous state.

4. The Fundus in Infantile Beriberi

The opinion was expressed by Burgess (1958) that there has never been an adequate assessment of the importance of beriberi as a cause of mortality in the infant. Funduscopic examination, although presenting its problems in the infant, would certainly provide valuable confirmatory evidence of the disease in such survey work. The changes consist of oedema of the fundus resulting in pallor, with the margins of the optic disc lacking in distinctness and the papilla itself being light in colour. The blood vessels, though dilated, are seen indistinctly (Naessens, 1930). Optic atrophy has been reported in infants suffering from beriberi (Ohta, 1930).

5. The Vitamin B Complex and Retinal Function

Riboflavin has been found in the retinae of many species but its function there is still not known (Section IC1). There does not seem to have been any recent investigation to confirm or clarify certain results reported some years ago, Kimble and Gordon (1939) found that some individuals with poor dark adaptation and low levels of vitamin A in the blood improved only when riboflavin as well as vitamin A was administered. It is not known whether riboflavin plays a part in absorption and utilization of vitamin A or whether it has a role in the retina. Pock-Steen (1939, 1947) claimed that patients with sprue had reduced visual acuity in dim light that was relieved by riboflavin but not by vitamin A, and that patients with riboflavin deficiency had impaired dark adaptation.

It is possible that the retina may reveal impairment of function in riboflavin deficiency long before the anterior segment shows any sign of

---

FIG. 59. Sections of brain from a 35-year-old man in whom Wernicke's disease became manifest during an attack of delirium tremens; death occurred 15 days later. (a) Coronal section through the cerebral hemispheres after formalin fixation. Lesions take the form of non-haemorrhagic "band necrosis" in walls of third ventricle; the centre of each mammillary body is also affected. Lateral ventricles are of normal size, third verticle slightly dilated. Cerebral cortex, caudate and lenticular nuclei, hippocampi and amygdaloid nuclei, and corpus callosum are intact. (b) Closer view of the same specimen. Note sparing of tissue immediately beneath the ependyma. The necrotic zone is grey and granular. In this case the fornices are normal. From Victor et al (1971).

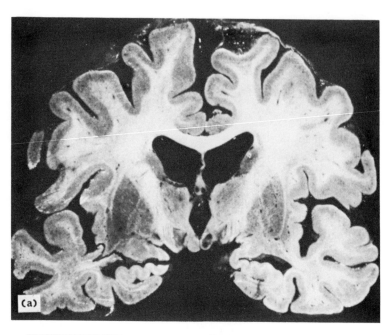

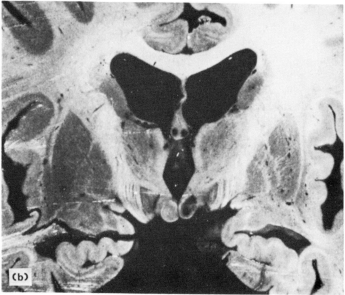

damage, just as is known to be the case for vitamin A deficiency. This is suggested by the prolonged human experiment carried out by Gordon and Vail (1950) (see Section A1, above) in mental patients who showed no evidence of corneal vascularization after 15 months on a diet severely restricted in riboflavin.

Horwitt et al. (1949) found no impairment of dark adaptation, but the threshold for flicker fusion was increased in most of their 15 male subjects maintained for periods of 9 to 17 months on a diet providing about 0.55 mg riboflavin daily, the minimum requirement. The test consisted of observation of a mercury bulb illuminated and extinguished at different controlled rates. The point at which light interruptions were first recognized was accepted as the threshold of flicker fusion.

Night blindness accompanying pellagra is usually regarded as being due to deficiency of vitamin A (Bietti, 1940). The role of nicotinamide as part of DPN in the oxidation of vitamin A to retinal provides theoretical grounds for a direct causal relationship, although there is at present no evidence that this occurs in man.

6. Retinal Haemorrhages in Megaloblastic Anaemias

Several workers have reported that retinal haemorrhage is more common in megaloblastic than in iron-deficiency anaemias (Cosnett and MacLeod, 1959; Adams and Hift, 1961) (see Chapter 5, Section IIBa). Lele et al. (1964) found 15 cases in 41 patients with megaloblastic anaemias, but only three cases in 259 patients with microcytic hypochromic anaemia. There was evidence of thrombocytopoenia in the megaloblastic anaemia group and this was also found in a series of 20 cases studied by Markar et al. (1969), with a significant rise of platelets on treatment.

Walsh (1957) states that retinal haemorrhages are the most frequent ocular complication of pernicious anaemia. They are usually flame-shaped

---

FIG. 60. Haemorrhagic necrosis of the fornices and mammillary bodies. The patient was a 72-year-old alcoholic man who died three days after the onset of a global confusional state. (a) Coronal section of formalin-fixed cerebrum. The frontal and temporal lobes are slightly atrophic (widened sulci) and both the lateral and third ventricles are enlarged. Haemorrhages are present in the right mammillary body and in both fornices. (b) Closer view of the same specimen. The third ventricular widening is not accompanied by visible lesions in the walls of the ventricles. Hippocampi, lenticular and caudate nuclei and internal capsules are intact. From Victor et al. (1971).

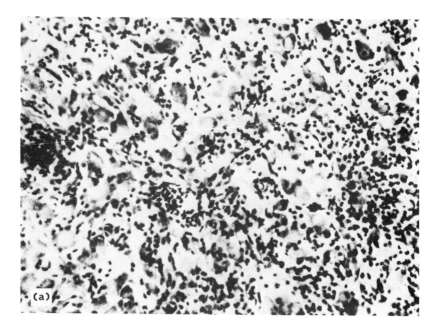

(a)

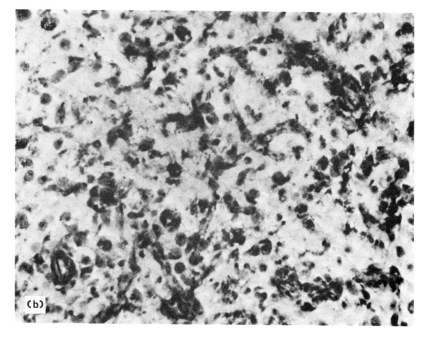

(b)

and in the posterior pole. In some instances there may be a white spot, composed of leucocytes, in the centre of the haemorrhage—the so-called Roth spot. Peripheral capillary microaneurysms, retinal oedema and papilloedema may occur.

7. Biotin Dependency

A number of children, some of them siblings, have been shown to have multiple carboxylase deficiencies which are biotin dependent. The symptomatology includes developmental regression, alopecia, dermatitis and immunodeficiency. One of three affected siblings had keratoconjunctivitis (Cowan et al., 1979). Biotin in large doses (5 mg twice daily) has resulted in dramatic improvement.

FIG. 61. (a) Recent lesions of the mammillary bodies (Nissl stain). Many of the neurones are still visible in regions where there is marked increase in cellularity (pleomorphic microgliacytes) (×180). Section is from a 52-year-old alcoholic who was admitted to the hospital with confusion, total external ophthalmoplegia, bilateral ptosis and miosis of abrupt onset. The neurologic signs subsided under the influence of thiamine, but he died 6 weeks later of Gram-negative sepsis. (b) A more severe and more chronic lesion shows prominence of small vessels ("vascular hyperplasia") in a region where disappearing nerve cells are replaced by histiocytes, some macrophages and astrocytes (×180). From Victor et al. (1971).

Chapter 4

Other Vitamins

I. Animal Studies

This chapter will perforce be very much of a miscellany. Unlike vitamin A or the vitamins of the B complex the remaining vitamins concerned in nutrition of the eye merit only a short chapter. If all the speculations, as opposed to scientific investigation, concerning the role of these factors were to be treated of here no doubt they would run to several lengthy chapters with ease. It is not the writer's intention to indulge in this stultifying pastime, but rather to stick to the facts as they are known, although it will be necessary from time to time to deal with some of the less well-documented material in a critical manner.

A. Vitamin C (Ascorbic Acid)

A deficiency of this vitamin in man and certain animals that are unable to synthesize it, notably other primates and the guinea pig, results in the disease known as scurvy. Shortly after the period 1928–33, during which the vitamin was isolated, identified, and synthesized, it was shown to occur in high concentrations in both the lens and the aqueous humour. Like glutathione, vitamin C occurs mainly in a reduced form, but it is also capable of being reversibly oxidized to ascorbone or dehydroascrobic acid, which is unstable. The usual method for its determination is by titration with the dye 2,6-dichlorophenolindophenol. Only the reduced form is measured by this method. The concentration of ascorbic acid varies in different parts of the body, tending as a rule to be higher in cells than in the extracellular fluids. However, the aqueous and vitreous humours are an exception to this, together with the lens having high concentrations of the vitamin. Generally speaking, the ascorbic acid level in the aqueous humour is much higher than that in the plasma—usually somewhere about 50 times. The level in the lens is higher still in some animals, but lower in others.

Although the aqueous humour and lens contain such a high concentration of ascorbic acid, and the levels fall rapidly in both experimental and human scurvy, cataract is not a feature of the scorbutic state. According to Duke-Elder (1946) Russian workers have claimed to have produced cataract in guinea pigs born from mothers fed a scorbutogenic diet, but this has not been substantiated. Furthermore the administration of large doses of vitamin C to both man and animals suffering from cataract has never resulted in reversal of the lens damage. There is also a consistent tendency for the level of ascorbic acid in the lens to decrease with cataract formation from any cause in both man and animals. Quite apart from cataract formation it has been shown that there is also a diminution of ascorbic acid in the lens with increasing age and within the lens itself the older part, the nucleus, has less ascorbic acid than the younger cortex. It is possible that ascorbic acid may have a pharmacological effect on the lens under certain circumstances for it has been claimed that large doses in rats delay the development of galactose-induced cataract (Bellows, 1936) and can arrest that caused by dinitrophenol. Claims to have demonstrated the synthesis of ascorbic acid by the lens are at variance with evidence that the concentration there is governed mainly by the rate of transfer of ascorbic acid into the eye and the permeability of the lens.

Turning from the lens, where deficiency of vitamin C seems to have remarkably little effect, to the cornea we find here a certain amount of evidence that this structure is affected in scurvy. It has been amply confirmed that collagen fibre formation in various parts of the body is reduced in scurvy. On the other hand the deposition of intercellular ground substance does not appear to be interfered with. Whatever the precise defect in connective tissue may be, the nutrition would seem to be impaired, for Campbell and Ferguson (1950) were able to show that vascularization of the cornea occurred with greater frequency following small standard heat injuries in scorbutic than in normal guinea pigs.

In a further study of this problem, Campbell et al. (1950) made superficial and deep heat injuries of the cornea of normal and vitamin C-deficient guinea pigs. They found that the healing of superficial lesions was not impaired but that the deeper lesions, involving the stroma, healed more slowly in deficient animals. Even after healing was complete, structural weakness of the wound persisted for as long as 3 weeks after injury. It seems rather paradoxical then to find that the concentration of vitamin C is much higher in the epithelium of the cornea than it is in the stroma. The wounded cornea of scorbutic guinea pigs also appears to react differently from that of the control animal under the influence of systemic cortisone. Barber and Nothaker (1952) showed that in control animals given cortisone wound healing was delayed due to the belated appearance of fibroblasts and prolonged immaturity of collagen. Similar treatment with cortisone of animals suffering from scurvy failed to alter the effects of vitamin C deficiency. That is to say that in these guinea pigs there was a definite increase in fibroblastic proliferation. A technique has been developed for the study of wound healing whereby polyvinyl sponges are implanted into the anterior chamber. It was found by Geever and Levenson (1960) and Sabatine et al. (1961) that collagen grew into the sponges even when the animal was scorbutic and that the ascorbic acid and dehydroascorbic acid concentrations decreased more slowly inside the eye than in the blood. Analysis for the amino acid hydroxyproline, among all proteins found only in collagen, and histological examination of sponges in the anterior chamber and also in the abdominal wall of scorbutic guinea pigs showed that deprivation of vitamin C has a much more marked retarding effect on the growth of connective tissue in the abdominal wall than it does in the anterior chamber. It would seem that the high concentration of ascorbic acid, even in the scorbutic animal, in the anterior chamber plays a part in permitting collagen formation to go on. How this high concentration is maintained is not known but there is some evidence that it is synthesized by the lens. Boyd (1955) found that wounds of the cornea in aphakic animals (without a lens) took 40% longer to heal than those in controls. The mean ascorbic acid concentrations of corneae and aqueous humour were significantly lower in aphakic than in control animals. These results are, however, at variance with work in man (Section IIA) in which the state of the lens, when present, or even its absence, failed to influence the concentration of ascorbic acid in the aqueous humour.

An electron microscope study of the cornea adds little to our understanding, with oedema and disruption of collagen being the main, and not unexpected, findings (Sulkin et al., 1972).

A careful study of the changes in the vitreous body in the scorbutic guinea pig (Cristiansson, 1957) has shown a lowered viscosity and raised glucosamine and water contents all of which return to normal on the administration of ascorbic acid. In the aqueous humour the fall in ascorbic acid was accompanied by a rise in glucosamine content. Glucosamine is the amino-sugar formed by the introduction of an amino group into glucose. It occurs extensively in nature in complex polysaccharides, usually in the form of its acetyl derivative N-acetylglucosamine.

Studies on the effects of experimental scurvy on other parts of the eye have been few. Orbital haemorrhage with proptosis was noted in a scorbutic monkey (Zilva and Still, 1920). It has been claimed (Terroine, 1953) that ascorbic acid protects against the spectacle eye produced by biotin deficiency in rats (see Chapter 3, Section IA2). Bessesen (1923) found the eyeballs to remain almost constant in absolute weight in scorbutic guinea pigs, in contrast to the loss of body weight. Finally, there was no alteration in size of the nuclei or staining of ganglion cells of the guinea pig retina in vitamin C deficiency (Müller and Nover, 1955).

B. Vitamin D (Calciferol)

The curative value of cod-liver oil in rickets had been known long before it became evident that this condition was a deficiency disease as a result of the production by Mellanby (1919) of rickets in puppies by feeding them on diets deficient in some factor present in certain animal fats. It was at first thought that this was the same as the growth factor isolated earlier and the "fat soluble A factor" necessary for the protection of the eyes. However, it soon became evident that there were two factors, not occurring in the same proportions in all the fats tested, for one fat might give good protection against rickets but not against xerophthalmia and another might give opposite results. It was also found that heat and oxidation destroyed more of the antixerophthalmic than the antirachitic factor. The importance of the balance of calcium and phosphorus in the diet in the prevention of rickets was shown by McCollum in experiment on rats. The long-known beneficial effect of sunlight was ultimately proved to be due to the irradiation of the animal body or of food; the ultraviolet light activating the provitamins 7-dehydrocholesterol in skin and ergosterol found only in the unsaponifiable fraction of fat.

A deficiency of vitamin D has been implicated in two ways in ocular pathology. The first was the early belief that rickets was responsible for the development of zonular cataract. However, it was later shown, and the evidence is given in Chapter 5, Section IA, that the hypocalcaemic state of tetany, which frequently accompanies but is only partly dependent upon rickets, is responsible. Secondly, on the basis of the weakening effect that a deficiency of vitamin D and calcium might have on the sclera the theory of "scleral rickets" as a cause of myopia has been propounded. In support of this, Knapp (1939, 1943) claimed to have produced prominence of the eyes, widening of the palpebral fissures, ectasia of the cornea, and deepening of the anterior chamber in dogs fed a diet deficient in vitamin D and calcium. These results have not been confirmed and the theory has little support at the present time.

Proptosis, similar to that occasionally seen in children (Section IIB) has also been noted in experimental animals (Yudkin et al., 1934).

The ocular damage resulting from hypercalcaemia due to vitamin D excess are described in Chapter 5, Section IIA*b*.

C. Vitamin E (Tocopherol)

This vitamin, found in abundance in green leaves and the germ of seeds, was shown to be necessary for the prevention of sterility in the male, and abortion, though not failure to conceive, in the female.

Demole and Knapp (1941) claimed to have produced keratoconjunctivitis consistently, and other lesions such as keratoconus, iridocyclitis, cataract, and serous retinal exudates occasionally, in rats. Unfortunately they did not give details of the diet used or their methods of examination, and such changes, some of which are obvious even to the casual observer, have not been reported by the many other workers in this field. Italian workers have reported retinal degeneration (Malatesta, 1951) and an alteration of histochemical staining for mucopolysaccharide in the cornea (d'Esposito, 1957)

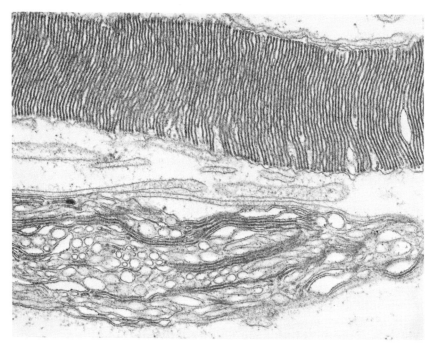

FIG. 62. Early stage of macular degeneration in vitamin E deficiency. An essentially normal rod outer segment (top) is adjacent to one undergoing degeneration (below). Disorientation and vesiculation of lamellae are apparent (×27 550). From Hayes, (1974).

in vitamin E-deficient rats. Prominence of the eyes was noted by Demole and Pfaltz (1940) and Lecoq and Isidor (1949) but this occurs in many deficiency states in which the eye tends to go on growing at an almost normal rate while the growth of the orbit is more severely affected. Devi *et al*. (1965) observed cataracts and ptosis in vitamin E-deficient rabbits. Bunce and Hess (1976) described lenticular opacity in young rats born to mothers deficient in either tryptophan or vitamin E.

Hayes (1974) maintained 12 New World cebus and 14 Old World cynomolgus monkeys on a diet deficient in vitamin E for more than 2 years. Focal macular degeneration resulted with disruption of the outer segments of rods and cones, probably caused by lipid peroxidation of these lipoprotein structures containing highly unsaturated fatty acids Fig. 62 (see Chapter 8, Section IC). He also studied the changes in vitamin A deficiency (Chapter 2, Section IC).

Interest has recently been revived in the possible role of vitamin E in oxygen-induced retinopathy or retrolental fibroplasia (RLF). Phelps and Rosenbaum (1977) using 75 kittens have developed a quantitative scoring system for measuring the retinal damage induced by oxygen therapy. They report beneficial effects when tocopherol was given daily from birth. As in the human disease, they found that with identical oxygen environments there were considerable differences between the eyes of the same animal and between animals of different genetic backgrounds.

D. Vitamin K

In the course of a period of 10 years, from 1929 to 1939, the existence of this vitamin, the disease in animals and man which results when it is deficient, the vitamin's mode of action, and its isolation were all discovered and achieved. It was first noted that chicks fed on a diet poor in fats developed a haemorrhagic disease, and shortly afterward the fat-soluble nature of the vitamin was proved. The haemorrhagic disease of chicks was shown to be due to a prolongation of the clotting time which was the result of hypoprothrombinaemia. In man and other mammals the deficiency state results, not from dietary lack, but in association with conditions in which there is an absence of bile from the intestine. Bile is essential for the proper absorption of the natural vitamin but synthetic analogues, particularly the water-soluble ones, do not need bile salts. As far as is known vitamin K has only one function in the body. It takes part in an enzyme system in the liver concerned with the formation of prothrombin, probably serving as the prosthetic group which complements the apo-enzyme system and does not form part of the prothrombin molecule.

Deficiency of vitamin K is not known to produce any ocular manifestations in animals. In view of the rather controversial nature of the retinal haemorrhage in newborn babies, believed by some to be due to vitamin K deficiency (Section II*b*), it is surprising that attempts do not seem to have been made to reproduce this condition in experimental animals. On the other hand, there is some evidence (Simonelli, 1950) that very large doses of the vitamin in the guinea pig fail to cause any ocular lesions even when severe degenerative changes have been produced in the liver, kidneys, and adrenals that lead to death.

II. Human Studies

A. Vitamin C

The older literature does not lack references to eye manifestations associated with clinical scurvy. Most of these are found to be haemorrhagic in nature. The sites of intraocular haemorrhage have included the conjunctiva (Kitamura, 1910), iris (Löwenstein, 1917), and the retina (Jacobsthal, 1900; Kitamura, 1910). Petechial haemorrhages into the skin of the lids have been noted in scurvy but are of no special significance. It would seem that in infantile scurvy intraorbital haemorrhage is a fairly common complication, for a collective investigation carried out by the American Pediatric Society (1898) showed that it occurred in more than 12% of several hundred cases. The extravasation of blood usually occurs between the periosteum and the bony roof of the orbit and causes the globe to be pushed forward, downward, and outward (Fig. 6.3).

During the first world war and after the long Lenten fasts in Russia before that time it used to be thought that night blindness was a feature of scurvy in adults. The fact that they showed in addition conjunctival xerosis and that both these symptoms were rapidly cured by liver or the oil makes it clear in retrospect that these people had a combined vitamin C and vitamin A deficiency.

Ever since ascorbic acid was discovered in high concentration in the lens in 1933 there has been speculation concerning its function there. Because cataract formation is accompanied by a fall in lens ascorbic acid many have tried to halt or even reverse the process by administering this vitamin. Their efforts have met uniformly without success. It would seem that the lens plays no part in the production or the maintenance of the high concentration of ascorbic acid in the aqueous humour but that it enters the posterior chamber in the reduced form from the ciliary body. Purcell *et al*. (1954) found that the concentration in the aqueous varied with that in the serum regardless of

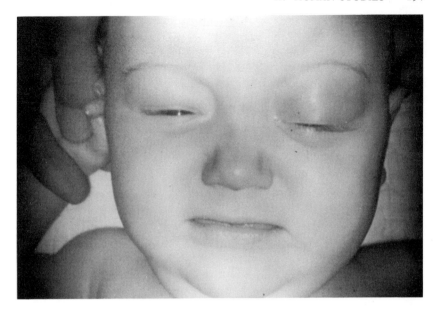

FIG. 63. Orbital haemorrhage in an infant with scurvy. By kind permission of Dr C. Woodruff, Columbia, Missouri.

whether or not the lens was cataractous. The high ratio of concentration in aqueous/plasma was maintained even in two aphakic patients several months after intracapsular extraction of the lens.

In a single report (Linnér, 1964) lowering of intraocular pressure in 12 volunteers given large doses of vitamin C (500 mg twice daily) compared with levels in 10 untreated controls has been claimed.

Hood and Hodges (1969) reported ocular lesions in a well-conducted human vitamin C-deprivation study in nine adult volunteers lasting 84 to 99 days. Subconjunctival haemorrhages occurred in four towards the end of the deprivation period (Fig. 64). Another subject showed conjunctival vessel congestion with telangiectasia after 74 days and xerosis was present on day 91 as measured by the Schirmer test, using a paper strip for measuring tear production. None of the subjects showed abnormality of permeability of retinal vessels or retinal blood flow by fluorescein angiography.

It has been claimed that there is a correlation between the level of vitamin C in the blood and the size of the visual field for green (Biernacka-Biesiekierska and Szczygowa, 1954). They found a contraction of the field in vitamin C deficiency and improvement with treatment. There is supposed to be a seasonal variation, with the field for green larger in autumn than spring, and this might be explained by the availability of fresh vegetables and fruits.

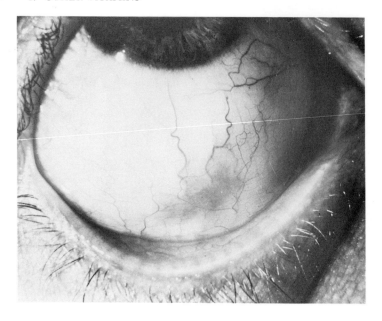

FIG. 64. Bulbar subconjunctival haemorrhage. From Hood and Hodges (1969).

Stewart (1941) reported an improvement in dark adaptation from 150 mg of vitamin C daily in subjects who had not previously shown any response to vitamin A alone. Good evidence that vitamin C plays any part in retinal function is, however, lacking.

B. Vitamin D

There is little evidence that the eye is seriously involved in rickets, at least as a direct result of deficiency of vitamin D. The association of zonular cataract with tetany and not with rickets has been appreciated for a long time and this matter is considered therefore under calcium (Chapter 5, Section IIA).

Proptosis has been recorded in rickets resulting from skull deformity in which the orbit is affected (Cohen, 1906) and this may be associated with haematomata and palpebral oedema (Rainess, 1930). It is not clear whether these latter features are distinct from the haemorrhages of scurvy. If they are rachitic the mechanism is quite obscure.

Osteomalacia is the adult equivalent of low calcium rickets modified by the absence of growth. It has been especially associated with pregnancy and famine. In its florid form it is a rare disease today in Europe and North

America, although it is possible that mild degrees may account for some instances of difficult labour with slight contraction of the pelvis occurring after several normal pregnancies. Osteomalacia still constitutes a problem in some parts of Asia.

The first account of cataract in osteomalacia is that of Meinert (1887). From northern China, Pi (1934) described four cases of subcapsular cataract complicating osteomalacia and Maxwell and Pi (1940) gave an account of a total of 13 cases. In the early stages the slit lamp is necessary for diagnosis and by this means the appearances are seen to resemble those in the cataractous lenses of postoperative tetany. It is said that treatment with vitamin D and calcium results in some improvement.

The conjunctival and corneal changes produced by an excessive intake of vitamin D are considered in Chapter 5 Section IIA*b*, for the underlying condition is hypercalcaemia, as it is in a variety of other diseases that have the same defects as part of their symptomatology.

C. Vitamin E

Before the role of oxygen was demonstrated it was thought that retrolental fibroplasia might be due to vitamin E lack. Owens and Owens (1949) claimed some improvement with tocopherol, but this was before its aetiology was understood. More recently Johnson *et al.* (1974) claimed it had a protective effect, but there is clearly need for much further study.

D. Vitamin K

Interest in the ocular complications of deficiency of vitamin K has centred around haemorrhage into the retina in the newborn. This phenomenon seems to have been reported for the first time 100 years ago by Jaeger (1861). There have been many confirmatory reports since then, most of them emphasizing the importance of the lesion but disagreeing as to its causation. In six series of cases, including that of his own in 100 newborn infants, Giles (1960) found an incidence varying from 2.6 to 59%. This worker suggested that these differences might be explained by the time after birth when the infants were examined. Those in his series were all examined within 1 hour of birth when the incidence was found to be 40%. This fell in subsequent examinations to 36% at 24 hours, 25% at 48 hours, and 20% at 72 hours. Giles studied the effect of various maternal and parturitional factors such as parity, weight of the infant, duration of labour, anaesthetic, and degree of cyanosis and felt these could not be definitely implicated. Rapid release of the increased intracranial pressure resulting from poor delivery of the head did play a significant part, in his opinion. Giles (1960) and Falls and Jurrow (1946) discounted any effect of vitamin K administered to the mother prenatally in lowering the incidence of haemorrhage into the retina in the newborn infant.

Several workers, however, have provided evidence that vitamin K therapy given to the mother some days before labour will lower the incidence of retinal haemorrhage. Thus Maumenee *et al*. (1941) found that prothrombin levels were lower in those infants who developed haemorrhage than in those who did not. By giving expectant mothers 2 mg menaphthone daily for 4 days before labour they were able to reduce the incidence of retinal haemorrhage in their series from 25% in controls to 4% in the treated. Pray *et al*. (1941) confirmed this and obtained their best results with 10 or 20 mg menaphthone before labour. Wille (1944) emphasized the importance of giving vitamin K before delivery and considered that it was necessary to do so every day for several months prenatally.

As in scurvy, so in those diseases of which vitamin K deficiency is a feature, the possibility of retinal haemorrhage should be guarded against.

Chapter 5

Essential Elements

Extensive analyses of the various tissues of the eye have been carried out many times and the main results of these have been summarized by Bellows (1944) and by Pirie and van Heyningen (1956). It will be quite unnecessary to repeat these here. A consideration of only those elements, an imbalance of which appears to have an effect on the eye, will be included here together with a few remarks about the physiological significance of the element where that seems appropriate.

I. Animal Studies

A. Calcium and Phosphorus

An increase in calcium content of tissues of the body is one of the most constant features of the process of ageing. It is also one of the most consistent findings in the lens in cataract formation. The significance of this rise in the calcium content of cataractous and ageing lenses is still disputed. Bellows (1944) in his discussion of the evidence came to the conclusion that in all probability calcium infiltration of the cataractous lens is secondary to degenerative processes comparable to aged or injured tissues elsewhere in the body. With Rosner he demonstrated the truth of this in experimental galactose cataract when it was found that the calcium concentration in the lens rose only after opacification had already commenced.

Phosphorus is present in the body in many forms: in carbohydrates, fats, proteins, and various inorganic salts, It is also essential in enzymatic processes. The calcium: phosphorus ratio is of importance in the maintenance of the transparency of the lens (see below).

Reference has already been made (Chapter 4, Section IB) to the association between zonular cataract and rickets and tetany. Long before critical animal experiments were carried out clinical evidence had been accumulating that the true association was between tetany, and not rickets per se, and these cataracts in young children. The clinical aspect of the story was discussed in Chapter 4, Section IIB, where it was seen that identical lens changes also result quite apart from any dietary deficiency or rickets in association with spontaneous or post-operative hypoparathyroidism.

Early attempts to produce cataract by feeding animals rachitogenic diets were inconclusive (Chapter 4, Section IB). Numerous workers had been successful in demonstrating lens changes similar to those occurring clinically by removing the parathyroid glands in animals including dogs, rats, and rabbits, and thus producing tetany. The first account was that of Erdheim (1906) in rats, with many confirmatory reports subsequently (Duke-Elder, 1940). One of the most thorough studies was that of Goldmann (1929), in which parathyroidectomized dogs were kept alive for 12 months. During this time he induced periods of tetany by withholding calcium in the diet. In this way he was able to produce subcapsular opacities during the periods of hypocalcaemia. In the intervening tetany-free periods new clear fibres were laid down in the lens, and by repeating this several times Goldmann was able to observe alternating layers of opaque and clear lens fibres in the cortex. He concluded that the cataractous changes resulted from an acute poisoning of lens fibres and not from a chronic state of hypocalcaemia.

Thus it seemed clear that cataract was frequently associated with tetany, but the role of rickets was not elucidated until the experiments of von Bahr (1936). The proportion of calcium to phosphorus in a diet designed to produce rickets had traditionally been 4:1. Like all other previous investigators von Bahr observed no cataracts in rats fed such a diet over long periods. However, when rats previously fed the rachitogenic diet were suddenly fed a normal stock diet, in which the calcium:phosphorus ratio was 1:1, lenticular opacities appeared. Of 109 rachitic rats 49 showed cataract and all but 1 of these had received the tetanogenic diet (Ca:P = 1:1). There were marked differences with regard to blood chemistry and neuromuscular sensitivity between the rachitic and tetanic animals. The former had little change in galvanic sensitivity and a normal blood calcium was accompanied by a fall in phosphorus, while the latter were hypersensitive and hypocalcaemic. Von Bahr further showed that there was a close relationship between the current necessary to provoke muscular response and the appearance of cataract. Only one rat with a normal sensitivity (1.2 milliamperes or over) developed cataract, 19 out of 35 rats reacting at 0.3–0.6 mA showed opacities, and all animals that reacted at less than 0.3 mA had cataract. Histologically the lens change was identical with that described in experimental parathyreoprival tetany, the opacity appearing first in the superficial cortex and forming a typical zonular cataract as fresh lens fibres were formed (see Fig. 65).

Further evidence for the primary importance of tetany and incidental role of rickets in the aetiology of this type of cataract was supplied by Bietti (1940) in experiments with the rat in which he demonstrated the appearance of cataract in uncomplicated tetany of dietary origin but not in uncomplicated rickets. Each of 49 rabbits fed from weaning a diet low in calcium (Swan and Salit, 1941) but with adequate vitamin D developed cataract.

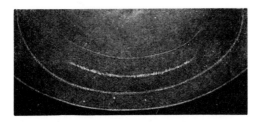

FIG. 65. Cataract associated with tetany in the rat. From Goldman (1929).

Clefts, vacuoles, and punctate opacities appeared in the equatorial region within 9 to 12 days, preceding the onset of tetany by about 4 to 7 days. They progressed subcapsularly from the equator toward the anterior and posterior suture lines. A striking finding was that there was no difference between the calcium content of the lenses of these hypocalcaemic rabbits and those of a group on a normal diet, although the mean serum calcium level was 4.2 and 10.8 mg/100 ml respectively.

Many theories have been advanced to explain the cause of this type of cataract, some rather fanciful, as those dependent upon mechanical influences associated with the convulsions of tetany. Others which attracted more credence have mostly been concerned with changes in the composition of the aqueous humour or in capsular permeability. Von Bahr (1940) was able to show a lowering of the calcium content of the aqueous humour in rats which developed tetanic cataract. He also produced opacities in the isolated rabbit lens incubated in a fluid low in calcium content when a haemolysate of blood was added to the medium, while control lenses remained clear. It was his contention that the lowered calcium content of the aqueous humour caused an increase in the permeability of the lens capsule and that this allowed the penetration of an unknown colloidal agent toxic to lens fibres. He postulated that this compound is normally present in red blood cells in high concentration and that traces could diffuse into the plasma and so into the aqueous. It would be prevented from entering the lens under normal conditions by the calcium content of the aqueous humour but when this fell then the barrier would be removed. It is well known that calcium plays an important role in cellular ionic balance but the precise mechanism of hypocalcaemic cataract is still unknown.

In an early paper it was claimed by Yudkin (1924) that the absence of both phosphorus and vitamin A from a diet led to a more rapid onset of keratomalacia in rats than when vitamin A alone was withheld. It is possible that this was due to greater oxidation of vitamin A in the phosphorus-deficient diet, as resulted from the substitution of ferrous for ferric sulphate in other experiments (see Chapter 2, Section IB).

B. Sodium, Potassium and Magnesium

The sodium and potassium contents of the aqueous humour are similar to those of plasma (about 300 mg and 20 mg/100 ml water, respectively). If the sodium content of a tissue is a measure of extracellular water, and potassium of intracellular water then the very low sodium content (46 mg/100 ml) and high potassium content (404 mg/100 ml) in the lens would indicate that most of the lenticular water is intrafibrillar. Potassium is in high concentration in the retina where it is of special importance, as it is in all nervous tissue, as changes in concentration take place on the passage of nervous impulses.

Diets deficient in these two elements are extremely difficult to devise as they are so universal in their distribution. Consequently a natural deficiency state can hardly ever arise. A diet containing only 0.002% of sodium was devised by Orent-Keiles et al. (1937). After 6 or 8 weeks on this diet rats began to show eye changes which consisted of "sanguinolent secretion", presumably porphyrin in nature, together with corneal ulceration, perforation, hypopyon, and keratinization. The histological changes were later described (Follis et al., 1942) as consisting of dilatation of the ducts of the tarsal and Meibomian glands, but with no changes in the lacrimal glands, and in the Harderian gland only just before the end of the experiment. The cornea showed vascularization, infiltration of the stroma with leucocytes, and keratinization of the epithelium. This work is of considerable interest in showing the severe degree of damage that can result in the anterior segment of the eye from a marked deficiency of sodium and suggests that it is possible that minor degrees of sodium lack, likely to be present in various states of inanition, might play a secondary role in the production of ocular lesions. In dogs fed diets deficient in sodium for a period of 8 weeks no eye lesions were observed by Turpeinen (1938).

Knopik and Stankiewicz (1972) and Stankiewicz et al. (1972) claimed to produce cortical cataract in all 50 rabbits fed a diet deficient in potassium and magnesium. K^+, Mg^{2+}, ATP and lactic acid concentrations fell, while Na^+ and Ca^{2+} accumulated. Knopik et al. (1973) also claimed to produce cataracts in rabbits with either deficiency separately.

C. Zinc

This element and copper occur in the highest concentrations in pigmented tissues and in the pigment fractions of these tissues in the eye. Up to about 100 times the concentration of both are found in the corresponding tissues of fresh water fishes as compared with mammals (Bowness et al., 1952).

Among mammals, Weitzel et al. (1954) showed a marked correlation between the structure of choroid, tapetum, and retina and zinc concentrations. Those with low zinc levels in the choroid were herbivores and had a fibrous tapetum, while those with high zinc concentrations were carnivores and had a cellular tapetum where zinc deposits were especially rich. Intravenous doses of the metal-chelating agent diphenylthiocarbazone (dithizone) caused gross loss of zinc from the tapetum with secondary retinal detachment and permanent blindness (Budinger, 1961).

Follis et al. (1941) described corneal vascularization, without keratinization, in two out of seven rats which were fed a daily diet supplying only 2 to 4 μg of zinc per day. In a study of the effects of zinc deficiency in suckling mice deprived of colostrum Nishimura (1953) reported changes in the eyelids in addition to pronounced skin lesions. In the palpebral conjunctiva the epithelial layer became squamous and occasionally the stratified cuboidal or columnar epithelium was transformed into a stratified squamous epithelium. Despite the poorer body growth as compared with controls the zinc-deficient pups showed a tendency for the eruption of the lower incisors and the separation of the eyelids to be accelerated. The mean difference for lid separation between the two groups was quite considerable, of the order of about 48 hours, with the eyes of the controls opening usually on the 16th day and those of the experimental group on the 14th day. Mention of retardation of lid separation is made in Chapter 1, Section IA2 and Chapter 9, Section IL.

Hubbard et al. (1969) used topical or oral zinc in a study of corned wound healing in normal rabbits. There was no increase in the mean tensile strength of the wounds in animals so treated compared with controls.

D. Chromium

This trace element has been shown to be an essential nutrient for some species. In 10 out of 60 rats fed a diet containing less than 100 parts per billion chromium, corneal opacities and congestion of iridal vessels developed (Roginski and Mertz, 1967). Two parts per million chromium in the drinking water prevented, but did not fully reverse, these changes (Fig. 66). In 13 out of 15 squirrel monkeys maintained for more than 6 weeks on a

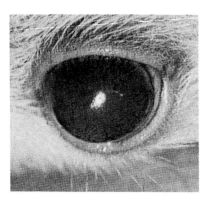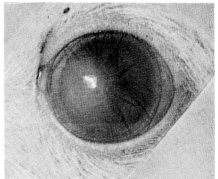

FIG. 66. Photographs showing both eyes of a rat *in vivo*, with congestion of the iridal vessels in both eyes, and corneal opacity in eye to the right. The small bright spots are reflections of the light used and are not related to the lesion. From Roginski and Mertz (1967).

low chromium diet, mid-stromal corneal opacities developed with neovascularization, maximal at 9–10 weeks (Martin *et al.* 1972).

E. Selenium

In rats fed a selenium-deficient diet with supplements of vitamin E, hypoplasia of the dermis and of the spermatic tubules, producing sterility, and cataract occurred (Sprinkler *et al.,* 1971). Selenium is an integral part of the enzyme glutathione peroxidase that is thought to destroy peroxides derived from unsaturated fatty acids. Peroxides also accumulate in vitamin E deficiency and the two states are known to have similar effects (see also Chapter 4, Section IC).

Selenium toxicity, selenosis, in farm animals is known as "blind staggers", an acute form, or "alkali disease" in chronic poisoning. The disease appears to be the same as that caused by locoweed (Chapter 10, Section ID) which contains as much as 1.5% selenium.

F. Silicon

This is known to be an essential trace element for the rat. Deficiency has been shown to result in abnormal bone structure, including distortion of the orbits (Schwarz and Milne, 1972).

II. Human Studies

A. Calcium and Phosphorus

a. Hypocalcaemia

Calcium deficiency, as evidenced by a lowering of blood calcium level (normal about 2.5 mmol/l), resulting in tetany in marked deficiency, occurs in nutritional rickets and osteomalacia due to vitamin D deficiency and in a variety of conditions in which there is defective production of one of the active metabolites of vitamin D, $25(OH)D_3$ or $1,25(OH)_2D_3$. It is also a feature of states in which there is lack of parathyroid hormone. It is unlikely that hypocalcaemia ever results from dietary deficiency of calcium alone, as under these circumstances marked increase in the efficiency of intestinal absorption occurs.

It is especially cataract of the zonular or lamellar type that has been found associated in many instances with tetany. This is an opacity lying between the centre and the periphery of the lens and covering the nucleus more or less completely. Some of these cataracts appear to arise as the result of an hereditary disposition and others may follow local eye disease or trauma, but many appear in the early years of life in relation to infantile tetany and others later on as a result of parathyroid deficiency. It is the infantile form associated with tetany and in a more indirect manner with the frequently accompanying rickets that gives justification for a consideration of this condition here.

Bellows (1944) has thoroughly reviewed the early literature on this subject and has summarized the evidence for the view, never challenged since that time, that the primary association is with tetany. From the data collected by von Bahr (1936) of many hundreds of cases with zonular cataract it is evident that the symptoms of both tetany and enamel hypoplasia occur more frequently than do those of rickets. The site of the enamel defect shows that the cause must have acted during the second 6-month period of life, and this corresponds to the period when infantile tetany is most common. Further support is gained from the observation that cataract is more frequently associated with mild or healing rickets than it is with the florid type. A possible explanation of this is to be found in the fact that the severe stage of rickets is characterized by a very low phosphorus blood level but the calcium content may be normal. It is only when the disease is in regression and the phosphorus retention by the healing skeleton draws upon calcium in the blood that the blood calcium level tends to fall in the absence of a high calcium dietary intake. The conclusive demonstration of this relationship in the experimental animal has been referred to in Section IA.

Although there is no report of other ocular symptoms attributable to the tetanic phase of rickets there is such an account due to parathyroid deficiency. Lyle (1948) described a case developing 4 years after thyroidectomy in which diffuse subcortical lens opacities were accompanied by raised intraocular pressure, papilloedema, gross constriction of the visual fields, and epileptiform convulsions. The general and visual symptoms improved following the administration of calcium lactate and dihydrotachysterol.

Ireland et al. (1968) reported an incidence of nearly 50% of cataract in chronic hypoparathyroidism after surgery.

As the treatment of renal failure has improved in recent years there have been numerous reports of eye changes. Berlyne (1968) noted microcrystalline deposition of calcium phosphate in the conjunctiva in both acute and chronic renal failure. These deposits occurred most commonly in the epithelial and subepithelial layers in the interpalpebral fissure, especially in the limbal area, and appeared to be unaffected by treatment. Harris et al. (1971) reported conjunctival and corneal deposits of calcium in 14 of 18 severely uraemic patients. All these patients had elevated serum phosphorus with normal or low serum calcium. Long-term haemodialysis had no effect on the deposits. Berlyne et al. (1972) described punctate stippling of the lens in half their patients in terminal renal failure or on dialysis and postulated persistent and severe hypocalcaemia as the cause. Similar conjunctival and corneal deposits have been reported by Ehlers et al. (1972), Demco et al. (1974) and Hanselmayer et al. (1974). These changes are very similar to those reported in hypercalcaemia (see below) and their precise relationship to calcium status is not at present clear.

A characteristic uraemic retinopathy following long-term dialysis was reported in 40 patients by Kobayashi and Mimuran (1974).

b. Hypercalcaemia

Vitamin D poisoning has, in common with a number of other disease states, a high blood calcium level, and it is this that is responsible for the damage to the eye. These other conditions include hyperparathyroidism, sarcoidosis, severe renal damage, and so-called "milk-alkali disease" resulting from an excessive intake of milk and alkali as part of the dietary treatment of peptic ulcer or some other digestive disorder. The first case reported (Meesmann, 1938) was due to vitamin D intoxication.

The ocular features consist of deposits in the conjunctiva of small glass-like, crystal-clear particles in the region of the palpebral fissure and a band keratopathy in the cornea. This latter is a superficial opacity in the palpebral area of the cornea starting peripherally, where it is separated by a clear zone from the limbus, as is seen in arcus senilis and fades off axially after about 3 mm, not extending far enough to interfere with vision (Cogan *et al.*, 1948). Calcified scleral nodules have also been demonstrated in two elderly patients with hypervitaminosis D (Gartner and Rubner, 1955). Many patients also have nephrocalcinosis and nephrolithiasis and it is considered that the process producing these changes in the kidneys is similar to that in the cornea.

In the 1950s a number of reports from parts of Europe, including Britain, described a syndrome or group of related syndromes in which hypercalcaemia in infancy had been the constant feature. There had usually been a history of a high calcium intake associated with a more than adequate amount of vitamin D. In the original report of Fanconi *et al.* (1952) both children affected had convergent strabismus. Some authors have made special mention of the corneae and conjunctivae showing no change in these infants and it would seem that hypercalcaemia results in calcium deposits in the eye only after a prolonged period, as was the case in most of the adults referred to above. In 12 patients with the benign form of idiopathic hypercalcaemia, six in infants and six in children aged from 4 to 8 years, Gerard-Lefebvre (1959) noted a peculiar slaty colour of the sclera with a yellow-grey appearance of the skin.

Lemp and Ralph (1977) reported the rapid development of band keratopathy in the dry eyes of three patients with lacrimal insufficiency. Hypercalcaemia was present and the deposits were of phosphate and carbonate salts of calcium in a non-crystalline form.

In marble bone disease (osteopetrosis) blindness results in some cases; two out of nine cases reported by Yu *et al.* (1971) were from optic atrophy caused by compression in small optic foramina. A low calcium diet from infancy has proved beneficial.

c. Hypophosphataemia

The syndrome of phosphate depletion is becoming more widely recognized as long-term therapy is being carried out. Phosphorus-low solutions may be infused as in parenteral nutrition and haemodialysis, accentuated in the latter by ingestion of large amounts of phosphorus-binding antacids.

Eye lesions do not appear to have been reported under these circumstances but should be looked for in view of the reported findings in familial hypophosphataemic (vitamin D resistant) rickets. These have included band keratopathy, conjunctival calcification, orbital malformations, blue sclerae, cataracts, proptosis and papilloedema (Lessell and Norton, 1964; Brenner *et al.*, 1969).

B. Iron

a. Iron Deficiency

Anaemia from any cause usually results in ocular manifestations only if of severe degree with haemoglobin less than 6 or 7 g%, and their incidence increases in proportion to the severity of the anaemia. The conjunctiva is pale, especially in the cul-de-sacs, which are normally mildly hyperaemic and pink in colour. The red reflex of the fundus, dependent on the choroidal vascular bed, is paler than normal. Retinal oedema and dilatation of retinal vessels occur, the former condition probably related to ischaemia and the latter to reduced intraocular tension.

Retinal haemorrhages tend to be from the arteriolar capillaries, and as they are usually confined to the nerve fibre layer they tend to be flame-shaped and rarely involve the avascular macula and cause no visual loss. Extraretinal haemorrhages into the vitreous, choroid, conjunctival space or lids are rare. Retinal exudates may be acute or chronic. The former are greyish-white "cotton wool" patches, probably representing ischaemic infarcts, usually occurring in the posterior pole and they disappear without visual damage. Chronic exudates or oedema residues of solid yellowish-white appearance are either scattered throughout the fundus or localized to the macula. Absence of arteriolar vasospasm helps to differentiate the latter from the "macular star" associated with severe hypertensive retinopathy. Resorption occurs slowly but often completely without visual impairment. Retinal detachment is very rare, but reattachment usually accompanies treatment of the anaemia (Kolker, 1966).

Chronic hypochromic microcytic anaemia responding to iron therapy is a well-documented cause of papilloedema (Lubeck, 1959; Beutler *et al.*, 1963). About 20 cases have been reported, most of them near the beginning of this century, mainly girls with retinal haemorrhages and exudates. A rise in cerebrospinal fluid pressure of obscure cause was sometimes demonstrated.

Eye lesions in association with nutritional megaloblastic anaemias were discussed in Chapter 3, Section IIB7, and as was mentioned then some workers have reported retinal haemorrhages to be much more common in these anaemias than in iron deficiency anaemia.

b. Iron Overload

This is characterized by excessive focal or generalized deposition of iron within tissues (haemosiderosis). When this is associated with tissue injury it is termed haemochromatosis. Primary or ideopathic haemochromatosis is a genetically determined error with increased absorption of iron from a normal diet. Secondary haemosiderosis or haemochromatosis results from prolonged exposure to abnormally high amounts of iron, as in repeated transfusions, in the diet, alcoholic beverages or oral therapy.

In primary haemochromatosis there is bronze pigmentation of the skin, cirrhosis, diabetes mellitus and cardiomyopathy. Roth and Foos (1972),

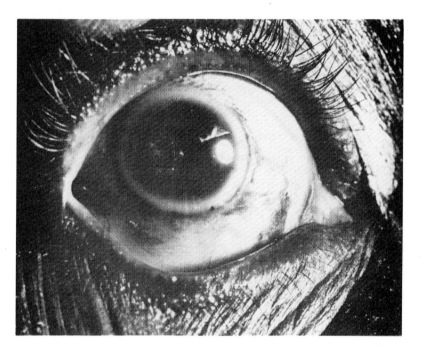

FIG. 67. Pseudo arcus senilis in haemochromatosis. From Gillman (1957).

examining the eye, detected iron deposition only in the ciliary epithelium and the sclera in contrast to local haemosiderosis bulbi in which all ocular tissues other than the sclera were affected. On the other hand, Davies *et al*. (1972) in 13 out of 44 cases of primary haemochromatosis found melanin deposition in the conjunctiva or lid margin and, at autopsy in three cases, iron within the corneal epithelium and in the ciliary body.

Diabetic retinopathy in primary haemochromatosis is rare, but one case has been reported (Galton, 1965).

Gillman (1957) described a golden-brown limbic ring, superficially resembling arcus senilis or the Kayser-Fleischer ring, in South African Bantu consuming large amounts of iron-rich beer and eating food cooked in iron pots. Incomplete arcus senilis-like changes due to local corneal disease have to be distinguished (Fig. 67 and Fig. 68).

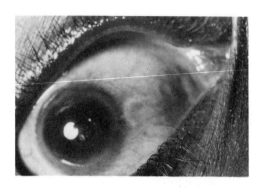

FIG. 68 Incomplete arcus from repeated paralimbal infection.

Wamoto and DeVoe (1976) studied under the electron microscope the brown pigmentary line around the base of the cone in keratoconus. It contained ferritin particles.

C. Zinc

Zinc is found in high concentrations in some parts of the eye in certain animals (Section IC). Zinc deficiency, resulting in growth retardation and hypogonadism, has been reported from the Middle East. Chelation of dietary zinc by soil eating and a high phytate or fibre diet are thought to be largely responsible. Zinc deficiency has also been associated with poor growth and loss of appetite in young children in the United States and Germany. Eye lesions have not been described.

In some patients with chronic impairment of liver function Vallee et al. (1959) found a defect in dark adaptation which did not respond to vitamin A therapy. Zinc concentrations in serum and liver were low and urinary excretion was high.

Further evidence for zinc dependency of dark adaptation was provided recently by Morrison et al. (1978). Six stable alcoholic cirrhotic patients were found to have low serum zinc and borderline levels of vitamin A in serum. Dark adaptation was impaired in all. In three patients zinc sulphate 220 mg/day for 1–2 weeks restored the final rod threshold to normal with no change in serum vitamin A. Two patients showed no response to vitamin A alone. One patient improved with both zinc and vitamin A.

Impaired retinal function has been reported in chronic pancreatitis and usually attributed to malabsorption of vitamin A (Chapter 2, Section IIIB). In patients without steatorrhoea Toskes *et al.* (1977) found there was no correlation between serum vitamin A levels and abnormalities in dark adaptation and ERG. Zinc levels were, however, significantly reduced in all patients with chronic pancreatitis, and in two patients with impaired retinal function but with normal fat absorption and normal serum vitamin A levels

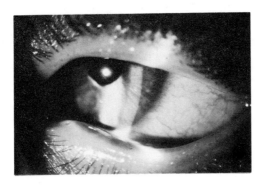

FIG. 69. Radiating linear superficial corneal opacities seen in patient with acrodermatitis enteropathica. From Warshawsky *et al.* (1975).

there was marked depression of zinc levels. The results of zinc therapy will be awaited with great interest.

Alcohol dehydrogenase is a zinc-dependent enzyme and in the visual cycle in the retina is responsible for converting retinol to retinal, and in the presence of TPNH and DPNH converts retinal to retinol.

Acrodermatitis enteropathica is an inherited, previously fatal, disorder recently shown to result from malabsorption of zinc. It is characterized by psoriasis-like dermatitis, hair loss, paronychia, growth retardation and diarrhoea. Zinc sulphate 30–150 mg daily results in complete remission. Eye involvement was first reported by Wirsching (1962). It consists of linear subepithelial corneal opacities (Matta *et al.*, 1975; Warshawsky *et al.*, 1975) (Fig. 69).

D. Copper

a. Copper Deficiency

Menkes' kinky hair syndrome is a sex-linked recessive disorder due to a defect in copper absorption. It presents with mental retardation, failure to thrive, depigmented steely hair, arterial lesions and scurvy-like bone changes. Copper given intravenously early in infancy (200 µg/kg daily) has alleviated the condition.

Microcysts of the iris pigment and progressive degeneration of retinal ganglion cells have been described (Wray et al., 1976) (Fig. 70). A

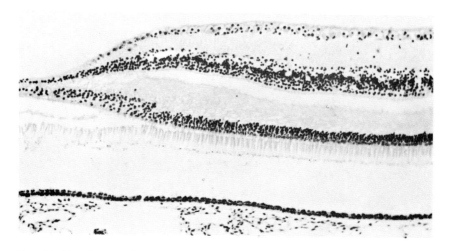

FIG. 70. Foveal zone of the retina. The number of ganglion cells has been decreased profoundly. Other layers of the retina appear to be normal. From Wray et al. (1976).

two-month-old baby was unable to fix and follow a light, and pupillary response was sluggish. Fundus vessels were tortuous and there was progressively decrease in the ERG amplitude and visually evoked response over three months, corresponding to a fall in serum copper, and there was no improvement after IV copper (Levy et al., 1974).

b. Copper Overload

Wilson's disease, hepatolenticular degeneration, is an autosomal recessive disorder of copper metabolism. There is a deficiency of the copper-binding plasma protein, caeruloplasmin, resulting in copper deposition in various tissues. This results in progressive neurological deterioration with extrapyramidal signs, cirrhosis and a renal tubular defect with aminoaciduria. Considerable improvement results with systemic penicillinamine which chelates copper and leads to its excretion.

The ocular lesions are pathognomonic. Deposition of copper in Descemet's membrane in the peripheral cornea produces a complete or incomplete brown to green ring near the limbus known as the Kayser-Fleischer ring (Fig. 71).

The deposition is most marked superiorly and inferiorly and is best observed in the early stages with the gonioprism (François, 1972). The ring was not observed in presymptomatic cases studied by Levi *et al*. (1967). Non-invasive quantitation of corneal copper by X-ray excitation spectrometry has been developed (Belkin *et al*., 1976).

Sunflower cataract, chalcosis lentis, is produced by radiating brownish spokes of copper carbonate on the anterior or posterior lens capsule. (Figs. 72–74.) It is not always a late development. Ocular motility is not affected,

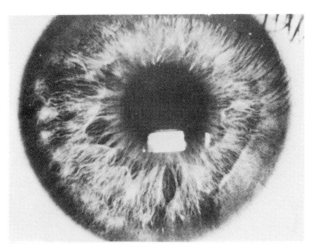

FIG. 71. Peripheral pigmented corneal Kayser-Fleischer ring is the hallmark of Wilson's disease. From Sugar and Podos (1975). *In* "The Eye and Systemic Disease (ed. F. A. Mausolf), Mosby, St Louis.

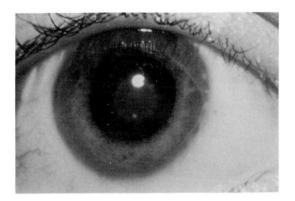

FIG. 72. 1963: Copper deposits in lens before treatment with penicillamine. From Cairns, Parry Williams and Walshe (1969). *Br. med. J.* iii, 95–96.

suggesting that the cortical fibres bypass the basal ganglia and extrapyramidal system (Goldberg and von Noorden, 1966).

Deposition of copper in the central cornea just anterior to the corneal endothelium and deep to the lens capsule has been reported in a case of multiple myeloma (Ellis, 1969).

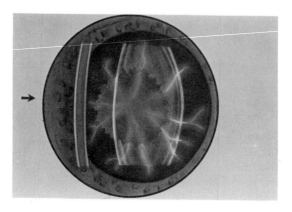

FIG. 73. 1966: Copper deposits in lens. Painting (Mr T. R. Tarrant) of anterior and posterior lens surfaces and optical section of lens (arrowed). From Cairns, Parry Williams and Walshe (1969). *Br. med. J.* iii, 95–96.

Very low plasma caeruloplasmin and increased urinary excretion of copper was reported in retinitis pigmentosa (Gahlot *et al.,* 1976), but this was not confirmed by Ehlers and Bülow (1977) in retinitis pigmentosa or in other tapeto-retinal degenerations.

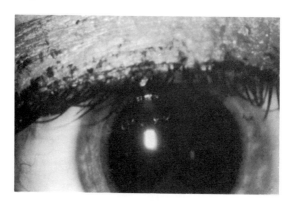

FIG. 74. December 1968: Lens, photographed as in Fig. 72, showing total clearing of copper deposits after treatment with penicillamine. From Cairns, Parry Williams and Walshe (1969). *Br. med. J.* iii, 95–96.

Although Kayser–Fleischer rings are generally regarded as being pathognomonic of Wilson's disease, as stated above, this has been challenged in a recent report (Frommer *et al.*, 1977) of identical rings in three patients with other liver diseases in which serum copper and caeruloplasmin were normal.

Chapter 6

Proteins and Amino Acids

Proteins are normal constituents of all animal cells and body fluids with the exception of urine and bile. They are essential components of both the protoplasm and nucleus of the cell. Many of the enzymes, hormones, and substances associated with immunological and antigenic reactions are known to be proteins. The molecular weights of proteins are of the order of tens or scores of thousands and even more but these large molecules or aggregates of molecules may be broken down by hydrolysis through various stages finally to a considerable number of amino acids. These amino acids are characterized chemically by the presence of a carboxyl (COOH) group with acidic properties and an amino (NH_2) group with basic properties, the two groups being attached to the same carbon atom. Amino acids are joined to each other in the protein molecule by what is known as a peptide linkage. In this the amino group of one acid is linked to the carboxyl group of the adjacent acid with the loss of a molecule of water. The arrangement of the amino acids on a peptide chain may vary and this results in isomers, all made up of the same units and having the same percentage composition but differing from each other in the spatial arrangement of these units. More than 20 amino acids are known to be of general occurrence in the protein molecule and the possible number of isomeric proteins is consequently very large indeed.

The amino acids are not all of equal importance in nutrition. Certain of them, designated as essential, cannot be synthesized by the animal body and have to be supplied in adequate amounts in the diet or nutritional failure results. There are 10 such amino acids for the albino rat, and among these arginine occupies a unique place in that it is required for optimal growth although some growth takes place in its absence. The amino acid requirements of different species vary somewhat. There are eight essential amino acids for man, both histidine and arginine not being necessary for the maintenance of nitrogen equilibrium in the adult.

Animals fed on diets devoid of all amino acids suffer generalized loss of body protein with consequent weight loss, anaemia, hypoproteinaemia, and muscular wasting. The susceptibility of the organism to infection is increased and the body is less capable of dealing with trauma and disease. One of the most striking effects of feeding a diet deficient in only one of the essential amino acids is rapid loss of appetite, the dietary intake falling within one day. The mechanism of this anorexia is not fully known. It is doubtful if there is any effect on taste, and tube-feeding in experimental animals of an incomplete amino acid mixture does not lead to an improvement of appetite, weight gain, or maintenance of nitrogen balance. It is most likely that the anorexia is related to some profound systemic effect.

Deficiency of certain essential amino acids results in rather specific and characteristic syndromes. Outstanding examples are afforded by tryptophan—a deficiency of which leads to corneal vascularization (Section C, below), lens cataracts (Section D, below) alopecia, anaemia, and dental disease, and in the chicken to an increased requirement for nicotinic acid—and by methionine, a deficiency of which, with that of several other methyl group donors, causes hepatic and renal damage, as well as corneal vascularization (Section C, below) and possibly lens opacities (Section D, below). However it is not surprising that many experimentally induced single amino acid deficiency states lack specific features because deficiency of any single essential amino acid has an effect on protein synthesis in general. Under other than experimental conditions in both man and animals amino acid requirements are invariably met by proteins and the development of single amino acid deficiencies is extremely unlikely. No attempt has been made to deal separately with the effects of deficiency of protein and of specific amino acids in this chapter but these will be considered together in the appropriate section.

I. Animal Studies

A. Growth of the Eye

Following upon his earlier researches into the effects of total inanition in the rat (Chapter 1, Section II) Jackson turned his attention in some of his last work to protein deficiency (Limson and Jackson, 1932; Jackson, 1936). Weanling rats were fed a basal diet consisting of 75% sucrose, 20% lard, and 4.5% salt mixture. An accessory diet of a mixture of brewer's yeast and dried wheat germ in equal parts was fed in amounts varying from 0.3 to

0.5 g daily. Vitamins A and D were also given. In the 11th week of the experiment 0.3 g of purified casein was given daily. The control rats were killed at weaning and the changes in weight of various organs were compared with the values for the controls after the experimental group had been on the protein-deficient diet for 17 weeks. During this period the mean body weight had increased from 40.75 g to 42.42 g only a 4.9% increase. The change in weight of the eyeballs over this same period was however +53.8% (0.2085 ±0.0044 as compared with 0.1355 ±0.0020), a further demonstration of the resistance of the eye to the adverse effects on growth of a deficient diet.

However, in a further experiment Jackson (1936) demonstrated that the eye is one of those organs in which catch-up growth is only partial on refeeding after prolonged suppression of growth. At weaning, rats were held nearly constant in weight for 15 weeks and then refed. At one year of age in the females only the eyeballs and skeleton among various organs were significantly less in weight than those of controls. In the males, in addition to the eyeballs and skeleton, body length, tail length, body weight, head and musculature were also significantly less in the refed.

The albino rat was also used by Lafon (1939) in a study of the effect of diets deficient in either lysine or cystine on the growth of various organs including the eye. After varying periods on the diets the rats were killed and the fresh and dry weights of the organs determined and compared with values for body-weight controls. The eyes, kidneys, and testicles showed conspicuous increase in weight on the deficient diets. The percentage dry weight of the eyes was greater in animals on either of the deficient diets than in the corresponding body-weight controls. A similar study was made on the organs of the offspring produced during a maternal deficiency of the same amino acids with comparable results. That there was no difference observed between the effect of the lysine- and the cystine-deficient diets is rather surprising in view of the fact that the latter but not the former can be synthesized by the rat. Cystine is known to exert a sparing effect on the requirement for methionine but is itself not essential.

The effects of protein deficiency on the growth and water content of the eyeball of the albino rat during the first 2 years of life have been studied by the writer (McLaren, 1958a). Three experimental groups of animals were employed, each fed on a different diet low in protein. Diet 1 had the following percentage composition: casein 3; salt mixture 3; yeast 1; maize starch 92. Diet 2 contained: whole wheat flour 80 parts; potato starch 10; haricot bean 5; lucerne meal 2; arachis oil 2; salt mixture 1. In order to obtain satisfactory litters and to rear them consistently it was found necessary to supplement this diet during gestation and lactation with 10% white-fish flour. Diet 3 consisted of brown cassava to which vitamins and minerals were added. In Fig. 75 is shown the very rapid growth of the eye that takes place between birth and weaning, amounting to more than a fivefold increase in weight. Before weaning the eyes of the low protein colony rats fed on diet 2 grew as well as those of the controls (Fig. 75) showing that the supplementation of this diet fed to the mothers during gestation and lactation brought the efficiency of the diet as far as growth of the eye was concerned up to

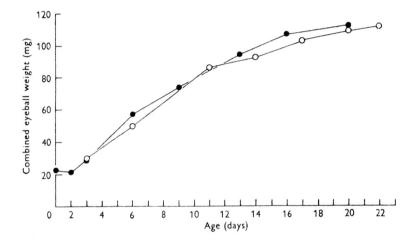

FIG. 75. Growth of the eyeball, before weaning, in rats from a colony fed on a normal diet, ●——● , and from a colony fed on a low-protein diet plus pre-weaning supplement, ○——○ . From McLaren (1958a).

normal. However, Fig. 76 shows that growth of the eyes of animals receiving diet 1, diet 2 without the supplement, and diet 3 was in every case inferior to that of controls. That the level of protein alone cannot account for differences in growth is shown by the almost identical curves for rats on diets 1 and 2 (Fig. 76) although the protein contents of these diets were 4 and 10.8%, respectively. It may be that the nature of the limiting amino acid is of special significance in this respect. In diet 1 it was methionine and in diet 2 lysine. Nevertheless the resistance of the eye to the adverse effects of gross quantitative and qualitative deficiency of protein is particularly well shown by the continued increase in the weight of the eye of rats on diet 3, despite a slow but steady loss of body weight from weaning. The values for these rats are only about 25 % less than those for age-controls. The main constituent of diet 3, cassava, contains only about 1% protein and this is deficient in almost all of the essential amino acids and especially so as far as the sulphur-containing amino acids, methionine and cystine, are concerned.

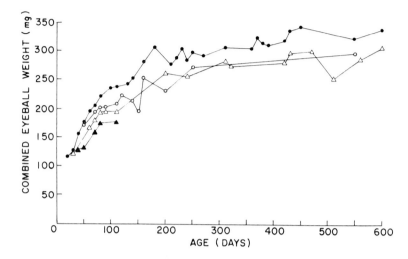

FIG. 76. Growth of the eyeball, after weaning, in rats fed on a normal diet, and on low-protein diets. ●——● , normal diet; △——△ diet 1; ○——○ , diet 2; ▲——▲ , diet 3. From McLaren (1958a).

Changes in the water content of the eye with age in both control and protein-deficient rats are shown in Fig. 77. It will be seen that after a steep fall before weaning there is a steady rise in the dry weight expressed as a percentage of the whole as seen already for the fresh weight of the eyes. Protein deficiency, even of the most severe degree, does not affect this trend

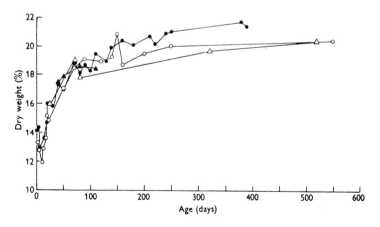

FIG. 77. Dry weight of the eyeball of rats fed on a normal diet and on low-protein diets. ●——● , normal diet; △——△ , diet 1; ○——○ , diet 2; ▲——▲ , diet 3. From McLaren (1958a).

materially. Donaldson and King (1936) suggested that the change in water content of the eye which they also found might be related to the opening of the eyes. The marked stability of the water content of the eye even under conditions of severe inanition shows that the suggestion of Jackson (Chapter 1, Section IA1) that the eye might continue to grow by increase in water content alone is not consistent with the facts.

Unpublished observations on the effect of a low protein diet on the growth of the eye, growth of the lens, and the dry weight of the lens in the rat showed that after about 50 days on the diet the growth of both the total eyeball and the lens had been slightly retarded but that the water content of the lens had not been altered.

Mention may be made here of the changes in the refractive state of the eyes of rabbits which Gardiner and Macdonald (1957) attributed to a low protein diet. Among the factors responsible for a change in overall refracting power of the eye are changes in refractive index of the media, curvature of the cornea and lens, and axial length of the eyeball. The mechanism of the refractive changes observed in the animals fed the deficient diet is quite obscure. Those in the experimental group received a diet containing about 5% protein for 2-, 4-, or 6-week periods, after which they were given the stock diet. Two main conclusions were drawn: first that the most striking refractive errors occurred after the resumption of the normal diet; and secondly that the magnitude of the error was proportional to the length of time the animal was fed the low protein diet. Several criticisms of this work need to be made and it is highly desirable that the claims should be confirmed. The numbers of rabbits used was small to begin with and was further reduced by deaths. Most of the animals contracted coccidiosis, and as one was reported to have died from this disease it is likely that the others were to some extent sick animals. There were quite wide variations in the refraction values and this examination is not of the kind permitting a very precise measurement. In our experience stock rabbits show very considerable variations in their refraction, tending to have quite a marked hyperopia.

In a further study Gardiner and Macdonald (1958) fed young rabbits a green food diet that was diluted with sucrose and found that they were more myopic than other animals receiving the green food diet alone. It is not clear exactly what the nutritional restriction was in the experimental group but protein was presumably a major factor.

Ward (1965) reported that in young protein-deficient rats the progressive tendency from myopia to hypermetropia was retarded, but this was not confirmed by Bardiger et al. (1968).

Buphthalmos has been reported to occur in chickens fed on a diet containing an excess of glycine, an essential amino acid for this species (Groschke et al., 1948). Helmsen et al. (1973) found that there was no abnormality in angle differentiation or aqueous inflow to suggest a rise in intraocular pressure as the cause, in contrast to buphthalmos induced in young chicks by continuous illumination where there is narrowing of the chamber angle and a shallow anterior chamber. The authors reported an abnormality of connective tissue development in glycine-induced buphthalmos.

B. The Ocular Glands and the Lids

The Harderian and lacrimal glands were examined from rats and pigs which had been fed for long periods since weaning on various diets low in protein. In the rat the cornea (Section C, below) and in the pig the lens (Section D, below) also showed characteristic changes (McLaren, 1959a). A total of 73 rats were reared from weaning on the cassava diet. These animals survived only a matter of weeks and in the terminal stages developed chemosis with incrustation of the lids with porphyrin secretion. In the Harderian (Figs 78 and 79) and to a lesser extent in the lacrimal glands there was shrinking down of the cytoplasm of the acinar cells. Pirie (1948) found similar changes in the Harderian gland of the tryptophan-deficient rat, Cole and Scott (1954) noted porphyrin material on the wrists, paws, and nose, and "spectacle eye" was described by Ferraro and Roizin (1947). Rats which received a protein-free diet from weaning also did not survive more than a few weeks and terminally showed chemosis with sticking together of the upper and lower lids but there was no porphyrin incrustation. Even more marked changes were seen in the glands, especially the Harderian (Fig. 80). The whole gland was atrophied with marked shrinking down of the cytoplasm of the acinar cells. There was infiltration with round cells, and in the case of the Harderian gland the acini were filled with granular debris, and actual degeneration of the acinar cells occurred.

The water and nitrogen contents of the Harderian glands of rats fed diets containing about 5% protein did not differ materially from the values for controls, but on the more deficient cassava diet the water content was increased and the nitrogen content of the dry substance of the gland was also raised. The most likely explanation of these findings is that the gland shared in the general increase of body water in these animals, many of which were clinically oedematous, and that the loss of cellular substance, as pictured in Fig. 79, affected cytoplasm more than nucleus and would thus lead to a relative increase in nitrogen.

Pigs that were on a low protein diet for several months did not show any histological changes in the Harderian and lacrimal glands but two animals that survived for more than 1 year on the diet, developing many of the clinical

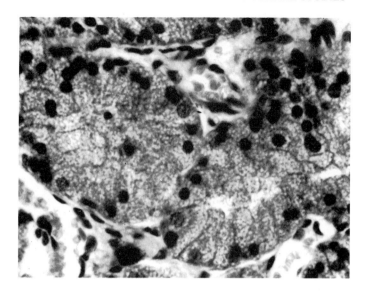

FIG. 78. Normal rat Harderian gland. (Hematoxylin and eosin. ×500.) From McLaren (1959a).

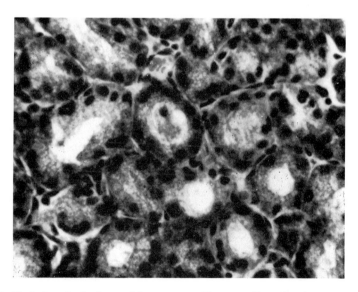

FIG. 79. Harderian gland of a rat fed on cassava. (Haematoxylin and eosin. ×500.) From McLaren (1959a).

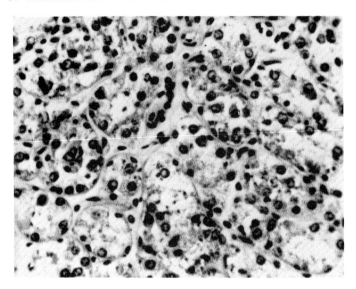

FIG. 80. Harderian gland of a rat fed on a protein-free diet. (Haematoxylin and eosin. ×500.) From McLaren (1959a).

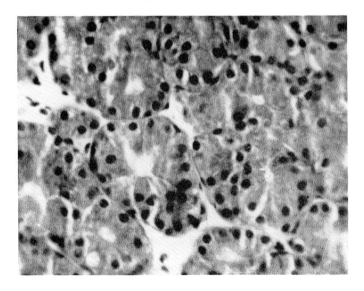

FIG. 81. Harderian gland of control pig. (Haematoxylin and eosin. ×500.) From McLaren (1959a).

signs of human kwashiorkor, had atrophic changes similar to those seen in the rats (Figs. 81 and 82).

The lids of rats are normally closed at birth and there is a distinct zone present between the edges of the lids at this stage filled with material, probably mucopolysaccharide in nature, staining strongly with periodic acid-Schiff reagent. This material also extends for some way along the inner

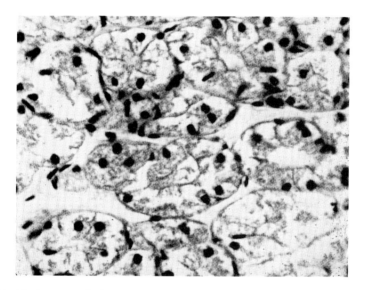

FIG. 82. Harderian gland of protein-deficient pig. (Haematoxylin and eosin. ×500.) From McLaren (1959a).

surface of the lids (Fig. 117a, Chapter 9). Absence of PAS staining in this area was one of the features observed in a litter born to a mother rat suffering from chronic protein deficiency (Chapter 9, Section L). A diet containing only 4% protein fed to mother rats in this laboratory during the last few days of pregnancy resulted in a delay in lid opening of 2 or 3 days compared with controls, until the 17th or 18th day of life.

C. The Conjunctiva and the Cornea

It is in the cornea in particular that the most significant ocular changes in protein and amino acid deficiency have been described. The first account of corneal vascularization due to an amino acid deficiency, in this case of either tryptophan or lysine, was given by Totter and Day (1942) in the rat and this has been repeatedly confirmed for this species. Corneal changes are not mentioned in the reports of Cartwright *et al.* (1945) on the pig and von Sallmann *et al.* (1959) on the guinea pig in tryptophan deficiency, and in these experiments the development of cataract was the main interest.

Subsequently, corneal vascularization has been reported to occur in the rat in deficiency of each of the other essential amino acids, i.e. leucine (Maun *et al.*, 1945a), methionine (Sydenstricker *et al.*, 1946), and valine, histidine, isoleucine, phenylalanine, arginine, and threonine (Sydenstricker *et al.*, 1947).

Experience varied to some extent from group to group. For instance, Maun *et al.* (1945b) found no vascularization at all in phenylalanine deficiency, while Sydenstricker *et al.* (1946) found it in all their phenylalanine-deficient rats and of a greater degree than in deficiency of any other amino acid. The same workers, Maun *et al.* (1946), found no changes in life and only doubtful evidence of corneal vascularization histologically in deficiency of histidine, while Sydenstricker *et al.* (1946) reported it in all their animals, although not of as marked a degree as in some other deficiencies.

The type of vascularization seems to vary to some extent, according to Ferraro *et al.* (1947) being deep in valine deficiency and superficial in tryptophan deficiency. These workers have also described a corneal dystrophy in their rats consisting essentially of epithelial keratinization with xerosis and keratitis.

Accompanying the ingrowth of vessels, Maun *et al.* (1945a) observed thinning of the corneal epithelium with keratinization of the surface. The cells of the basal layer stained more deeply with haematoxylin and showed an increased number of mitoses. The substantia propria appeared to have lost its fibrillar structure and to have become more homogeneous. Around the dilated blood vessels in the adjacent stroma were small collections of granulocytes. Descemet's membrane appeared slightly thickened. The vascularization and epithelial metaplasia were more marked near the limbus. In methionine deficiency (Berg *et al.*, 1947) the vessels were rather small and not very numerous. Histologically the most constant finding was oedema of the epithelium and substantia propria. In the epithelium the oedema was both intra- and intercellular. Karyorrhexis, or swelling of the cells with granular disintegration of the nuclear chromatin, was present, almost always confined to the cells of the outer three layers of the epithelium. Bowman's membrane was rarely affected and when it was it was usually slightly displaced in a wavy fashion. Vascularization was most frequently subepithelial in situation.

Diets deficient in, or devoid of, protein have also produced corneal vascularization in the rat (Sydenstricker *et al.*, 1946). The vascularization was very similar to that described in vitamin A and riboflavin deficiency, but Hall *et al.* (1946) found that in protein deficiency, but not in the other states, the newer portion of the injected capillary near the centre of the cornea appeared larger in diameter than the rest of the capillary. In their study, 23 rats aged 50–62 days old developed vascularization in 9–20 days and three adult rats took respectively 24, 38, and 59 days to show vascularization. These results were confirmed (McLaren, 1959b) in rats fed a protein-free diet from weaning. Using the same diet a small experiment was designed to show whether the initial level of protein affected the time of onset of vascularization. A litter of six rats was divided into three pairs, one male and one female in each. Each pair was weaned when 21 days old on to a different diet, differing only with regard to protein level (4, 11, or 18%) and adequate in all other respects. When 50 days of age all the rats were fed the diet devoid of protein. In each pair one rat developed corneal vascularization and the other died without showing it. Table IX summarizes the results and

TABLE IX. *Onset of Corneal Vascularization and Survival Times of Rats on Vitamin A-Free and Varying Protein Content Diets[a]*

Animal no.	Sex	Initial diet (per cent protein)	Day of onset of vascularization	Day of death if no vascularization
1	M		138	—
		18		
2	F		—	174
3	M		—	127
		11		
4	F		99	—
5	M		—	74
		4		
6	F		65	—

[a] From D. S. McLaren (1959b)

shows that the order of appearance of vascularization and that of death without vascularization both occurred in inverse relation to the protein content of the diet. It would seem then that, during the period when no protein was being consumed, the onset of vascularization was an indication that a certain stage of body protein depletion had been reached, the animals with the larger stores taking longer to reach this state.

It was claimed by Kaunitz *et al.* (1954) from a series of experiments in which many dietary factors were varied that vascularization occurs in rats fed a diet containing 5% protein from casein. However, it would seem that this was not due solely to the low level of protein in the diet, for many rats kept by the writer for 2 years and more since weaning on a diet in which the protein level was 4% supplied by casein without exception failed to develop vascularization.

Marked corneal changes, including vascularization, have been observed in rats fed three other low protein diets. These appearances varied quite considerably from diet to diet, although most of the animals on any given

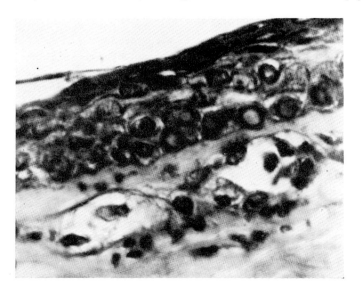

FIG. 83. Keratinizing epithelium and subepithelial vascularization of cornea in a rat fed on a protein-free diet. (Haematoxylin and eosin. ×1200). From McLaren (1959a).

diet showed the same type of lesion. The protein-free diet produced, besides vascularization to which reference has already been made, a haziness of the epithelium giving a "snowstorm" appearance under the slit lamp similar to that seen in the xerosis of vitamin A deficiency. There was a thinning of the layers of the epithelium with marked loss of cytoplasm and degeneration of the nuclei of the deeper layers and keratinization of the superficial cells (Fig. 83).

In contrast to this the cornea in the rats fed on the cassava diet had a quite different and very characteristic appearance (Figs. 84 and 85). The normal rat corneal epithelium is about five or six layers thick but in these animals there were only three or sometimes even two layers of cells. The fault would seem to lie with the basal cell layer, for these cells were markedly abnormal. They

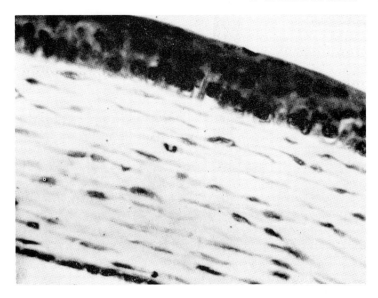

FIG. 84. Normal rat cornea. (Haematoxylin and eosin. ×500). From McLaren (1960).

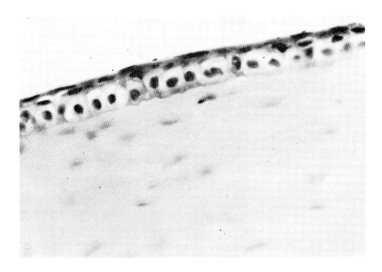

FIG. 85. Epithelium only two cells thick with ballooning of basal cells in rat fed on cassava. (Haematoxylin and eosin. ×500). From McLaren (1960).

appeared blown up, with large bladder-like areas of cytoplasm, and the nuclei were dense and pyknotic. These basal cells closely resembled the appearance of the corresponding cells in the human disease known as bullous keratitis and also in human cases dying from starvation reported from Greece (Chapter 1). These same cells in the normal rat take on a similar appearance when the cornea has been cauterized.

A much less marked degree of swelling occurred in the basal cells of the cornea of rats fed a diet in which arachin replaced casein, and accompanied the vascularization of the cornea that resulted without exception within 1 month of the animals being weaned onto the diet. Two or three weeks after the first ingrowing vessels were visible under the slit lamp they had extended inward to reach almost the centre of the cornea. The basal cells were swollen in the neighbourhood of the invading capillaries and it is probable that this change was responsible for the elliptical area of haziness that was seen around the vessels. Although the level of protein in the casein and arachin diets was the same, and methionine was the limiting amino acid in each case, the concentration of methionine in arachin is approximately half that in casein. This difference would seem to have been the determining factor that caused the ready appearance of corneal vascularization in the arachin-fed animals but none developed it from the group on casein. This conclusion was borne out by the prevention of vascularization by supplementing the arachin diet with DL-methionine and by causing regression of the vessels once vascularization had occurred by the same means.

There have been reports of the adverse effects of diets containing a high level of tyrosine or, to a lesser extent, of phenylalanine in the diet. Niven *et al.* (1946) observed retardation of growth and corneal vascularization in rats receiving a moderately low protein diet (10% casein) to which 1% of each of these amino acids had been added. It is known that phenylalanine is converted to tyrosine. The addition of relatively large amounts of either nicotinic acid or tryptophan appreciably diminished the effects of these amino acids. Hueper and Martin (1943) reported much more severe lesions of the cornea in which vascularization was accompanied by ulceration of the epithelium with a higher concentration of tyrosine, namely 11.7%, added to a diet containing 18% casein. The eye lesions occurred within 1 week of the commencement of the diet and most animals were dead within 3 weeks. Bowles *et al.* (1950) produced similarly severe damage to the cornea with 10% L-tyrosine and very much less severe lesions with 10–20% DL-phenylalanine.

Schweizer (1947) reported conjunctivitis, keratitis and corneal vascularization in all albino rats receiving L-tyrosine as 1.5% of the diet. It has been noted (Rich *et al.*, 1973) that similar damage to the cornea results in human tyrosinaemia (Section IIB*f*).

This is one example of the phenomenon of toxicity resulting from imbalance of amino acids, the only one known to affect the eye. The mechanism is not fully understood. It has been shown (Alam *et al.*, 1966) that the lesions are abolished by an additional supplement of the essential amino acid L-threonine. However, if this diet is continued for 2 months cataracts develop unless an additional supplement of 0.2% L-tryptophan is given. The additional threonine has clearly caused an imbalance with tryptophan. These workers showed that although threonine did not increase the excretion of tyrosine it did enhance its utilization in protein synthesis. David (1976) obtained evidence that the cytochrome *p*-450 enzyme system of the microsomal fraction of the liver converts tyrosine to a toxic metabolite.

The role of vitamin C in the healing of wounds of the cornea was discussed in Chapter 4, Section IA, and the effects of a deficiency of vitamin A and riboflavin on mitotic activity and wound healing were touched upon in Chapter 3, Section IB*1*. Protein and amino acids have received some attention too in this regard. Kobak *et al.* (1947) found a lowering of tensile strength in skin wounds of protein-depleted adult male albino rats, which they attributed to diminution in the number of fibroblasts, decrease in their maturation, and a failure to organize along the lines of stress. Soon after this Localis *et al.* (1948) showed that parenteral methionine (150 mg subcutaneously) shifted the curve of wound healing toward the normal. Further evidence of the importance of the sulphur-containing amino acids was brought forward by Williamson and Fromm (1952, 1955), who found that both methionine and cystine accelerated to some extent the healing rates of wounds in both the presence and absence of protein. Udupa *et al.* (1956) showed that on a protein-free diet less mucopolysaccharide accumulated in wounds and conversion to collagen was slower than normal. On the addition of methionine to this protein-free diet less mucopolysaccharide accumulated in wounds and conversion to collagen was slower than normal. The addition of methionine to this protein-free diet resulted in wound healing which was indistinguishable from that of control animals. It would seem that a redistribution of the sulphur-containing amino acids takes place during wound healing (Fromm and Nordlie, 1959). In the animal on a protein-free diet, after wounding, there is a preferential degradation of the more labile proteins in liver and extrahepatic tissues to supply amino acids, especially methionine and cystine, for protein formation in the wounds. Cystine freed in this way is immediately mobilized and methionine behaves similarly, being converted by the liver and kidneys into more cystine.

It is not known whether the above work on wounds of the skin is equally applicable to those of the cornea but what little evidence there is does point to the importance of sulphur-containing amino acids. In guinea pigs and rabbits Schaeffer (1946) made wounds in the cornea by means of a Castroviejo double knife with blades 2 mm apart. Healing of the wounds was assessed by the appearance on staining with fluorescein. The animals were consuming a normal dietary. Wounds were treated with amino acid mixtures as drops or ointment which included cystine, proline, asparagine, and glutamine in differing concentrations. The greatest effect was with cystine, which appeared to have a local stimulatory effect on the epithelialization of the cornea. In this respect methionine could not be substituted for cystine, which is interesting in view of the conversion of methionine to cystine by the liver and kidneys in the study above. This was also in agreement with tissue culture work in which it has been demonstrated that methionine has no stimulatory effect on the proliferation of isolated cell colonies. The corneal cells are also in a way isolated by injury and for them cystine appears to be the essential sulphur-containing amino acid. The disulphide (—SS) and not the sulphydryl (—SH) group would appear to be of major importance in wound healing, for only the former is present in cystine. On the other hand cysteine (with an—SH group) was found by McDonald (1954) to protect the cornea against the harmful effects of radiation. The subcutaneous injection of a total of 1 ml of 7% cysteine in two areas protected the epithelium, stroma, and endothelium against the application of 40 000 rep of β radiation 1 hour later.

Some work of the writer on the healing of corneal burns in the protein-deficient rat is referred to below (Section F). The main interest of this study was in the effect of a combination of protein and vitamin A deficiencies and is more conveniently dealt with there.

D. The Lens

Curtis *et al*. (1932) in their account of tryptophan deficiency in the rat mentioned a "white opaqueness of the eye and loss of the characteristic colours of the eye". This account in itself would hardly justify the conclusion that these workers were observing cataract but the photographs they published leave no room for doubt. Their results have been repeatedly confirmed since for the rat, notably by Totter and Day (1942), who also gave the first account of corneal vascularization in tryptophan deficiency (Section C, above). According to Buschke (1943) there are two types of tryptophan deficiency cataract, the acute and the chronic (Fig. 86). The first consists of feathery opacities in the posterior cortex with accentuation of the suture lines. This is followed by perinuclear and nuclear opacification, and the whole lens becomes opaque within 3 weeks of the onset of the first changes. In the chronic type the opacities consist of fine dots in the superficial portion of the cortex, the deep cortex and nucleus remaining clear. The cataracts did not mature during the 9 weeks that the animals were kept under observation. In the pig fed a diet characterized primarily by lack of tryptophan, in which protein was represented by an acid hydrolyzate of casein or by zein, cataract was one of the more constant features (Cartwright *et al.,* 1945). Von Sallmann *et al.* (1959) studied the evolution of tryptophan deficiency cataract

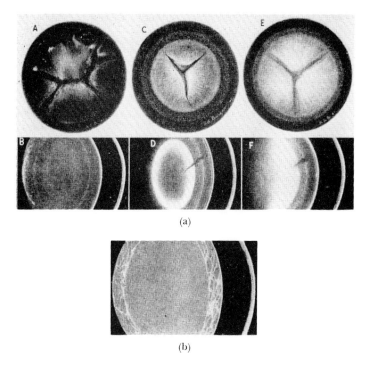

(a)

(b)

FIG. 86. Tryptophan deficiency cataract in the rat; (a) acute; (b) chronic. *A*, composite drawing of the posterior cortex and, *B*, optical section in the first stage. *C*, composite drawing of the posterior cortex and, *D*, optical section in the second stage. *E,* composite drawing of the posterior cortex and, *F*, optical section in the third stage. From Buschke (1943).

in the guinea pig. According to these workers the changes produced in this deficiency consist of hydropic degeneration of lens fibres beneath the capsule near the suture lines, with a subsequent proliferation of the overlying epithelium. The normal morphology of the equatorial region is preserved even in advanced cataract, in contrast to cataract produced by ionizing radiation, radiomimetic drugs, and mimosine.

In order to decide whether tryptophan plays a specific role in lens metabolism, or whether the development of cataract in tryptophan deficiency arises as a result of interference with protein synthesis, Schaeffer and Murray

(1950) fed rats on a diet deficient only in tryptophan but gave the amino acid by the method of delayed supplementation. It is known that all the essential amino acids must be simultaneously available for optimal utilization. In this experiment despite the relatively large quantities of tryptophan ingested by the rats cataract developed, indicating that the unavailability of tryptophan at the right time for protein synthesis was responsible for cataract formation. No difference was found between the tryptophan contents of lenses from normal and tryptophan-deficient animals.

The precise mechanism of cataract formation in tryptophan deficiency is obscure. It is possible that the disturbed tryptophan metabolism, particularly the reduction in the conversion of tryptophan to N'-methylnicotinamide, that occurs in alloxan diabetic rats (Chapter 7, Section ID) and riboflavin deficiency (Chapter 3, Section IB1) may play a part in the cataract formation seen in these states.

Lenticular damage in amino acid deficiencies, other than that of tryptophan, has been not nearly so thoroughly investigated and it is evident that if it does occur consistently it is much less marked. Sydenstricker and his colleagues, who attributed corneal vascularization in the rat to a deficiency of each of the essential amino acids, also described some degree of lens damage in a deficiency of all except arginine and in protein deficiency (Hall *et al.*, 1948). The most marked changes occurred in rats deficient in histidine or phenylalanine and were similar to those in tryptophan or riboflavin deficiency. They consisted of a general haziness of the lens, separation of the superficial fibres, widening of the sutures, diffuse and granular opacities in the cortex, granular degeneration of the superficial cortex, the appearance of a refractile line separating nucleus and cortex, and a dense nuclear opacity of varying extent. Some of these appearances are of rather doubtful significance and the very small eye of the rat makes detailed examination of the lens in life very difficult.

None of the rats fed on low-protein diets by the writer developed any lens changes that were attributable to the diet. The report of Rezende and De Moura Campos (1942) that cataract developed in four litter-mate rats as a result of their being fed on a diet containing 10% casein cannot be accepted. They stated that the first sign of lens change appeared at 50 or more days of age, but it is well known that, due to genetic factors, cataract develops quite frequently in members of certain litters of laboratory rats at about this time. Bagchi (1959a, b) found that in rats fed on a low-protein diet there was a consistent lowering of both GSH (glutathione) and PSH (protein-bound sulphhydryl) in the lens. He was able to produce cataract by injecting animals on this diet with methionine sulphoximine. Both the biochemical lesion and the early structural changes could be reversed by dosing with methionine or cystine, suggesting that the low sulphur-containing amino acid content of the diet was responsible for the former changes, and that methionine sulphoximine was acting as a methionine antimetabolite.

The most striking ocular lesion produced in the pigs fed on a low-protein diet was cataract (McLaren, 1959a). Most of the animals did not survive sufficiently long to develop blinding cataract, but the two that lived more than 1 year did so in both eyes (Fig. 87). The earliest changes consisted of a swelling of the lens fibres in the region of the equator, with separation of the

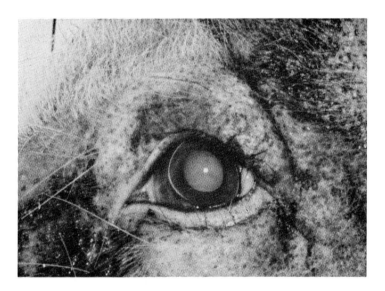

FIG. 87. Cataract in a protein-deficient pig. From McLaren (1959a).

fibres by vacuoles of varying size. This process gradually extended until all the fibres were involved, complete degeneration of fibres resulting in the filling of interfibrillar clefts with amorphous debris. Near the equator the fibres were affected in a characteristic manner, previously described by other workers, in various forms of injury to the lens, as "hydropic cells", "bladder cells", "bubble cells", etc. (Fig. 88). The presence of a nucleus in some of the cells and of a double line in the common boundary between two cells showed that these were hydropic cells, and not merely interfibrillar accumulations of fluid. In what was probably a lesser degree of protein restriction Kauffman and Norton (1966) reported normal lens growth and nitrogen content in the pig.

Besides the accounts given above of cataract quite clearly attributable to deficiency of protein or of one of the essential amino acids there is a number of reports of cataract having been observed under conditions in which the nutritional status was not clearly defined. Larvae of the tiger salamander *(Amblystoma tigrinum)* were reported to develop cortical cataract when fed diets deficient in cystine (Patch, 1934, 1941, 1943). The lens changes appeared to be of two kinds: the first, produced by diets of prepared casein and powdered milk, or muscle protein treated with dilute alkali, were

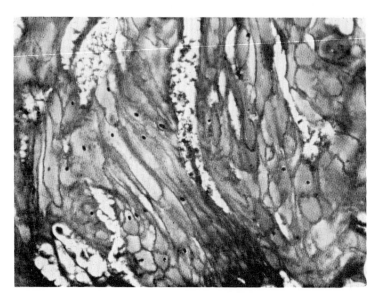

FIG. 88. Histological appearance of same lens as shown in Fig. 87. The fibres are completely disorganized, many have the appearance of "bladder" cells and cellular debris lies in the interfibrillar clefts. (Haematoxylin and eosin. ×95). From McLaren (1959a).

prevented by cystine; the second, associated with a diet of a high haemoglobin content, not prevented by cystine, but in which the feeding of the three amino acids of glutathione, namely glutamic acid, cysteine, and glycine, reduced the early symptoms and halted the development of cataract but did not bring about complete prevention. The further study of the amino acid requirements of this species, especially with regard to the need for cystine, would be worthwhile. The effectiveness of cystine in preventing cataract in the salamander recalls the report of Day *et al.* (1934) that they were able to prevent it completely by substituting egg albumin, rich in cystine, for casein in the diet of their riboflavin-deficient rats and chicks. Furthermore, Bourne and Pyke (1935) had no cataracts in 12 rats whose diet was supplemented with cystine, while in their experience, a riboflavin-deficient diet without that supplementation gave a 39% incidence of cataract (see Chapter 3, Section IC2).

According to Mitchell *et al*. (1940) an abundance of protein in the diet decreases the incidence and rate of development of galactose cataract in rats, and a deficiency has the reverse effect. It is probable that the cataracts produced by Vozza (1957) in rats by feeding them on human milk are of this nature. Human milk has only 1.2% protein as compared with 9.2% in the rat, and the lactose content is higher (7.0%/3.3%). It has been claimed that cataract may be produced by a disorder of tyrosine metabolism resulting from a high intake of sodium butyrate (Uyama *et al.*, 1955), large doses of tyrosine in diabetic rats (Uyama *et al.*, 1956), or certain combinations of tyrosine and the sugars glucose, galactose, or xylose in scorbutic guinea pigs (Ogino and Tojo, 1956).

Although the precise aetiology of the widespread occurrence of cataract in trout reported by Hess (1937–38) has never, to the writer's knowledge, been explained, mention may be made of it here as appropriately as anywhere. It was found that cataract developed in nearly all trout fed over 6 months exclusively on pig spleen in many hatcheries of New York State in 1931. There were also degenerative changes in the fins and iris associated with darkening of the skin. These lesions were totally prevented by adding liver and heart to the diet. Parasitic invasion of the lens, a common finding in fish, heredity, and exposure to light were excluded as aetiological factors.

Recent work (Poston *et al.*, 1977) suggests that this may have been an example of an amino acid deficiency cataract. These workers report that methionine, but not lysine, prevents cataract in lake trout fed isolated soy bean as the only source of protein.

Another interesting form of amino acid related cataract has been reported by Gunter *et al*. (1972). A model for human phenylketonuria was said to be produced in immature rats by the injection of parachlorophenylalanine and lenticular opacities resulted.

Until the nature of the fundamental change in senile cataract formation is understood the aetiology of this condition will continue to elude us. Much is known about the alterations that take place in the concentrations of water, various minerals, and organic constituents of the normal lens when it becomes cataractous but none of these seems to be of fundamental importance. In view of the high protein content of the lens and the denaturation of protein that is such an integral part of the cataractous process it has been thought that it might be possible to demonstrate alterations in the amino acid composition or protein nature of the lens beginning to undergo cataractous change. In aging there is a gradual loss of soluble proteins, especially from the nucleus, but this does not of itself result in opacification of the lens. No such changes have been demonstrated yet in human cataractous lenses (Schaeffer and Shankman, 1950; François and Rabaey, 1959). In weanling rats fed on a diet containing 5% protein for 6 months from weaning in our laboratory no alterations in tyrosine or tryptophan concentration could be demonstrated in the lenses of the experimental animals, although the soluble protein concentration fell in the usual way with increasing age.

E. The Retina

An analysis of the amino acid content of the retina in man, cat, dog, cow, horse, pig, rabbit, guinea pig, rat, hen, and carp revealed relatively large amounts of the non-essential amino acid taurine but was not otherwise notable (Kubíček and Dolének, 1958).

Aurbach *et al*. (1964) have reported impairment of the ERG in the albino rat on a protein-free diet for 4 to 5 weeks similar in magnitude to that found in vitamin A-deficient animals in 6 to 8 weeks. The animals were pair-fed so any effect of inanition can probably be excluded.

Several groups have described nutritional retinal degeneration in the cat (Scott *et al.*, 1964; Morris, 1965; Rabin *et al.*, 1973). The work of Hayes and his colleagues appears to have revealed the cause.

Hayes *et al*. (1975a) produced retinal degeneration in cats fed casein as the protein source. Casein is low in total sulphur amino acids and particularly in cystine, which is the precursor for taurine synthesis. Replacement of casein by egg albumin in early cases resulted in reversal of the changes (Hayes *et al.*, 1975b). In the casein-fed animals plasma and retinal taurine levels decreased selectively. The retinal appears to have a special requirement for taurine as its level there is three times that of any other free amino acid.

Supplementation with methionine or cystine was ineffective but animals given taurine were normal (Berson *et al.*, 1976a). They conclude that the

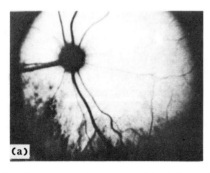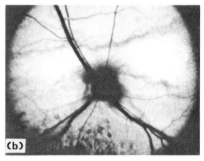

FIG. 89. Fundus photographs of the left eye of a control cat fed a normal commercial diet (a) and that of a cat fed the semipurified diet showing moderately advanced changes (b). From Rabin *et al.* (1973).

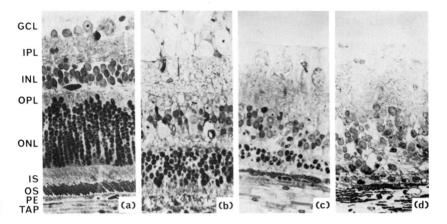

FIG. 90. Photomicrographs of the retina from a control cat fed a commercial formula (a) and three cats fed the semipurified diet (b, c, d). Anatomic layers are identified for the control only: GCL, ganglion cell layer; IPL, inner plexiform layer; INL, inner nuclear layer; OPL, outer plexiform layer; ONL, outer nuclear layer; IS, inner segment; OS, outer segment; PE, pigment epithelium; TAP, tapetum. Early (b), moderately advanced (c) and advanced (d) stages of the degeneration are represented. From Rabin et al. (1973).

deficiency may relate to a low level of decarboxylase in the liver in the cat (and in man) resulting in a slow rate of synthesis of taurine from either cysteine sulphinic acid or cysteic acid. The retinal changes consisted of granularity with a hyper-reflective white zone in the area centralis, photoreceptor cell degeneration and a non-detectable ERG (Schmidt et al., 1976) (Figs. 89 and 90).

A survey of 41 patients with various hereditary retinal diseases revealed no lowering of plasma taurine levels that might suggest a human counterpart to the condition in experimental animals (Berson et al., 1976b).

F. Protein and Vitamin A

The interrelationships of vitamins and relationships of vitamins to protein, carbohydrate, and fat have received increasing attention as the complexities of animal nutrition have been more fully realized. Outside the laboratory deficiency disease states are always multiple and correction of only one deficiency or over-correction of a deficiency may be actually harmful.

In an experiment designed to investigate the interrelationships of protein and vitamin A (McLaren, 1959b) a diet free from vitamin A was devised and the protein content, supplied by egg albumin, was varied with an appropriate change in the wheat starch content also. Other vitamins, except vitamin

E because of its vitamin A sparing effect, were added in the diet or fed by mouth. Rats were divided according to sex and litter and fed from weaning on one of the diets supplying 18, 11, 6, or 4% protein. Careful watch was kept on the animals for the onset of xerophthalmia as observed under the slit lamp, and the growth and survival time were noted. All animals fed on the diets containing 18 and 11% protein, but none of those on the 6 and 4% diets, developed xerophthalmia. While some of these latter animals died before those on the higher levels of protein were beginning to develop eye signs, nevertheless many lived sufficiently long for xerophthalmia to have developed if the low level of protein had not been exerting a restraining influence. Vitamin E deficiency has been shown to result in early death of animals fed on diets deficient in protein. That this might have been partly responsible for the early deaths of low protein animals in this experiment was shown by a further group, fed 4% protein from weaning with added vitamin E, which survived for 120 days on the diet, when they were killed, without having developed xerophthalmia. The rats fed on the 6 and 4% protein diets showed no growth whatsoever, while the others grew steadily until about 70 days of age, males more than females and those on the 18% more than those on the 11% protein diet, and thereafter lost weight with the deterioration in the general condition and onset of xerophthalmia.

The results of this work would seem to lend support to the contention that vitamin A is important for tissue protein growth although not for its maintenance (Brown and Morgan, 1948). That the rate of growth is closely related to the expenditure of vitamin A was shown by Johnson and Baumann (1948). Rats deprived of vitamin A and restricted in growth by inadequacy of calories, or of tryptophan or thiamine, were shown by these workers to use up their stores less rapidly than those which were lacking vitamin A alone. In the experiment described above there was no evidence that protein deficiency hastened the development of xerophthalmia; on the contrary in those animals fed on the very low protein diets (4 and 6%) the onset of eye signs was actually delayed. It was in these animals too that growth did not take place, thereby possibly causing the demand on liver stores of the vitamin to be very low indeed. This effect of growth was also seen to some extent in the rats on the 18 and 11% protein diets, those which grew less well developing xerophthalmia later.

Another approach to the same problem was made by studying the healing of standardized thermal burns of the cornea in different deficiency states (McLaren, 1960). The cautery consisted of a loop of 28 SWG platinum wire through which a constant current was fed. A relay in the circuit allowed the current to flow for any period between $\frac{1}{2}$ and $2\frac{1}{2}$ seconds with $\frac{1}{2}$ second intervals. Burns about 1 mm in diameter situated in the centre of the cornea were produced in this way. Within a few hours the cornea had become hazy, this appearance spreading out centrifugally from the burn. After about 24 hours this had become maximal, reaching in most cases to the limbus, which was congested. The pupil was dilated and in a few instances "cotton wool" exudates were present in the anterior chamber. The burn itself was dense white and was surrounded by a narrow zone of cornea which was quite clear and transparent. Outside this was a zone of haziness, which was in turn surrounded by a second clear zone and then beyond that again the generalized haziness extended toward the limbus.

After about 48 hours vascularization of the cornea was apparent, extending for not more than about 1 mm into the cornea. At about this time the burn usually became dome-shaped and had the appearance of a blister containing some exudate. From this time onward the haziness became progressively less, and usually by about the 5th to the 7th day the cornea had resumed its normal transparency and the only evidence of the burn was a very faint nebula. The burn was then regarded as healed.

Histological examination of the corneae with burns showed that the loss of transparency was probably due to a combination of two factors. Firstly, the basal cells of the epithelium were swollen and appeared to be filled with fluid, closely resembling the appearance they had in extreme protein deficiency (see Section C, above). Secondly, the whole thickness of the stroma, but more particularly subepithelially, showed a cellular infiltration.

TABLE X. *Time Taken to Heal by Corneal Burns of Rats on Different Diets*[a]

Rat no.	Litter no.	Type of diet	Healing time in days
1	1	Control	6
2	1	Control	6
3	1	Deficient in vitamin A and protein	12
4	1	Deficient in vitamin A and protein	17
5	1	Deficient in vitamin A	6
6	1	Deficient in vitamin A	6
7	1	Deficient in protein	7
8	2	Control	6
9	2	Deficient in vitamin A and protein	9
10	2	Deficient in vitamin A	6
11	2	Deficient in protein	6
12	3	Deficient in vitamin A and protein	14
13	3	Deficient in vitamin A	6
14	3	Deficient in protein	7

[a]Table 2.2 from D. S McLaren (1960).

The time taken for the burns to heal and the changes in the cornea as observed by the slit lamp microscope were studied in various groups of rats. In comparison with control animals, both mature and immature rats fed on the diet containing 4% protein from casein showed no delay in healing of the burn but there was consistently a greater intensity of corneal haziness. Identical changes were seen with rats fed the diet providing 4% protein from arachin. Similarly, in young rats on a vitamin A-free diet there was no delay in the healing of the burn.

In a small experiment using 14 rats from three litters the healing of the burn was compared in four groups, i.e. controls, protein-deficient, vitamin A-deficient, and both protein- and vitamin-A deficient. The results are given in Table X. In all but those in the combined deficiency group the burns never took longer than 6 or 7 days to heal, whereas in the presence of a deficiency of both protein and vitamin A it took at least half as long again and usually twice as long.

II. Human Studies

A. Protein-Energy Malnutrition

Ocular involvement is one of the most common and serious complications of the syndrome of protein-energy malnutrition (kwashiorkor and marasmus) in children in certain parts of the world (McLaren, 1958b). All the evidence pointed to the conclusion that this is primarily due to deficiency of vitamin A, and that protein deficiency is concerned only in so far as it may affect the metabolism of vitamins. These aspects of the subject have been considered in Section IF and Chapter 2, IIIA7a. Cataract and other ocular complications of fetal malnutrition are discussed in Chapter 9, Section IIA.

Emiru (1971) examined the eyes of 200 children suffering from kwashiorkor and found corneal involvement in only four. The mean serum vitamin A in this group was reported to be 33 μg/100 ml, within normal limits, which would seem to rule out xerophthalmia, the main cause of eye lesions in protein-energy malnourished children (see Chapter 2, Section IIIA7a). No mention is made of measles and it is probable that this was the cause rather than protein deficiency per se (Chapter 11, Section C).

ERG changes have been reported in undernourished children (Khetarpal, 1964). In 40 cases b potentials were depressed, in proportion to weight deficit. The depression was greatest if vitamin A deficiency was also present (see Chapter 2, Section IIIA4b).

Halasa and McLaren (1964) examined the refractive state of malnourished children. The subjects were 110 severely marasmic and 93 healthy children aged between 1 and 24 months. There was a highly significant myopic trend in the marasmic group (mean 1.55 D) compared with mean 2.85 D in the controls. Five marasmic infants were refracted throughout a 3-month period of rehabilitation during which the refractive state returned to normal in all patients. Serum vitamin A levels were markedly lower in the marasmic than the control group but clinical eye signs of xerophthalmia were absent. It should be noted that the marasmic form of malnutrition is more of an energy deficit than of protein.

In a further study of marasmic infants Halasa (1969) found no alteration of intraocular pressure. Sood and Gupta (1966) confirmed the myopic tendency in marasmus and found improvement with dietary treatment but refraction was not normal after 4 to 6 weeks.

Kwashiorkor may occur in an acute and in a chronic form in young adults, although much less commonly than in infants (Trowell *et al.*, 1954). Most accounts do not mention the eye, but as part of an interesting syndrome of which calcification and fibrosis of the pancreas are the main features, Zuidema (1955) reported a high incidence of senile-type cataract from Indonesia (Chapter 11 Section B).

In man protein deficiency is such an ill-defined concept inevitably complicated by deficiency of other nutrients, that it is not possible in a single instance to give an account of ocular lesions which may be attributed with confidence to it alone. Bietti (1950), in one of the few papers on the subject, dealt with what he called the ophthalmic aspects of protein deficiency and disordered protein metabolism but there is no real evidence that this was the basis for the symptoms described. Some of the instances cited are accounts of undernutrition in prisoners of war and cannot be clearly differentiated from other reports, mentioned in Chapter 1, where starvation was thought to be of prime importance.

For instance, subconjunctival haemorrhage is said to have occurred in 5% of hunger oedema cases during the first world war (Bürger, 1920). Weekers (1942) reported faulty dark adaptation in 15 Belgian cases of nutritional oedema where lack of vitamin A could be excluded, and found no rise in intraocular tension in this condition. In Germany, Klemens (1948) observed night blindness and optic atrophy in chronic nutritional oedema, and Balcet (1948) thought that there was an increase of myopia. Another report of night blindness responding to treatment other than vitamin A concerns a study carried out on 24 prisoners of war returning to Germany from Russia (Niedermeier, 1950). Cysteine by mouth or intravenous injection caused the dark adaptation to return to normal in 22 cases within a period of 3 weeks. The author believed that cysteine acted by improving the small intestine's ability to absorb proteins and other substances, but gave no real evidence that this did in fact occur.

Patients suffering from various diseases giving rise to malabsorption of nutrients may show some ocular changes. It was reported by Zivkov and Teoharov (1958) that in a series of 81 such patients, some had greatly diminished visual acuity and retinal oedema. The latter was confirmed histologically in some who died and was localized particularly to the disc area (Chapter 1).

The work of Sydenstricker and his colleagues, in which they produced vascularization of the cornea in the rat by deficiency of each of the essential amino acids, and protein deficiency will be recalled (Section IC). They mention that they looked for this sign in 20 protein-malnourished human subjects but with negative results (Sydenstricker *et al.*, 1946).

Schaeffer (1950) followed up earlier work (Section IC) on healing of experimental corneal wounds by testing the effect of different amino acids on corneal wounds in man. In this work too, he found that cystine was the most effective, and could not be replaced by methionine.

B. Aminoacidopathies

In recent years a great variety of disorders of amino acid metabolism have been described. Those selected for discussion here have two characteristics in common; they have ocular manifestations and they are also responsive to a varying extent to dietary management.

a. Cystinosis

This is an autosomal recessive disease in which cystine deposition may occur in most tissues. The classic infantile nephropathic variety is characterized by fever, growth retardation, rickets, polyuria and progressive renal failure. In a milder form of the disease deposits may be mainly in the bone marrow and the eyes, and expectation is not reduced (Giles and Wong, 1969).

The ocular findings are of diagnostic importance but do not interfere with vision. On slit-lamp examination fine cystine crystals may be observed in the cornea, mostly at the periphery, in the conjunctiva and dusting the iris. On a histological cross-section of the cornea they are easily missed (Cogan and Kuwabara, 1960). They have been studied with the electron microscope (Kenyon and Sensenbrenner, 1974). Photophobia may occur. Peripheral pigmentary retinal degeneration is frequent (Wong *et al.*, 1967) (Figs. 91 to 93).

Cystinosis should not be confused with the relatively benign condition, cystinuria, which does not involve the eye. Nutritional treatment includes vitamin D and phosphate for the rickets; vitamin C 200 mg/kg daily may remove cystine deposits and in a diet containing only 35 mg/kg daily

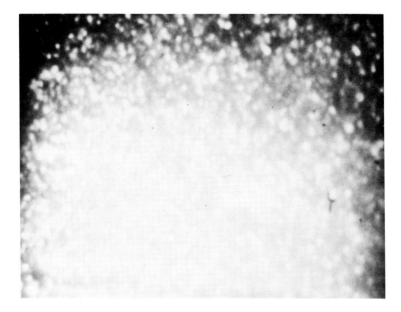

FIG. 91. High-power view of multiple, refractile, birefringent cystine crystals in cornea of patient with infantile cystinosis. From Sugar and Podos (1975).

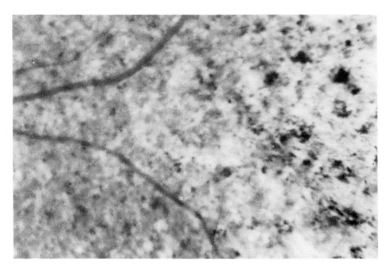

FIG. 92. In cystinosis, peripheral retinal pigment splotches and mottling are a frequent occurrence. From Sugar and Podos (1975).

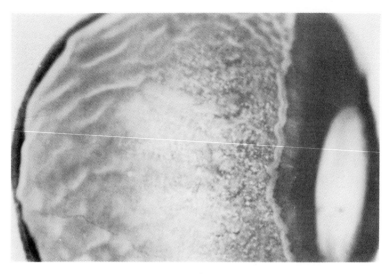

FIG. 93. Gross pathologic demonstration of cystinotic eye with peripheral pigmentary disturbance. From Sugar and Podos (1975).

methionine should be used but it is unpalatable and results in malnutrition if there is further restriction, so careful monitoring is essential.

b. Homocystinuria

The metabolic defect appears to be a recessively inherited deficiency of cystathionine β-synthase, necessary for the metabolism of methionine. Most of the patients have been mentally retarded children, but the condition has been described in adults of normal intelligence. Typically, patients have a fair complexion, malar flush, red blotchy skin and fine, sparse blonde hair. Mental retardation and seizures are frequent, as are skeletal deformities and hepatomegaly, Thromboembolic phenomena are common, sometimes following ocular surgery, and increased platelet adhesiveness has been demonstrated.

The ocular manifestations have to be distinguished from those of Marfan's syndrome (Figs. 94 and 95). Dislocated lenses and glaucoma are the most common (Lieberman et al., 1966). Glaucoma occurs when the partially dislocated lens blocks the pupillary space. Other ocular features include cataracts, optic atrophy (Presley et al., 1969), retinal artery occlusion (Wilson and Ruiz, 1969), high myopia (François, 1972) and pigmentary mottling near the ora serrata. There may be peripheral retinal degeneration, and PAS-positive deposits on the ciliary body are zonular fragments (Ramsey et al., 1975).

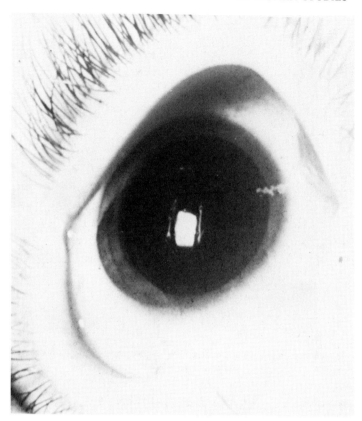

FIG. 94. Lens is dislocated down and into anterior chamber of this patient with homocystinuria. From Sugar and Podos (1975).

Diets restricted in methionine are used in treatment in order to reduce the accumulation of methionine, homocysteine and their metabolites. The diet is supplemented with L-cystine to provide some cysteine, which is an essential amino acid for patients with this disorder. Some cases have responded to large doses of pyridoxine (vitamin B_6) and this is probably dependent upon the existence of some residual cystathionine β-synthase activity.

c. Hyperlysinaemia

This is a rare group of disorders. Smith *et al.* (1971) studied three sibs and a cousin who were affected. One patient had bilateral subluxated lenses and lateral rectus palsy. Another had spherophakia.

Diets low in lysine have been devised but their value remains in doubt at present.

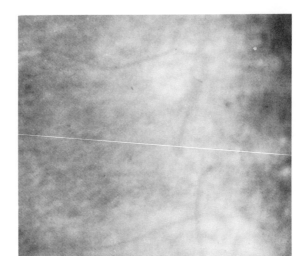

FIG. 95. Pigmentary mottling near ora serrata in a young girl with homocystinuria. From Sugar and Podos (1975).

d. Hyperornithinaemia

This progressive genetic disorder, resulting from lack of ornithine ketoacid aminotransferase activity, leads to blindness by the age of 40 or 50 due to gyrate atrophy of the choroid and retina (Simell and Takki, 1973). The enzyme is vitamin B_6 dependent but large doses of the vitamin have shown neither biochemical nor clinical improvement. However, recently (Shih *et al.*, 1978) the possibility of response to long-term treatment has been indicated by the finding of increased enzyme activity in cultured skin fibroblasts from one of five patients when increased amounts of pyridoxal phosphate were added to the medium.

e. Maple Syrup Urine Disease

In its classical form the disease occurs as an autosomal recessive trait in which there is failure of decarboxylation of the three branched-chain amino acids, valine, leucine and isoleucine. Failure to thrive, mental retardation, convulsions and early death result in the absence of treatment.

Ocular involvement is uncommon but has consisted of delayed optic nerve maturation, nystagmus, ptosis, strabismus and lens opacities (Roy and

II. HUMAN STUDIES 251

Kelly, 1973). Zee et al. (1974) reported ophthalmoplegia in a 3-week-old infant.

Dietary management is very difficult as three amino acids are involved and there is no simple method for their analysis. Most foods are rich in these amino acids. Treatment with a diet low in the branched-chain amino acids should be started within the first few days of life if mental retardation and death are to be prevented. Natural foods should be gradually introduced early.

f. Phenylketonuria

This relatively common aminoacidopathy results in mental retardation in the absence of adequate dietary control. Eye involvement is very rare, and besides the common light-coloured irides there is only one report of bilateral lamellar cataracts in a 2-year-old child (Park and Schwilk, 1963). Cataracts were produced experimentally by an antimetabolite of phenylalanine (Section ID).

Dietary treatment of this condition is the most successful of any aminoacidopathy. A regulated diet low in phenylalanine, commercially available, should be initiated as soon after birth as possible. It is still undetermined when the diet may be discontinued but most agree to late in childhood.

g. Sulphite Oxidase Deficiency

The first case was reported by Irreverre et al. (1967) of an infant with many neurological disorders present at birth. In the second year of life bilateral dislocation of the lens, nystagmus and blindness were noted and death occurred at $2\frac{1}{2}$ years. Shih et al. (1977) studied a case at 4 years with acute infantile hemiplegia and dislocated lenses. Large amounts of abnormal sulphur-containing metabolites (sulphite, thiosulphite and S-sulphocysteine) occurred in the urine. Sulphate oxidase activity in skin fibroblasts was undetectable in the patient and was reduced in both parents, compatible with autosomal recessive inheritance.

Treatment with a low sulphur amino acid diet produced a good biochemical response but no clinical improvement, for which treatment may have to be started much earlier. Sulphite oxidase is molybdenum-dependent and this trace element might prove useful in treatment.

h. Tyrosinaemia

The disease is described in two forms. In hereditary tyrosinaemia (Baber's syndrome, cirrhosis and the Fanconi syndrome) there is deficiency of p-hydroxyphenyl-pyruvic acid oxidase. This enzyme is responsible for the production of homogentesic acid in the degradative pathway of phenylalanine. Hepatosplenomegaly, cirrhosis, renal defects and rickets are characteristic. In one case cataracts developed in youth (La Du and Gjessing, 1972).

In another form of the disorder there is tyrosine aminotransferase deficiency. Mental deficiency, palmar and plantar keratosis, and bilateral superficial stellate central corneal ulcers occur (Fig. 96) Burns, 1972; Buist *et*

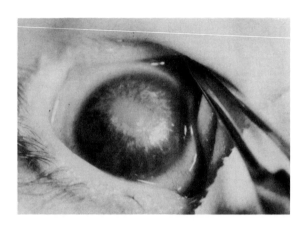

FIG. 96. Right eye, fluorescein-stained central corneal ulcer with very irregular margins at one month of age. The appearance of the ulcers in both eyes was the same. From Burns (1972).

al., 1973). Zaleski *et al.* (1973), reporting another case, stated that the corneal erosions may be an early manifestation and often eventually clear without scarring, probably unrelated to treatment. Similar lesions have been produced by high tyrosine diets in rats (Section IC).

In a few cases a diet restricted in phenylalanine and tyrosine has led to healing of the renal tubular lesion, cure of rickets, growth spurt and general improvement.

Chapter 7

Carbohydrates

The main interest in the possible effects these substances in the diet may have on the eye lies not so much in states in which they are deficient in large amounts but in the harmful results they are known to have when circulating in the blood or deposited in the tissues of the body. Diets rich in certain carbohydrates, some of which are normal dietary constituents and some of which are not, consistently interfere with the metabolism of the lens. Considerable attention has been devoted to the mechanism of the resulting cataract, and the nature of the fundamental change in this type of cataract is perhaps better understood than most.

Glucose is one of the monosaccharides of which a high concentration in the blood is associated with cataract. This never arises, either in experimental animals or in man, merely by ingestion of large quantities of glucose, but only as a result of damage to the pancreas. Diabetogenic cataract in animals and true diabetic cataract in man are therefore not due to malnutrition as it has been defined in the introduction to this work but are due to a disturbance of metabolism.

The lens may also be damaged in hypoglycaemia, and cataract is a prominent feature of the human disorders of galactose metabolism, galactosaemia and galactokinase deficiency.

A brief review of the normal metabolism of the lens is essential for the understanding of the biochemical changes that lead to the formation of the sugar cataracts. The lens capsule is permeable to glucose, amino acids, salts, vitamins, and other substances present in the aqueous humour. The cells of the lens epithelium actively transport amino acids into the lens against a concentration gradient, and are also responsible for maintaining an ionic balance. These cells contain adenosinetriphosphatase which, activated by sodium and potassium, maintains an excess of potassium and a deficiency of sodium within the lens fibres compared to the aqueous humour.

The energy required for this is supplied by glucose. The level of glucose in the aqueous is closely related to that in the blood and is about 70 mg/100 ml. The level of glucose in the lens is about one-tenth of this and probably enters the lens by diffusion. The mechanism of entry of glucose into the lens fibres is not clear, but it has been suggested that the rate of glucose utilization and the rate of entry into the lens are equal, so that at normal levels of glucose in the blood and aqueous the lens fibres are essentially glucose free. The limiting factor in glucose utilization is phosphorylation of glucose by hexokinase.

Most of the carbohydrate metabolism of the lens is by way of anaerobic glycolysis. This has the advantage for the lens in that it can be carried on in the absence of oxygen. Under physiological conditions glycolysis proceeds at the maximum possible rate. This was shown by Lou and Kinoshita (1967), who found that if a lens is cultured in a medium containing 200 mg or more of glucose per 100 ml the rate of glycolysis does not increase although the concentration of glucose in the lens increases.

The end product of glycolysis is lactic acid, the greater part of which (70–90%) diffuses into the aqueous humour. The rest is broken down aerobically in the cells of the epithelium to CO_2 and water.

It has never been determined with certainty what fraction of the lens' need for energy is met by the aerobic breakdown of glucose, but all evidence suggests that less than 30% of the energy requirement of the lens is derived by oxidation of glucose and most of this is available through the monophosphate shunt, very little entering the Krebs cycle.

Insulin has no effect on glucose entry into the aqueous humour either in the normal or in the diabetic rabbit. Moreover, the consensus of opinion is that insulin has no effect on glucose uptake by the lens, either *in vivo* prior to culture or *in vitro*.

Van Heyningen (1962) has described the sorbitol pathway of glucose metabolism which is unique to the lens, and although not operative under normal conditions becomes active in hyperglycaemia. The lens contains an enzyme, aldose reductase, which with the reduced coenzyme nicotinamide adenine dinucleotide phosphate ($NADPH_2$) catalyses the reduction of glucose to sorbitol:

$$Glucose + NADPH_2 \rightleftharpoons Sorbitol + NADP$$
$$Aldose\ reductase$$

Another enzyme in the lens, polyol dehydrogenase, will oxidize sorbitol in the presence of the coenzyme NAD to form fructose and $NADH_2$:

$$\text{Sorbitol} + \text{NAD} \rightleftharpoons \text{fructose} + \text{NADH}_2$$
$$\text{polyoldehydrogenase}$$

It has been suggested that these two reactions help to maintain the balance of oxidized and reduced forms of the nicotinamide coenzymes. A change in the ratio of oxidized and reduced coenzyme may stimulate or retard a particular reaction. For example, reduction of glucose to form sorbitol is accompanied by oxidation of the reduced coenzyme $NADPH_2$. This stimulates the metabolism of glucose through the monophosphate path with concomitant reduction of NADP.

The accumulation of sorbitol and/or fructose in the lens depends on two factors: (1) the ratio of the activity of the enzymes of the sorbitol pathway to the activity of hexokinase, the starting enzyme for both the aerobic and anaerobic breakdown of glucose, (2) the rate of diffusion of the substances sorbitol or fructose through the cell membranes. Most cell membranes are slightly permeable to sorbitol.

Although it has been shown that the activity of lens hexokinase to lens aldose reductase measured under optimal conditions is about 1–1, yet the avidity of hexokinase for glucose is 200 times greater than the avidity of aldose reductase for glucose. Thus at the normal concentration of glucose in the lens, lens hexokinase is almost saturated whereas lens aldose reductase will show only 2% of its maximum activity. Put more precisely, the concentration of glucose at which hexokinase shows half its maximum activity is 1.8 mg/100 ml, while aldose reductase has half its maximum activity at a glucose concentration of 500 mg/100 ml. As a result of the difference in the activity of the two enzymes, the rate of phosphorylation of glucose by hexokinase and therefore the rate of glycolysis will not change when the blood sugar rises as in diabetes, but the reduction of glucose to sorbitol by aldose reductase will increase with increasing blood sugar.

I. Animal Studies

A. Galactose

This monosaccharide has a wide distribution in the animal kingdom, especially in milk lactose and in the cerebrosides of nervous tissue. It occurs in minute quantities in the eye as a constituent of mucoprotein in the cornea and the capsule of the lens. Before absorption lactose is hydrolysed into its component monosaccharides galactose and glucose. As long ago as 1860 Weir Mitchell reported the production of cataracts in pigs by the administration of sugar. Diets with a high content of lactose produce cataract because of the galactosaemia that results (Mitchell, 1935; Mitchell and Dodge, 1935). So far this type of cataract has mainly been described in the rat. Young animals are much more susceptible than older, strains vary to some extent in susceptibility, and lens opacities have been reported in the young of mother rats fed galactose during pregnancy (see Chapter 9, Section M). The time taken for the opacities to develop is inversely proportional to the level of galactose in the diet. Thus Mitchell and Dodge (1935) found that diets containing 70, 50, and 30% lactose resulting in early cataractous changes in young rats in 1.3, 2.4, and 3.6 weeks, respectively. Dietary levels of galactose from 25 to 70% have been consistently found to produce cataract in young rats.

The clinical and histological appearances of galactose cataract have been fully described (Gifford and Bellows, 1939; Patz, 1953) and would seem to

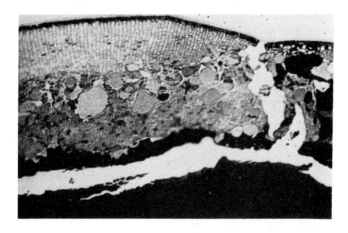

FIG. 97. Galactose cataract in a rat which had received 25% galactose in its diet for 18 days after weaning. The massive degeneration of the cortical zone is seen. From Patz (1953).

be similar in most respects for all the sugar cataracts. The earliest change apparent on clinical examination is the appearance of vacuoles in the cortex, usually anteriorly, but posterior polar or nuclear opacities may also develop before the cataract is mature. On histological examination it is seen that the equatorial region is the first affected. Here the lens fibres disintegrate into granules and fluid accumulates around these. The nuclei of the lens fibres degenerate and the epithelium may proliferate into a layer many cells thick (Fig. 97).

Young rats fed on diets with about 80% galactose die fairly soon. Coincident with the rise in blood galactose there is a fall in the glucose content and the liver becomes depleted of glycogen. It is not known just how the lens is affected, whether directly by a high concentration of galactose in the aqueous humour or whether secondary to some general effect. There was an appreciable loss of amino acids in the urine in young rats fed a diet containing 70% galactose (Craig and Maddock, 1953) and it was suggested that protein deficiency might account for most of the changes, but as Pirie and van Heyningen (1956) pointed out, on lower levels of galactose there are no other changes apart from cataract even after long periods on the diet. These authors have reviewed the biochemical aspects of galactose metabolism as it affects the lens in both experimental and human galactosaemia.

The dietary level of protein has been shown to affect the development of galactose cataract. Mitchell and Cook (1937) employing a diet containing 25% galactose showed that the time taken for opacification to develop was reduced from 26.3 days to 15 days on the average by diminishing the casein content from 15% to 5%. A very high protein diet seems to have the reverse effect to a slight degree but addition of various amino acids and some vitamins has had no effect. When a diet containing 35% galactose was fed to rats on alternate days, with a normal diet fed on the intervening days, cataract did not develop (Patterson, 1953). If the normal diet was replaced by days of starvation, cataracts developed in an average of 40 days. He postulated that the lowering of galactose blood levels at regular intervals might remove a cellular blockage and allow the entrance of some "essential" metabolite. Patterson (1953) found that the cataractogenic effects of galactose feeding and diabetes were additive and suggested that the basic mechanism was the same for the two types of cataract.

Hörmann (1954) claimed to have prevented cataract in rats consuming diets containing either 70% lactose or 30% galactose by repeated injection of cocarboxylase. This is the pyrophosphoric ester of thiamine and is concerned in the metabolism of pyruvic acid, an intermediate product of carbohydrate metabolism. Without cocarboxylase the rats survived only 12 or 14 days, but this coenzyme extended their survival to the full experimental period of 100 days, without the development of cataract. On the basis of these results he concluded that these sugars cause cataract by interfering with carbohydrate metabolism in some way. It is difficult to reconcile these findings with those of the majority of other workers who have not found these levels of lactose and galactose in the diet to bring about the rapid death of even very young rats.

Paper electrophoresis of the water-soluble lens proteins in rats with different degrees of cataract formation induced by galactose feeding was reported by François et al. (1954). The mean percentage of water-soluble proteins was diminished in proportion to the degree of clinical change. All fractions were affected so that there was no appreciable change in the concentrations of the different lens proteins. These results are also found in other types of cataract and do not, unfortunately, help toward an understanding of the process.

Schwarz and Golberg (1955) reported approximately 10 times the normal concentration of galactose-1-phosphate in the capsule of the lens in rats fed a diet containing 30 % galactose. This sugar is not normally present in the lens fibres but is found in the capsule. In the animals fed on the high galactose diet glucose-1-phosphate was not found in the lens fibres but was confined to the capsule. Only those lenses showing cataractous change contained the ester, indicating that accumulation of this substance was closely related to structural damage.

Lerman (1959) demonstrated that glucose-6-phosphate dehydrogenase activity in the lens, part of the hexose monophosphate shunt shown by Kinoshita (1955) to be of considerable importance in lens metabolism, is specifically inhibited by galactose-1-phosphate both *in vivo* and *vitro*. This inhibition appears to take place before there is any alteration in soluble protein synthesis. The same worker has subsequently shown (Lerman and Heggeness, 1961) that the hexose monophosphate shunt is especially active in the lens of the young rat, at the time when the lens is most susceptible to galactose and xylose feeding, and that this activity diminishes with age.

Van Heyningen (1959a) demonstrated that the polyol dulcitol (galactitol) accumulated in the lens and suggested that cataract was caused by the resulting osmotic imbalance. This was confirmed by Kinoshita *et al.* (1962). He later showed (Kinoshita *et al.,* 1968) that galactose cataract in the rabbit was prevented by the aldose reductase inhibitor tetramethyleneglutaric acid. Also from Kinoshita's laboratory comes the report of inhibition of polyol accumulation in the lens of galactosaemic and diabetic rats by the aldose reductase inhibitor AY–22, 284 (Dvornik *et al.,* 1973). Aldose reductase is probably the initiating factor in sugar cataract production. The order of effectiveness of causing changes in lens water and polyol levels, D-xylose, D-galactose, D-glucose, is consistent with substrate specificity properties of lens aldose reductase and the activity of the sugars as substrate (Obazawa *et al.,* 1974).

Like other sugar alcohols, dulcitol is not metabolized further, does not penetrate the membrane of lens fibres and is trapped within the cells where it is produced. Water is drawn into the cells to maintain osmotic balance. This leads to diminution of amino acids in the lens, arrest of protein synthesis, depression of glycolysis and ATP generation, and failure of the cation pump as shown by a decrease in the capacity to take up tracer potassium and exclude sodium.

Patterson and colleagues (Patterson and Bunting, 1965; Patterson and Patterson, 1965) reported that a high fat diet delayed the onset of mature galactose cataract, as it does in experimental diabetes (Section ID). A low level of corn oil in the diet altered the long chain fatty acid composition of the lens (Hatcher and Andrews, 1970).

In Australia kangaroos are often reared as pets on cow's milk and may develop cataract. They lack the enzymes galactokinase and galactose-1-phosphate uridyl transferase necessary for galactose metabolism. Kangaroo milk contains almost no lactose (Stephens *et al.*, 1974).

B. Xylose

Xylose is a pentose found in plants, and like arabinose, but unlike glucose and galactose, does not occur naturally in animals. Darby and Day (1939, 1940) produced cataract in young rats fed a diet containing a high proportion of xylose (Fig. 98). Certain strains appear to be more susceptible than others

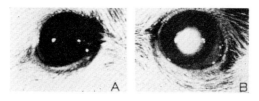

FIG. 98. (a) Normal eye of rat fed glucose. (b) Cataract in xylose-fed rat. From Darby and Day (1940).

and only very young animals develop cataract. The changes in the lens are similar to those described in galactose toxicity but have the unusual feature of spontaneous reversibility with continuing ingestion of high concentrations of xylose. In susceptible strains of rats vacuoles appear in the equatorial region of the lens after 5 days of xylose feeding. They steadily increase in size and in the extent of the lens involved until the 12th or 15th day when they begin to regress, and by the 21st day only a few vacuoles remain in the periphery. Even in these susceptible strains only about 10% of the animals develop actual opacification. While the changes are progressing there is a loss of potassium from the lens, found also in galactose cataract, but in the case of xylose potassium reaccumulates as the lens changes regress. Van Heyningen (1958) has shown that there are certain differences in the way in which these two sugars are dealt with by the calf lens. Both penetrate the isolated lens to some extent. Galactose is phosphorylated and yields lactic acid, but xylose does not. In the intact lens xylose inhibits the formation of lactic acid but galactose does not have this effect.

In a comparison of the cataractogenic effect of xylose, galactose, and alloxan diabetes (Sterling and Day, 1951), in which a dietary level of 35% of the sugars was fed and two degrees of severity of pancreatic damage were employed, xylose was slightly more effective than galactose and much more so than the diabetes. The blood sugar level was higher in the alloxan treated rats, especially those receiving the larger dosage (Table XI) and this seemed to indicate that the type of sugar played a part, independent of the level of reducing sugar in the blood.

A clearer understanding of the biochemical changes that occur in this and the other sugar cataracts resulted from the studies of Van Heyningen (1959a, b). The polyol xylitol, corresponding to the sugar xylose, accumulates in the lens when the latter constitutes 35% of the diet. This takes place before clinical signs of cataract are evident. Sorbitol, the corresponding polyol of glucose, also accumulates to some extent. Both these polyols are found in the lenses of adult rats fed xylose, although these animals do not develop cataract. In young rats, after the cataracts have disappeared these polyols are still present in high concentration in the lens, but are not found in other tissues. Another approach to the causation of xylose cataract was made by Heggeness and Lerman (1960). It has been shown (Heggeness, 1960) that weanling rats fed diets with a high carbohydrate content show a transient rise in metabolic rate which is self-limiting. This so-called "calorigenic" response occurs at the period of greatest susceptibility to cataract formation. This response is abolished by feeding the animals sufficient of the high carbohydrate diet to permit only maintenance of body weight for several days, this process being termed "adaptation". Balance studies showed that the lens changes regressed without any alteration in the xylose intake or excretion. Furthermore, the especial susceptibility of the weanling rat to xylose cataract did not depend upon the calorigenic response it shows, and lens damage was even more severe in the adapted animals in which this response had been abolished.

Van Heyningen (1969) has shown that the regression of xylose cataract in the weanling rat and the resistance of the older rat to this form of cataract are due to a decrease in the concentration of blood xylose and a greater decrease in the ratio of blood xylose to blood sugar which causes a steep decrease in the concentration of xylitol in the lens and hence in the recovery from cataract.

Xylose readily penetrates the blood-aqueous barrier and enters the lens, resulting in the accumulation of xylitol and then sorbitol which gives rise to the same osmotic effects as previously described for dulcitol in galactose cataract. When the cataract begins to disappear in the young animal there is a resumption of monophosphate shunt activity and ATP synthesis.

C. Arabinose

Bellows and Chinn (1941) reported the development of cataract following

TABLE XI. *Blood Sugar Levels and Cataract in Alloxan Treated, Galactose Fed, and Xylose Fed Weanling Rats*[a]

| Group | No. of rats | Appearance of cataracts | | | | | | Blood sugar | |
| | | Incipient cataract | | Gross cataract | | No. of determinations | | |
		Average time (days)	Incidence (%)	Average time (days)	Incidence (%)			Level (mg/100 ml)
I Control	10	—	0	—	0	70		117.8 ±0.4[b]
II Galactose fed	10	4	100	20	90	80		244.5 ±3.9
III Xylose fed	9	3	100	7.5	90	77		301 ±32.1
IV Alloxan diabetics (150 mg/kg)[c]	9	17.6	77.8	—	0	82		292 ±88
V Alloxan diabetics (200–250 mg/kg)[c]	7	9.6	100	56	30	43		522.2 ±82.9

[a]From Sterling and Day (1951).
[b]Standard error of the mean.
[c]Size of single injected dose of alloxan.

the intravenous injection of arabinose. L-Arabinose is cataractogenic while the D-form of the other sugars has this property. It is, however, L- and not D-arabinose that has the configuration common to all the cataractogenic sugars. As a supplement to a D-galactose diet it was less effective in enhancing cataract formation than either xylose or galactose.

D. Experimental Diabetes Mellitus

Diabetes mellitus has been studied experimentally or spontaneously in at least four species of animal—monkey, dog, rat and Chinese hamster. As in humans, long duration of the diabetic state is necessary for ocular lesions to be produced.

Bellows (1944) mentions that turbidity of the lens was described more than 100 years ago following immersion of freshly removed lenses in strong hypertonic glucose solutions. He also refers to early claims that cataract could be produced by subcutaneous, intraperitoneal, subconjunctival, intra-ocular, and intravenous injection of glucose, but it has usually been found that a permanent raising of the blood sugar level is necessary. This has been done in a number of ways. Removal of the pancreas resulted in cataract formation in eight out of 10 dogs (Chaikoff and Lachman, 1933) as did almost total pancreatectomy in the rat (Foglia and Cramer, 1944). In a group of nine dogs made permanently diabetic by injections of anterior pituitary hormone one developed cataract (Dohan et al., 1941).

With the discovery in 1943 that alloxan causes almost complete necrosis of the beta cells of the islets of Langerhans without damaging the other parts of the pancreas a simpler method has been available for the production of permanent diabetes. Alloxan diabetes in rats and rabbits resulted in cataracts indistinguishable from those caused by pancreatectomy (Bailey et al., 1944). Anterior segment haemorrhages and corneal vascularization have also been observed frequently in rats with severe chronic diabetes (Janes and Ellis, 1957). More recently the same type of cataract has been produced by injections of ascorbone (oxidized ascorbic acid) (Patterson, 1952) in rats, and of diphenylthiocarbazone in rabbits (Butturini et al., 1953).

The early lens changes in alloxan-induced cataract in the rat have been studied under the biomicroscope and histologically (von Sallmann et al., 1958). Within a week or so after the injection of alloxan two types of lesion were observed under the slit lamp. The earliest change usually consisted of a complete or partial ring of densely packed short radial striae close to the equator. These striate opacities shortly gave way to typical subcapsular vacuoles. At this stage the ring of vacuoles resembled that seen in galactose cataract but in the following weeks the vacuoles tended to disappear, leaving a fine diffuse opacity behind. Another early appearance, less constant than the first, was a diffuse haze or greyish patch that assumed a star, Y, or circular shape near the surface portion of the anterior suture system. These opacities gave way later to spoke- or sector-shaped opacities of the anterior cortex, as in advanced stages of other experimental cataracts.

The histological changes were limited to the anterior cortex at first and comprised hydropic swelling of the lens fibres with cytoplasmic disintegration and epithelial proliferation (Fig. 99). Damage occurred most readily in

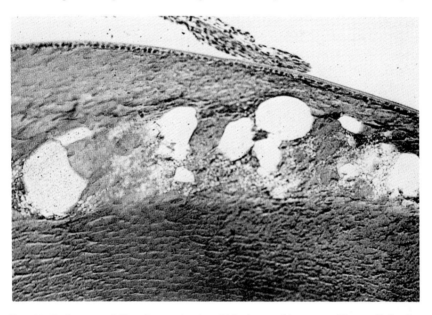

FIG. 99. Early stage of fibre destruction in middle layers of bow area. The small droplets confluate to larger vacuoles. Some of them are filled with granular debris. From von Sallmann *et al.* (1958).

deeply seated portions of the fibres near the lens bow and at the anterior endings of fibres near the suture system. Even when the anterior and posterior cortex were the seat of advanced cataract new fibres were being formed. At the anterior pole and sometimes elsewhere in the cell layer patchy areas of epithelial cells were seen which were apparently unrelated to the fibre pathology and were considered to distinguish this type from all other types of experimental cataract.

Various factors play a part in the development of diabetogenic cataract. One of these appears to be the severity of the diabetes itself. Thus it was found that rats which had had about 95 % of the pancreas removed developed cataract within 50 days, while less marked lens changes took more than 200 days to appear when only 80% of the pancreas was removed (Foglia and Cramer, 1944). In both alloxan- and ascorbone-induced cataract an inverse relationship has been found between the degree of glycosuria and hyperglycaemia and the time taken for the cataract to develop (Charalampous and Hegsted, 1950; Patterson, 1952). Further evidence for the importance of the blood glucose level is provided by delay in or prevention of cataract formation by insulin (Patterson, 1952). In the alloxan diabetic rat there is a disturbance of tryptophan metabolism (McDaniel *et al.*, 1956). Tryptophan deficiency readily results in cataract in the rat (Chapter 6, Section ID).

A study of lens metabolism with the reversible cation shift (Harris, *et al.*, 1954) has shown the importance of the optimum concentration of glucose. It appears that a high concentration of glucose has a deleterious effect on the lens, not due to osmotic pressure changes, but to some interference with the adenosine triphosphate (ATP) available to the lens for they showed that the effect of large amounts of glucose can be counteracted if adenosine triphosphate is added. There are grounds for believing that ATP mediates in the initial phosphorylation of all sugars and it has been suggested that the high blood sugar prevents either the absorption of a substance essential for the production of ATP or that it prevents the participation of ATP itself in the intracellular metabolic processes. In support of this is the report of the decreased ATP content of tissues of diabetic rats (Charalampous and Hegsted, 1950).

That the effect of insulin is due to lowering of the blood glucose and not by a direct effect was suggested by the results of Patterson (1953) in an experiment in which phlorizin prevented cataract. This substance does not relieve the symptoms of diabetes, but lowers the blood sugar by interfering with the reabsorption of glucose by the kidney tubules. Other means of lowering the blood sugar in the diabetic animal are also effective in alleviating the formation of cataract. These include the feeding of diets with a high fat (Charalampous and Hegsted, 1950) (see Chapter 8, Section IA) or high protein (Roderiguez and Krehl, 1951) content. The reduction in the blood sugar level and the associated protection against the development of cataract in diabetic rats starved for periods amounting to 40 hours per week has already been referred to (Chapter 1, Section A2).

On the other hand, the results of another experiment carried out by Patterson (1955) suggested that a high glucose blood level in itself was not responsible. He found that galactose-fed rats following unilateral carotid ligation developed cataract on the side with the better blood supply. However, this did not apply when the procedure was repeated on diabetic rats. These results led to the suggestion that the prevention of cataract by the measures adopted previously might be due to the provision of some other source of energy than glucose. This occurs in the ketosis that accompanies the administration of phlorizin, in starvation, and in the consumption of diets containing large amounts of fat or protein providing non-carbohydrates substrates for energy. Unfortunately in all these instances there is an accompanying lowering of the blood sugar. In a further experiment (Patterson, 1955) a high-fat diet (85% corn oil) and 50% fructose, with no glucose, was fed to diabetic rats with initial blood sugar levels in excess of 350 mg/100 ml blood. On this diet acceleration of the growth rate occurred and the blood sugar was maintained at this high level, despite which the development of cataract was prevented.

A diet rich in highly unsaturated fat from maize oil was reported to reduce the incidence of cataract and moderate the long-term effects of diabetes in streptozotocin-induced diabetes in rats (Hutton et al., 1976). Polyol intermediates were, however, only slightly increased as compared with controls.

The work of Van Heyningen (1959b) strongly suggested that the osmotic effects of sorbitol accumulation in the lens lead to the initial lesion in diabetic cataract. Sorbitol accumulation also causes irreversible change in the configuration of α-crystallin and brings to a halt activity of the hexose monophosphate shunt and protein synthesis (Patterson and Bunting, 1965).

Retinopathy developed more than 4 years after commencement of experimental diabetes in three out of 10 dogs (Engerman and Bloodworth, 1965). In two spontaneously diabetic, related, dogs on histological examination dilatation of retinal arterioles was present in one and diabetic retinopathy with typical micro-aneurysms of the capillaries in the other (Sibay and Hausler, 1967). Retinopathy has been described in rats receiving 72% of a diet as sucrose from the time they were 70 g in weight until 10–12 months of age (Cohen et al., 1972; Yanko et al., 1972a, and b). There was looping of retinal capillaries and micro-aneurysms, loss of both segments of rods and extensive loss of nuclei in the outer nuclear layer.

E. Hypoglycaemic Cataract

Greiner and Chylack (1976) studied the mechanism of formation of cataract in the isolated rat lens exposed to a low level of glucose. Cataract and other ocular abnormalities have been reported in the human newborn (Section IID). In an incubating medium with less than 2.0 mM glucose thin lamellar opacities occurred on the anterior and posterior lens surfaces. Wet weight and sodium concentration increased, while potassium, ATP and hexokinase activity fell. Nuclear cataract occurred after 48 hours deprivation of glucose. Thermal deactivation of hexokinase follows rapidly upon depletion of its substrates, ATP and glucose. The hexokinase competitive inhibitor,

2-deoxyglucose, blocks the entry of glucose into the glycolytic sequence and cataract results.

II. Human Studies

A. Galactosaemia

This is an autosomal recessive condition in which there is deficiency of the enzyme galactose-1-phosphate uridyl transferase involved in the conversion of galactose to glucose. It can be measured in erythrocytes and tissue culture.

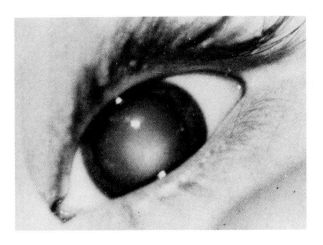

Fig. 100. Complete opacification of lens in patient with untreated galactosaemia. From Sugar, A. and Podos, S. M. (1975). *In* "The Eye and Systemic Disease" (Ed. F. A. Mausolf), Mosby, St Louis.

Galactose-1-phosphate and its reduction product dulcitol (galactitol) accumulate in tissue, the latter seeming to be more important in cataract formation (Gitzelmann *et al.*, 1967). Galactose comes from lactose in milk. Features include failure to thrive, hepatosplenomegaly, hypoglycaemic convulsions, jaundice, aminoaciduria and mental retardation.

Cataract occurs in about 70% of cases (Fig. 100). Vacuolar "oil droplet" changes occur early and may be present in the first week of life. Lens changes have even been reported in the fetus, in which the defect was diagnosed by amniocentesis and tissue culture (Vannas *et al.*, 1975). Later lens changes may be anterior cortical, zonular, lamellar, or posterior cortical. It is not established whether heterozygotes have an increased incidence of cataracts (see Chapter 11, Section B). Variants are described; the "Duarte" variant being asymptomatic (Gitzelmann *et al.*, 1967), but the "Indiana" variant is associated with nuclear cataract (Chacko *et al.*, 1971).

Treatment of all forms of galactosaemia consists in dietary elimination of galactose and if instituted early in infancy may prevent cataract formation and progression, and even lead to regression of early changes (Kinoshita, 1965). Experimentally the enzyme deficiency may be corrected in skin fibroblast culture from galactosaemic patients by transduction with a bacteriophage containing the transferase gene, suggesting the possible treatment with genetic engineering in the future (Merril *et al.*, 1971).

B. Galactokinase Deficiency

The first step in glactose metabolism is dependent upon this enzyme, a deficiency of which produces cataracts similar to those in transferase deficiency. In contradistinction to galactosaemia, patients are usually otherwise healthy. Beutler *et al.* (1973) studied 106 patients developing cataract in the first year of life. Two had a total deficiency of galactokinase and there was a significant lowering of the enzyme in the others, but not in patients developing cataract later in life. Levy *et al.* (1972) found early onset of cataract in 1 out of 7 heterozygotes for this enzyme deficiency. Many mothers of children with unexplained cataracts have low galactokinase activity although the children had normal levels (Harley *et al.*, 1974).

Galactose restriction is indicated for both patients and carriers and regression of lens changes may occur under treatment (Levy *et al.*, 1972).

C. Diabetes Mellitus

The eye is among the organs most seriously affected by this condition and there is an extensive literature on the subject. The ocular manifestations are summarized here and more detailed information is to be found in the monograph of Caird *et al.* (1969).

Transient visual symptoms include a myopic change as a common initial occurrence and, less commonly, a hyperopic change which characteristically develops a few days after the institution of insulin therapy. There may be the rapid onset of a diminution in the brightness of the red reflex when the blood sugar becomes elevated and an increase in brightness after insulin. Slit-lamp examination revealed that the anterior part of the lens was the site of reversible opacification (Vere and Verel, 1955). The refractive changes may be related to lens swelling consequent upon sorbitol accumulation and its spread to the nucleus in the reflex changes (Huggert, 1954).

It has been known for many years that the diabetic patient is prone to develop cataract (Fig. 101). Patterson (1952) has shown that the speed of development of cataract is directly related to the degree of hyperglycaemia and therefore to the concentration of glucose in the aqueous humour. Two morphological forms of cataract occur in the diabetic patient: one form is senile cataract, in which the changes are indistinguishable from those usually met in aged subjects; however, in diabetes they occur more frequently, at an earlier age, and tend to progress more rapidly. The second form is true diabetic cataract, first described by O'Brien et al., (1934), is invariably bilateral and characterized by dense bands of white spots in a subscapsular position—"snowflake cataract" in the anterior and posterior cortex. There are also fine needle-shaped opacities of uniform diameter located in the

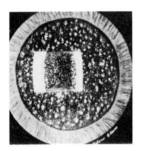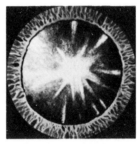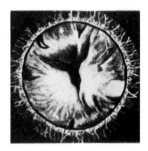

FIG. 101. The true diabetic cataract (left) with numerous white, flaky opacities in the cortex gives the appearance of a snowstorm. The more common type of true diabetic cataract (centre) is a posterior subcapsular opacity with radial striae extending into it from the equatorial zone. In more advanced stages (right) lens fibres become distorted with the formation of vacuoles and clefts between them.

posterior subcapsular area, with vacuoles and water clefts and separation of the sutures. The snowflake type of opacity may occasionally be the first manifestation of diabetes. This type of cataract is rare in occurrence. It may appear at an early age in infantile diabetes, is more common in adolescents, and gets less frequent in middle and old age. Characteristically, the cataract matures rapidly, especially in the young, sometimes within a few hours. It may be preceded by the development of myopia of sudden onset.

Corkscrew-like appearance of the conjunctival vessels was reported in 75% of 100 diabetic patients, with 100% incidence in those who had the disease for 11 years and more (Mesropian, 1970). Diminished corneal sensitivity, as measured by an aesthesiometer, seemed to be related to the duration of the disease rather than the age of the patient (Schwartz, 1974).

Safir and Rogers (1970) measured intraocular pressure in 65 patients with juvenile-onset diabetes; aged less than 25 years, with sudden onset and insulin dependency. In 10% the pressure was definitely raised and only 7%

had a pressure less than 15 mmHg. Using applanation tonometry and tonography in 390 patients Armaly (1967) found no abnormality of intraocular pressure. In a study of 45 patients under 20 years and 211 over 20 years of age Armaly and Baloglou (1967) found a greater incidence than in non-diabetic subjects of conjunctival micro-aneurysms (8%), deposition of pigment on the posterior surface of the cornea, anterior iris and in the trabecular meshwork (32%), and ectropion uveae (72%). In a postmortem study of 57 diabetic patients, Smith and Glickman (1975) found a lace-like vacuolation of the iris pigment epithelium with similar changes in renal tubules in 19 out of 23 of those with a blood glucose greater than 200 mg/100 ml before death. This change was absent in those with lower blood glucose.

There is an association between diabetes and asteroid hyalitis (Benson's disease) and also synchisis scintillans affecting the vitreous (Bankes, 1971).

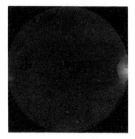

FIG. 102. Diabetic retinopathy. The vascular changes are predominantly at the posterior pole of the eye with "dot and blot" haemorrhages and hard exudates arranged side by side. There are minimal arteriovenous changes. By kind permission of Mr Ching, Oxford Eye Hospital.

Ophthalmoplegia and optic atrophy have only occasionally been reported but there is a high frequency of lipaemia retinalis accompanying diabetes (Chapter 8, Section IIA).

Retinopathy is the most serious ocular complication of diabetes (Fig. 102). Caird et al. (1969) describe seven features of the clinical picture: micro-aneurysms, abnormalities of retinal veins, haemorrhages, exudates, new vessel formation, glial proliferation, and vitreous detachment. The relationship of the development and progress of the condition to control of the diabetic state is not finally settled, but it is probable that good control, at least in the young, reduces the frequency and delays the appearance of retinopathy. Lundbaek et al. (1970) claimed that hypophysectomy in juvenile diabetics inhibited the development of retinopathy by lowering growth hormone.

The effect of alteration of diet on diabetic retinopathy is clearly difficult to study. King et al. (1963) reported their findings in 40 patients with exudative changes which took three main forms: clusters of small deposits, ring formation, or a large waxy-looking plaque. Twenty-five patients received their usual diet and 17 patients (26 eyes) consumed over 3 years a diet of 20 g animal fat and 60 g unsaturated vegetable fat per day. The groups were matched for age, sex, duration of diabetes, and treatment. The blood cholesterol fell in the group receiving the diet high in unsaturated fat. In 21 of the 26 eyes of the patients of this group there was a significant acceleration of disappearance of exudates. However, visual acuity was not improved, probably because its impairment was related to neuronal degeneration which was unaffected by treatment.

In the 1950s there were several reports of abnormal vitamin B_{12} metabolism in diabetic retinopathy (see McLaren, 1963) but these were not confirmed by others and there was no obvious improvement with vitamin B_{12} therapy (Keen and Smith, 1959).

D. Neonatal Hypoglycaemia

Severe hypoglycaemia may occur in the first few days of life, especially in the infant small for gestational age, as a result of deficient glycogen stores or hyperinsulinism, accentuated by fasting.

The ocular findings include cataract, esotropia, nystagmus and optic atrophy and are often associated with disorders of the central nervous system (McKinna, 1966). Ketosis usually accompanies these changes (Wilson, 1970). The mechanism probably resembles that seen in the comparable state in experimental work (Section IE).

Chapter 8

Lipids

An overall deficient dietary intake of fat does not result in disease. Energy deficit may be made good from carbohydrate or protein. The essential fatty acids have to be provided by the diet, and although deficiency has been shown in experimental animals to affect the eye (Section IC) ocular dysfunction has not been reported in the few instances of deficiency in man.

An excessive intake of saturated fat and cholesterol predisposes to lipid deposition in tissues and the eye is among the organs affected. Some disorders of lipid metabolism may result in ocular manifestations and those that are amenable to dietary management will be considered here.

I. Animal Studies

A. Dietary Fat

Analyses of the lipid content of various ocular tissues have been done (Pirie and van Heyningen, 1956). As might be expected, the retina, anatomically part of the brain, has a high concentration.

The effect of varying the fat content of experimental diets has been observed on the development of corneal vascularization induced by the riboflavin antagonist galactoflavin (Kaunitz *et al.,* 1954). A fat-free diet was found to delay the onset of galactoflavin-induced vascularization and would seem to indicate some role of fat in riboflavin metabolism. A fat-free diet also delayed the appearance of cataract in the diabetic rat (Charalampous and Hegsted, 1950) but high fat diets caused even greater protection, preventing the development of cataract for as long as 120 days. Delay in the development of experimental diabetic cataract also resulted from high dietary levels of fat in the work of Roderiguez and Krehl (1951) and of Nieman (1955), and also of Busulfan (1,4-dimethanesulphonoxybutane) cataract (Light *et al.,* 1956).

B. Cholesterol

Cholesterol is obtained from the diet and also synthesized in the body for production of bile acids and steroid hormones. Diets high in cholesterol fed

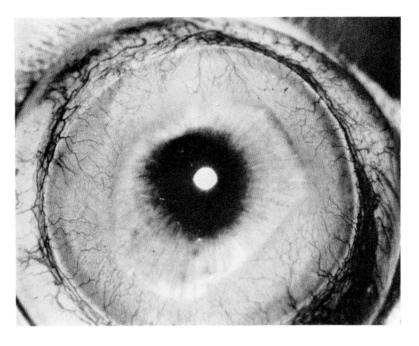

FIG. 103. Arcus of hypercholesterolaemic rabbit. From D. G. Cogan and T. Kuwabara (1959a).

to rabbits induce atherosclerotic lesions more readily in the aorta than in coronary, cerebral or ocular arteries (Suga, 1960) and the relevance of this state to human atherosclerosis is doubtful.

Cogan and Kuwabara (1959a) studied experimental and human corneal arcus (see Section IIA) and have shown that the two conditions differ materially.

After several months on a high-cholesterol diet albino rabbits show yellowish masses between the root of the iris and the pupillary margin on the posterior surface of the iris. The corneal changes consist of an arcus continuous with the limbus and involving only the anterior part of the stroma and vessels invading it from the limbal plexus (Fig. 103).

Janes (1964) found fatty lesions in all parts of the eye except the lens in 2–6 months feeding of a diet containing 0.75% cholesterol to rabbits. Aortic transplants in the anterior chamber led to greater accumulation of cholesterol in the operated eye, especially in the uveal tract and sclera, in the hypercholesterolaemic animal (Rubenstein *et al.,* 1967). Experimentally induced atherosclerotic retinopathy undergoes some improvement as judged by the ERG and planimetry of retinal blood vessels in response to essential phospholipid dosing in the form of polyunsaturated phosphatidylcholine (Samochowiec, 1976).

One report (Lijo Pavia, 1954) described arterial constriction in four dogs fed a milk diet with additions of from 1 to 6 g of cholesterol daily. This arterial constriction gradually intensified until the end of the experiment, which lasted 16 weeks, and was reversed when ingestion of cholesterol was stopped. After 3 or 4 weeks on the diet cholesterol crystals appeared in the retina, disappeared in 3 to 5 weeks when cholesterol ingestion was stopped, and appeared again when it was resumed 3 weeks later. In one dog given injections of a lipotropic substance, the crystals did not reappear.

These workers were able to produce a lesion resembling arcus senilis by injecting hypercholesterolaemic plasma into the cornea of rabbits. They conclude that in arcus senilis the fat is probably not the result of active lipogenesis by the cornea but a deposition of blood fat in the stromal extracellular spaces.

Lipaemia retinalis, comparable to that in man (Section IIA) has been the subject of single case reports of the condition occurring spontaneously in a cat and a dog with elevated serum lipids (Wyman and McKissick, 1973).

C. Essential Fatty Acid Deficiency

Rigid exclusion of fat from an otherwise adequate diet results in skin changes and death. Polyunsaturated fatty acids linoleic acid ($18:2\omega6$), the major dietary source, and arachidonic acid ($20:4\omega6$), made from the former in the liver, prevent the disease. Linolenic acid ($18:3\omega3$) promotes growth, prevents death but does not affect the skin lesions. The formulae indicate the number of carbon atoms, the number of double bonds, and the position of the double bond nearest the methyl terminus, counting from the same, indicated by the symbol ω.

Hands *et al.* (1965) reported impaired visual acuity in rats fed a diet free from fat. In essential fatty acid deficiency an abnormal metabolite of oleic acid, $20:3\omega9$ accumulates. Anderson and Maude (1972) found that this metabolite accumulated in all tissues examined except the retina and photoreceptor membranes in essential fatty acid deficiency. As these membranes are renewed every 9 days they suggested that the retina has a mechanism for preserving the linolenic acid family ($\omega3$) of polyunsaturates, of which $22:6\omega3$ is dominant in rod outer segment membranes. Wheeler *et al*. (1975) studied the effect of the precursors of linolenic acid and linoleic acid on the ERG of deficient rats. The former had a greater effect than the latter, consistent with the known composition of rod outer segment membrane phospholipids.

Dudley *et al*. (1975) found that there was no decrease in rhodopsin content, phospholipid—rhodopsin ratio, or protein content of outer segment membranes and no electron microscopic changes in photoreceptors or membranes. Yet it was also shown (Anderson *et al.,* 1976) that outer segment disc renewal almost ceases in the deficient albino rat, suggesting that the removal of photoreceptor membranes by new disc formation is a function of polyunsaturated fatty acid availability and that they provide the proper viscosity for events associated with visual excitation or a unique hydrophobic environment.

Futterman *et al*. (1968) found that the synthesis of polyenoic fatty acids was depressed in the retina of diabetic animals. In a subsequent study of rats fed a diet deficient in essential fatty acids Forrest and Futterman (1972) came to the conclusion that this deficiency was probably not responsible for the loss of intramural pericytes from capillaries in the posterior pole of the retina characteristic of diabetes mellitus (see Chapter 7, Sections ID and IIC).

II. Human Studies

A. Hyperlipoproteinaemias

This complex group of disorders is determined by many factors both genetic and environmental. Heredity and diet predispose to hyperlipidaemia, especially hypercholesterolaemia, and through the development of atherosclerosis and hypertension, and accentuated by such factors as heavy cigarette smoking, physical inactivity and stress a variety of diseases affecting primarily the cardiovascular system occur (Connor and Connor, 1972).

In the familial hyperlipoproteinaemias, as classified by Fredrickson *et al*. (1978) ocular involvement varies considerably. In type I (familial lipoprotein lipase deficiency) lipaemia retinalis and palpebral eruptive xanthomas occur. Less frequently iris xanthomas, lipid keratopathy and adult onset Coats' syndrome are found (Vinger and Sachs, 1970). In the common disorder type II (familial hypercholesterolaemia) xanthelasmas are common and xanthomas may occasionally be seen in various ocular tissues. Arcus senilis occurs in 10% of patients under 30, and 50% of patients under 50 years of age (Berman, 1974). This is the only type of lipoproteinaemia in which lipaemia retinalis does not seem to have been reported. Type III is associated with tuberous or eruptive lid xanthomas, arcus senilis and Schnyder's crystalline corneal dystrophy. Lipaemia retinalis and of the limbal vessels is described (Bron and Williams, 1972). In type IV (familial hypertriglyceridaemia) palpebral eruptive xanthomas and lipaemia retinalis may occur. Bolmers (1975) reported two patients with progressive diminution of visual acuity: one had coarse granular macular pigmentation and the other had macular degeneration sicca and a narrow arterial system. Type V carries a very high incidence of palpebral eruptive xanthomas and lipaemia retinalis. Kurz *et al.* (1976) reported multiple retinal haemorrhages in a fatal case and another patient in whom vision was low due to occlusion of many retinal arteries by lipid.

In lipaemia retinalis all the retinal vessels have a creamy-opalescent appearance and the whole fundus takes on an orange hue. It is said to occur only when serum triglyceride levels exceed 2500 mg% (Vinger and Sachs, 1970).

Xanthelasma, or xanthoma planum, usually appears in the third or fourth decade, developing symmetrically on the inner third of the upper lids. It consists of slightly elevated, indurated, yellowish-brown plaques in the skin. Larger, darker and more elevated lesions, xanthoma tuberosum, may affect the limbs and also the viscera. There is a more frequent association with cardiovascular disease than there is for xanthelasma.

Human arcus senilis contrasts in a number of ways with the arcus produced experimentally (Cogan and Kuwabara, 1955, 1959b) see also Section IB; as shown in Table XII.

Arcus senilis seems to depend to some extent on the presence of proximal blood vessels but spares the immediate environs of these vessels (Cogan and Kuwabara, 1959a). It thus frequently occurs in an irregular fashion in relation to paralimbal vascularization and must be distinguished from the arcus due to chronic local infection (Fig. 68).

The correlation between serum lipid levels and degree of arcus senilis formation was studied by Forsius (1954) in 165 individuals of various ages. In those below the age of 50 there was a direct relationship between the degree of arcus and the serum cholesterol and phospholipid values. In this age group the mean cholesterol concentration was 44% higher for those with arcus than those without. After the age of 50 arcus formation depended not on altered fat metabolism but was related to local senile changes. Friedman

TABLE XII. *Comparison of Experimentally Induced Arcus and Arcus Senilis in Man*[a]

Hypercholesterolaemic rabbit	Human arcus senilis
Clinical features	
Directly related to blood cholesterol level	So related before 50, after this to local senile change
Almost entirely in superficial cornea	Throughout depth of stroma and including Bowman's and Descemet's membranes
No sparing of paralimbal region	Paralimbal region spared
Always vascularized	Not vascularized but depends on presence of proximal vessels
Scintillating crystals present	No crystals
Pathological changes	
Bowman's and Descemet's membranes not involved preferentially	Diffuse sudanophilia in periphery of Bowman's and Descemet's membranes
Only most superficial layers of stroma affected by globular intracellular lipid and accompanying histiocytosis	Granular sudanophilia of limbal portions of entire thickness of stroma with lipid extracellular and no accompanying changes

[a]After D. G. Cogan and T. Kuwabara (1959b).

and Rosenman (1959) found a threefold increase of arcus senilis in a group of men with chronic "excessive and competitive drive and an enhanced sense of time urgency" in comparison with men of the opposite type of behaviour.

Patients with hypercholesterolaemia have been treated with low-fat diets in the past with only moderate success. It may be that a diet high in polyunsaturated fatty acids and perhaps the use of substances which interfere with the synthesis of cholesterol, such as δ,4-cholesterone, will give better results in the future. The report (Laughlin, 1962) of a toxic type of cataract developing after the use of one of these blood cholesterol-lowering agents sounds a note of warning. In any case there is sufficient evidence of the value

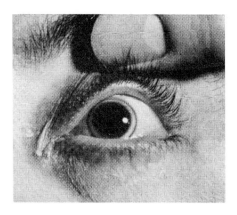

FIG. 104. Arcus of familial hypercholesterolaemia. From Cogan and Kuwabara (1959a).

of these ocular signs as possible indications of disturbed lipid metabolism to justify a general examination of subjects in whom they appear.

The terms arcus senilis and gerontoxon are inappropriate for those lesions seen in the hyperlipoproteinaemias (Finley *et al.*, 1961; Macaraeg *et al.*, 1968) and premature arcus is more suitable (Rifkind, 1972).

Hollenhorst (1961) first reported the presence of bright, orange-coloured plaques at the bifurcations of retinal arterioles in about 10% of patients with occlusive disease within the carotid and vertebral-basilar arterial systems (Fig. 105); he suggested that they were cholesterol emboli. Russell-Ross (1963) reported three similar cases. Hollenhorst in 1966 reported on 208 consecutive cases with cholesterol emboli in the retina: 63% had new or old strokes or transient ischaemic attacks, 59% had clinical ischaemic heart disease, 42% moderate to severe peripheral arteritis obliterans, 16% aortic abdominal aneurysms, and 12% retinal arteriolar occlusions.

Dietary management varies with the type of hyperlipoproteinaemia. In type I chylomicronaemia is reduced to a minimum by a very low fat diet (40–60 g daily for an adult). Degree of saturation is unimportant. Medium-chain triglycerides, absorbed by the portal tract, are a useful supplementary source of energy. Type II responds partially to limitation of total cholesterol daily intake to 300 mg for adults and 150 mg for children. Saturated fat should be reduced and polyunsaturated fat increased. Other measures may also be necessary to restore the blood cholesterol to normal, such as cholestyramine, parenteral nutrition, portacaval shunt surgery or plasma exchange.

Diet is most effective in type III. Calories are restricted until initial body

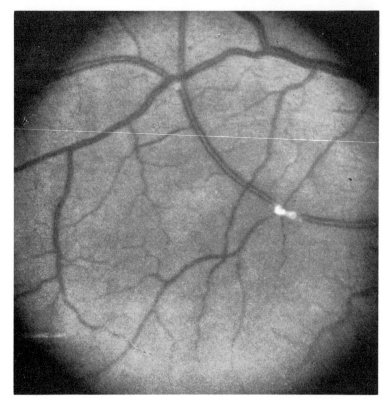

FIG. 105. Two plaques of cholesterol on retinal arterioles. From Hollenhorst (1961).

weight is attained, if indicated. Alcohol intake is restricted. Energy should come from carbohydrate (40%) and fats (40%), much of the latter from polyunsaturated acids. Type IV usually responds to weight reduction and carbohydrate restriction; and type V to strict energy balance and limitation of dietary fat to 30–50 g daily.

B. Abetalipoproteinaemia

This autosomal recessive disorder is also known as the Bassen-Kornzweig syndrome. There is a failure in lipid transport. Malabsorption, steatorrhoea, ataxia and posterior column disease, and misshapen erythrocytes (acanthocytes) are features in childhood. Cardiovascular disease appears in early adulthood.

Nystagmus, strabismus and ptosis are common. There may be a blue-yellow colour vision defect (Khachadurian *et al.*, 1971). Three patients with ophthalmoplegia were reported by Yee *et al.* (1976a): electronystagmography in one patient revealed abnormally slow voluntary saccades and slow or

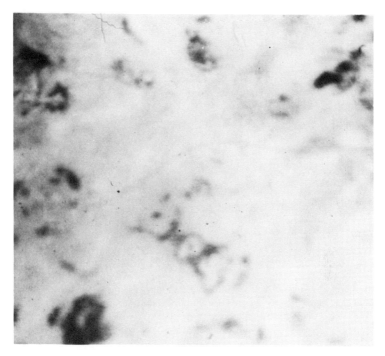

FIG. 106. Typical blotches and spicules of pigment in periphery of retina in patient with abetalipoproteinaemia. From Sugar, A. and Podos, S. M. (1975) *In* "The Eye and Systemic Disease" (Ed. F. A. Mausolf), Mosby, St Louis.

absent fast components of vestibular nystagmus, opticokinetic nystagmus and jerk-type dissociated nystagmus. They postulated that these findings may be accounted for by changes in the centres that generate saccadic eye movements.

The major eye changes are retinal pigmentary degeneration with arteriolar narrowing and pigment clumping in the midperiphery or with areas of pigment atrophy (Figs. 106 to 108). The picture sometimes resembles retinitis punctata albescens. Optic nerve pallor and posterior pole degeneration may be seen (Jampel and Falls, 1958). Abnormal fields, impaired dark adaptation and abnormal ERG findings are usual (Sperling *et al.*, 1972). Histopathology shows loss of rods, cones and the outer granular layer and deposition of rounded bodies in the optic nerve (von Sallmann *et al.*, 1969).

Improvement of the retinal changes has been observed with parenteral vitamin A therapy (Gouras *et al.*, 1971; Sperling *et al.*, 1972). Due to failure in transport there is vitamin A deficiency which is known to damage the retina in experimental animals and in man (Chapter 2, Section IC and III4*i*).

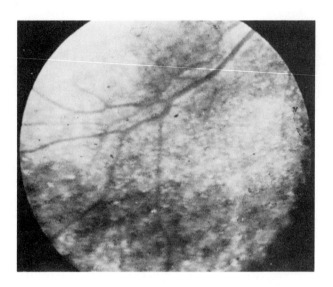

FIG. 107. Flecked retina similar to retinitis punctata albescens in abetalipoproteinaemia. This patient demonstrated greatly reduced electroretinogram amplitude, contracted fields, and night blindness. From Sugar, A. and Podos, S. M. (1975). *In* "The Eye and Systemic Disease" (Ed. F. A. Mausolf), Mosby, St Louis.

Vitamin A therapy should be instituted as soon as diagnosis is made but it is not known yet whether retinal damage can thus be prevented.

A recent study (Muller *et al.*, 1977) of eight patients followed from 3.4 to 15.8 years provided evidence of delay in the progression of retinal and neurological lesions in the three oldest patients that may have been related to large oral doses of vitamin E. The diet was restricted in fat, and vitamin A was also given.

C. Familial Hypobetalipoproteinaemia

This is a genetic disorder considered to be distinct from abetalipoproteinaemia. Some homozygotes may develop retinal degeneration indistinguishable from that of abetalipoproteinaemia (Yee *et al.*, 1976b). Heterozygotes may have asymptomatic retinal changes.

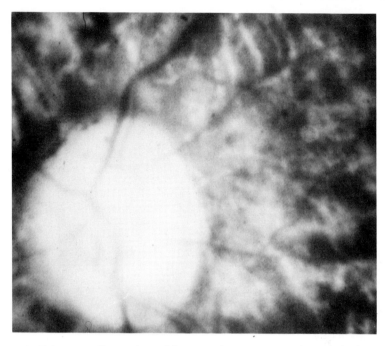

FIG. 108. Pale, waxy disc, and arteriolar narrowing accompany the retinal pigmentary degeneration in abetalipoproteinaemia. Note pigment splotches near the macula. From Sugar, A. and Podos, S. M. (1975) In "The Eye and Systemic Disease" (Ed. F. A. Mausolf), Mosby, St Louis.

D. Refsum's Disease

This recessively inherited defect is due to the absence of phytanic acid α hydroxylase. As a result there is failure in the α oxidation of certain exogenous fatty acids, especially phytanic acid, which accumulates in tissues and damages them. Fish oils and ruminant products are especially rich.

Clinical features include cerebrellar ataxia, peripheral polyneuropathy, tremors, paresis and sensory loss. Heart disease, deafness and ichthyosis also occur. The onset may be from childhood until the fifth decade. Periods of exacerbation and remission are typical.

Nystagmus is usually present. Night blindness is often the presenting symptom. It is associated with a pigmentary retinopathy of mottled salt and pepper or bone spicule appearance (Figs. 109 and 110). Retinal arterioles are often narrowed and the ERG may be diminished or extinct. Visual field loss is common. Posterior cortical or subcapsular cataracts are present in about

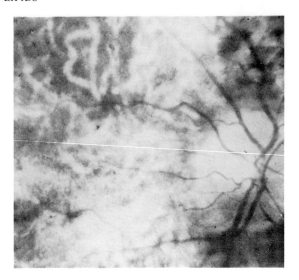

FIG. 109. Posterior pole in Refsum's disease demonstrating pallor of optic nerve head, arteriolar narrowing, and retinal pigmentary disease. From Sugar, A. and Podos, S. M. (1975) *In* "The Eye and Systemic Disease" (Ed. F. A. Mausolf), Mosby, St Louis.

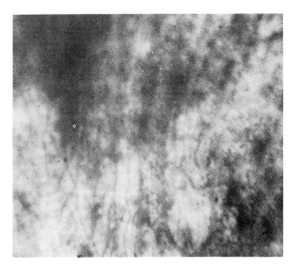

FIG. 110. Retinal periphery in Refsum's disease may show mottling, salt-and-pepper pattern, or bone spicule pigmentary degeneration. From Sugar, A. and Podos, S. M. (1975). *In* "The Eye and Systemic Disease" (Ed. F. A. Mausolf), Mosby, St Louis.

35% of cases (Steinberg, 1978). Pathologic examination has shown lipid deposition in the retinal pigment epithelium, iris and trabecular meshwork, with degeneration of photoreceptors (Toussaint and Danis, 1971).

Baum *et al.* (1965) reported a single case of supposed Refsum's disease with bullous keratopathy. However, it is doubtful that this was a correct diagnosis as phytanic acid could not be identified in the corneal button removed at surgery, nor in the urine, serum, or liver.

Dietary management is designed to prevent the intake of those foods rich in phytanic acid. These include fat meat and fish, whole dairy products and foods made from them such as chocolate; most vegetables, and nuts. Permitted items include skimmed milk and lean cheese, potatoes, one orange per day, lean meat and fish, all cereals and butter-free cakes, sugar, sweets and all kinds of drinks. Considerable improvement has resulted from prolonged dietary treatment but this does not apply to the ocular manifestations so far studied.

Chapter 9

Pre-natal Influences

There is good reason for devoting a special chapter to malformations of the eye arising as a result of nutritional deficiency *in utero*. Ocular lesions were among the first reported to occur in this way (Section IA*1*) and as the spectrum of nutrients involved has been broadened in later years the eye has continued to figure prominently in the accounts of organs affected in a variety of deficiency states.

Various factors will determine the level of requirement of nutrients. Among these must be considered the bulk of the new living material to be formed, the actual amounts of nutrients that will be used, and the varying rates at which they will be utilized. It has been shown that the nutrient requirements, the intensity of metabolism, and the speed of synthesis of tissue all decrease with the age of the fetus so that by birth almost the entire original power of growth has been expended.

Malformations are not the only harmful effects that malnutrition may have in association with the origin and intrauterine development of mammalian life. Reproduction itself may be prevented. Resorption or abortion of the fetus may take place depending upon the species. These occur if the deficiency state is such that life cannot be created or maintained under its malevolent influence. Malformations are characteristic of the embryonic stage and may or may not be associated with death of the fetus, depending upon the intensity of the deficiency and to some extent upon the nature of the malformation. Less marked deficiency may lead to no malformations but result in underdevelopment. It is also possible for lesions to appear in the fetus similar to those found after birth. Thus in fetal rickets the bone changes are identical with those in the young, and keratinization of the epithelium of the urinary tract has been observed in the vitamin A-deficient fetus as is characteristic of the deficiency state *ex utero*.

It is evident that the interrelationship of nutrients is of very great importance before birth. An imbalance of vitamins brought about by absence of a specific vitamin in the presence of normal amounts of the others has been found to be more harmful than a generalized deficiency. It has been suggested by Millen and Woollam (1958) that the teratogenic effects of hypervitaminosis A may be brought about by inducing a deficiency of vitamins of the B complex, for adding these vitamins prevented malformations due to excess vitamin A. Similarly a general deficiency of protein or starvation do not appear to have teratogenic effects.

The type of congenital malformation produced is influenced by the nature of the deficiency. Thus, vitamin A deficiency affects particularly mesodermal tissue and its derivatives, while deficiency of riboflavin produces micromelia, syndactyly, and cleft palate; and of pantothenic acid defects of the brain and eye. If a vitamin antagonist is employed to induce the deficiency state the abnormalities are much more varied and the characteristic syndromes are obscured.

Of equal importance on the type and incidence of the malformations induced by dietary deficiency is the effect of the stage of embryonic development. This has been demonstrated most clearly in work where antivitamins have been employed to create a sudden deficiency at various stages throughout gestation. This relationship will be illustrated later in connection with the production of some of the ocular abnormalities.

Little is known concerning the precise mechanisms whereby the various deficiency states have their teratogenic effects. Many of the vitamins are components of enzymes and may be implicated in this way, while lack of specific amino acids would interfere with protein synthesis. It is also possible that deficiency states in the mother may have an indirect effect on the fetus through disturbances of the endocrine glands.

In this connection mention may be made of the high percentage of eye defects that occurred in the rat embryo after thyroidectomy in the mother animal (Langman and van Faassen, 1955). These malformations consisted of all degrees of lens opacity, sometimes giving the strange appearance of several small lenses having been formed within one larger lens. Other defects observed were peripheral and central folding of the retina and some cases had coloboma and even anophthalmos.

That the teratogenic effect of nutritional factors may be modified by the presence of hormonal and other influences was shown by the potentiation of the teratogenic effect of hypervitaminosis A by cortisone, although it did not itself cause malformations (Millen and Woollam, 1957). A similar enhancing of the effect of hypervitaminosis A has been found to result from immobilization stress (Härtel and Härtel, 1960) In both these experiments deformities of the brain and calvaria were especially studied and eye lesions were not recorded. However, these are known to occur in hypervitaminosis A in the rat (see below, Section IA2) and in the figure in Millen and Woollam's paper it appears that at least two of the animals have ocular defects.

It is now recognized that pathological regression of previously well formed parts is an important process in the production of congenital malformations (Gruenwald, 1958). Necrosis is a normal factor in the development of the embryo and it is possible that some defects may arise merely as an exaggeration of the normal mechanism. The results of this work as they affect the eye are presented below, Section IJ.

Genetic factors have been shown to play a role in malformations induced by dietary deficiency as well as in those of different aetiology. Species differences have already been referred to and are of particular practical importance when the possibility of human maternal malnutrition being responsible for congenital defects is considered. That similar defects may arise in different ways in different species is exemplified by conditions of the retina in the mouse and rat (Grunëberg, 1943). In the mouse the condition known as "rodless retina" develops as a hereditary trait during the early postnatal period as the result of an arrest of development. In the rat a similar trait follows degeneration of a normally formed retina somewhat later in postnatal life (see also Chapter 2, Section IC). Due caution must be exercised to avoid the dangers of extrapolation of results in experimental animals and their application to the human situation. The evidence in this regard is considered in Section II.

I. Animal Studies

A. Vitamin A

1. *Vitamin A Deficiency*

Soon after the identification of the vitamin it was shown that the changes due to the oestrus cycle in the uterus of the rat do not take place in the absence of vitamin A and keratin scales are found continuously in the vaginal smear. Later it was found that testicular degeneration occurs in the male. The first demonstration of congenital malformations induced in the offspring by a maternal dietary deficiency was by Hale (1935) in the vitamin A-deficient pig. He fed sows on diets low in vitamin A for from 150 to 200 days before breeding and during the first few days of gestation. Some fetuses died and others were born puny. Prominent among the defects observed was arrested development of the eyes, amounting in some instances to complete anophthalmos. Other deformities included accessory ears, harelip and cleft palate, subcutaneous cysts and horseshoe kidneys.

Later, working with the rat, Warkany and Schraffenberger (1946) produced many congenital defects in vitamin A deficiency with the eye again being constantly affected. This time the structure of the eye was examined in detail. Out of 140 female rats that were raised and then mated on a diet low in the vitamin, and that were given no vitamin A at all during gestation, seven produced litters at term. All the eyes of the young were abnormal, the changes consisting of absence or maldevelopment of the anterior chamber, the iris, and the ciliary body; failure of the vitreous body to form, its place being taken by connective tissue which entered the eye through a coloboma

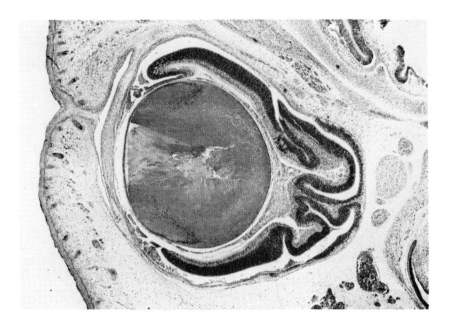

Fig. 111. Folding and eversion of the retina in the newborn rat due to maternal vitamin A deficiency. From Warkany and Schraffenberger (1946).

or cleft in the lower part of the retina; and folding and disorganization of the retina which had the appearance in some instances of cerebral tissue (Fig. 111). In the normal rat the eyelids have fused by the 18th day of intrauterine life but in some of these fetuses the condition of "open eye" was present, the eye being exposed on the surface of the body due to the failure of the lids to fuse in the normal way.

Palludan (1966) carried out an extensive study on the effect of vitamin A deficiency on the progeny of 36 gilts or sows. Of the 299 young born, 251 showed microphthalmos. Some had anophthalmos and abnormalities of rods and cones.

It was further demonstrated (Warkany, 1954) that the duration and timing of the vitamin A deficiency state were important in influencing the incidence of eye lesions. When there was a deficiency throughout pregnancy 92% of fetuses showed ocular malformations. This was reduced to 68% by giving the vitamin from the 15th day onward. A much greater reduction was obtained when supplementation began only 2 days earlier, when only 15% developed eye defects. By comparing these results with similar work carried

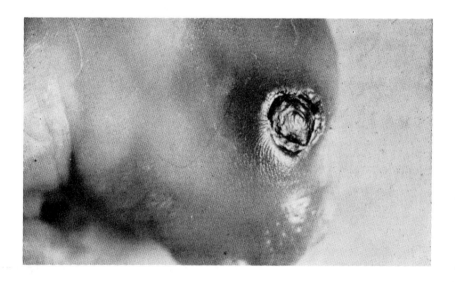

FIG. 112. "Open eye" in the rabbit. From Lamming *et al.* (1954).

out with folic acid (see below, Section IC) it will be seen that vitamin A deficiency has its most marked teratogenic effect on the eye several days later than does deficiency of folic acid.

In the newborn calf, as well as in young calves fed on a diet low in vitamin A (Chapter 2, Section IC), Moore *et al.* (1942) found blindness from another cause, namely compression of the optic nerve in the optic foramen. Identical changes were described in rabbits born of vitamin A-deficient mothers (see Section IC) by Millen *et al.* (1953) and "open eye" occurred in some Fig. 112) (Lamming *et al.*, 1954).

In contrast with the results in other species, O'Toole *et al.* (1974) found no congenital malformations in the offspring of 10 rhesus monkeys maintained on a vitamin A-deficient diet throughout pregnancy. Two of the young were born with xerophthalmia and one developed it after 2 years of deficiency.

2. Hypervitaminosis A

Just as the teratogenic effects of a deficiency of a vitamin were first demonstrated in the case of vitamin A, so was it this vitamin that was first shown to have similar effects when in excess. Cohlan (1953) reported gross defects in the development of the eye, among other malformations, in about half of the offspring of female rats dosed with 35 000 i.u. (international units) of vitamin A between the 2nd and 16th day after mating. The most common abnormality was anencephaly, and other defects included hydrocephalus, macroglossia, harelip, and cleft palate. This work was confirmed by Giroud and Martinet (1955), who studied in further detail the effect of altering the days upon which a dose of 60 000 i.u. of vitamin A was given. This had a very marked effect upon the type of defect produced. As far as the ocular lesions were concerned the grosser changes, such as anophthalmos and microphthalmos, occurred when the dosing took place in the earlier organogenetic period. Later dosing resulted in the less severe defects of "open eyes" and cataract.

In the rabbit it has been shown (Giroud and Martinet, 1959) that hypervitaminosis A may result in haemorrhages into the lens, retinal haemorrhages and detachment, and considerable fibrosis of the vitreous body.

Pelagalli (1963) inoculated fertile chick embryos of 4–8 days incubation with 5000–10 000 i.u. vitamin A. The lens studied on day 18 showed degeneration of fibres and interfibrillar material in capsular and subcapsular regions. The cytoplasm and nuclei of the epithelium showed degenerative changes.

Kalter (1964) showed that a large single dose of vitamin A to pregnant mice resulted in retinal coloboma in some of the offspring. In one instance all structures in the anterior segment of one eye were missing. The teratogenic effect in mice of retinoic acid is much greater than that of other vitamin A compounds (Kochhar, 1967). Microphthalmos, anophthalmos and exophthalmos were the eye defects observed and many other tissues were affected.

B. Riboflavin

Earlier accounts of riboflavin deficiency-induced malformation in birds and the rat did not include ocular defects. Warkany (1945) noted cerebral and eye defects only rarely. Using the riboflavin antagonist galactoflavin, Nelson *et al*. (1956) induced in the rat multiple congenital deformities including a fairly high incidence of "open eyes" and microphthalmos. Depending on the length of the deficiency and the dose of galactoflavin, cerebral and eye defects together were found in 7 and 9% of two of their groups.

C. Folic Acid

Multiple congenital abnormalities were induced by Nelson and her colleagues (Nelson *et al.,* 1955) in the rat by feeding a diet deficient in pteroylglutamic acid (PGA, folic acid) together with 1% succinyl sulphathiazole and 0.5% "crude" PGA antagonist (*x*-methyl PGA) (see Fig. 113). The deficient diet was given for 24, 48, and 72 hours only at varying periods during the first 14 days of gestation and the young were removed by Caesarean section on the 21st day. These workers point out that implantation normally takes place on the 7th day in the rat. A 2- or 3-day period of deficiency instituted after implantation markedly affected fetal development but a single day of deficiency had little or no effect, as did a 3-day period before implantation. It will be seen that folic acid deficiency has its maximum effect on the eye several days earlier than that of vitamin A deficiency (Section A1, above).

D. Pantothenic Acid

French workers have studied the teratogenic effects of pantothenic acid in considerable detail (Giroud and Boisselot, 1947; Lefebvres-Boisselot, 1951, 1965; Potier de Courcy, 1966) in the rat. Two typical abnormalities have been produced, namely exencephaly and microphthalmos. Both lesions occur very early on in development. The ocular defects (Fig. 114) may consist of complete absence of the eye, that is anophthalmos, without optic cup or crystalline lens. In the less severe degree of damage, microphthalmos, there is anything from a small residue of ocular tissue with gross disorganization to an eye slightly smaller than usual, more or less normal in structure. Whatever the degree of damage to the eye itself the extraglobal structures such as the eyelids and lacrimal glands are not affected.

E. Nicotinic Acid (Niacin)

The essential amino acid tryptophan is known to be a precursor of nicotinic

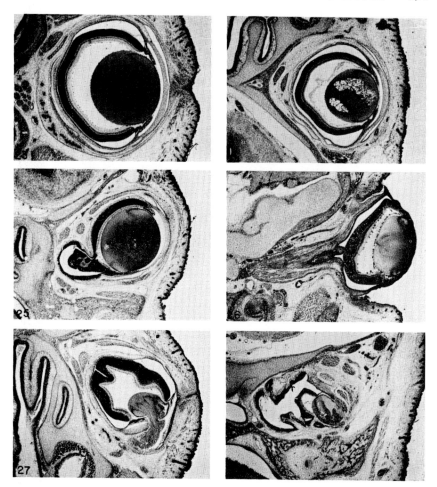

FIG. 113. Folic acid deficiency and congenital malformations of the eye in the rat. From M. Nelson: *AAAS Symposium on Antimetabolites and Cancer, 1953*, p. 124.

acid. The results of an experiment in which rats were fed various tryptophan and nicotinic acid supplements suggested that nicotinic acid deficiency might result in congenital cataract (Pike, 1951). The numbers of animals were rather small and the results not clear cut. Cataract did occur in the control group and it was considered that the extremely low food consumption of animals fed two of the diets in which the highest incidence of cataract was observed, might have led to multiple deficiencies. It was concluded that supplementation of tryptophan at the level of 0.2 % did not prevent cataract

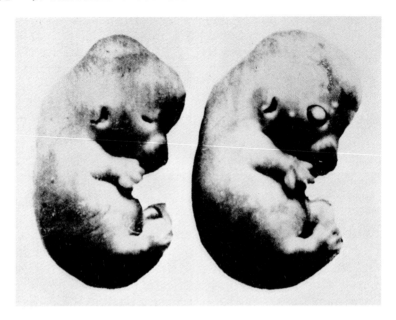

FIG. 114. *Left:* Anophthalmos in 18th day fetus deficient in pantothenic acid. *Right:* Normal. From A. Giroud and J. Lefebvres (1951). *Bulletin de la Société ophtalmologie* 9, 916.

but did so when accompanied by a further supplement of 10 mg/100 g of nicotinic acid. When the tryptophan supplement was reduced to 0.025% and the nicotinic acid was unchanged cataract occurred.

Chamberlain and Nelson (1962) briefly reported eye defects and other malformations resulting from a single intraperitoneal injection of 6-aminonicotinamide during the second and third weeks of pregnancy.

F. Vitamin B_{12} (Cobalamin)

In a study of reproduction in vitamin B_{12}-deficient rats in which special attention was paid to intrauterine injury, Lepkovsky *et al.* (1951) failed to find any congenital defects in the embryos. However, shortly afterward it was reported that rats fed on a corn-wheat gluten diet, known to be deficient in riboflavin and vitamin B_{12} as well as rachitogenic, produced young with a high incidence of hydrocephalus, skeletal abnormalities, and eye defects (Grainger *et al.,* 1954). Supplementation of the diet with riboflavin had no appreciable effect on the incidence of eye defects but these were virtually abolished by vitamin B_{12} supplementation (Table XIII). Details were not given of the nature of the ocular abnormalities but they were described as "small or missing eyes". Ferguson and Couch (1954) reported a few instances of "absent eyes" in their study of vitamin B_{12} deficiency in the chick embryo.

TABLE XIII. *Vitamin B_{12} Deficiency and Eye Defects*[a]

Group no.	Vitamin supplement		Offspring born (No.)	Malformations		
	Riboflavin[b]	B_{12}[c]		Eye defects (%)	Bone defects (%)	Hydro-cephalus
6	−	−	94	0.0	16.0	0.0
7	+	−	375	6.7	14.4	11.7
8	−	+	112	2.7	24.1	0.0
9	+	+	399	0.5	1.8	0.0

[a]From Grainger *et al.* (1954).
[b]Supplement supplied 1.6 mg of riboflavin per 100 g of ration.
[c]Supplement supplied 3 µg of vitamin B_{12} per 100 g of ration.

Special attention was paid to the nature of the eye defects by Ransdell (1956) in the embryos of vitamin B_{12}-deficient rats. No changes occurred in the 16-day-old embryos but all of the 18-day-old ones had abnormal eyes, varying in extent from a decrease in the size of the optic cup to great distortion of the lens and retina. In the newborn there were two instances of anophthalmos, one unilateral and one bilateral. The usual findings, however, were various degrees of coloboma, retention of the cavity of the old optic stalk, and extension of everted retinal tissue into the optic nerve. Of the newborn 57% had abnormal eyes, and of these 87% were in the same rats as also had hydrocephalus.

G. Vitamin E

There is a number of reports of vitamin E deficiency being responsible for congenital defects, among which the eye has been one of the organs affected. Callison and Orent-Keiles (1951) found that some of the offspring of rats deficient in this vitamin had smaller eyes than normal, that the eyelids sometimes failed to open, and that behind the pupil there was an opaque membrane. This last structure was suggestive of the changes that take place in the disease in newborn infants known as retrolental fibroplasia. Cheng *et al.* (1957) reported "open eyes" among a number of other defects in the rat.

Many of the embryos obtained from turkey hens fed on a practical-type diet of low vitamin E content or on a synthetic diet deficient in the vitamin developed ocular defects (Ferguson *et al.*, 1956). The cornea showed a prominent bulging appearance similar to that of keratoconus and this was associated with a degeneration of the cells in the stroma of the centre of the cornea. There was intraocular haemorrhage in two of the embryos. The main

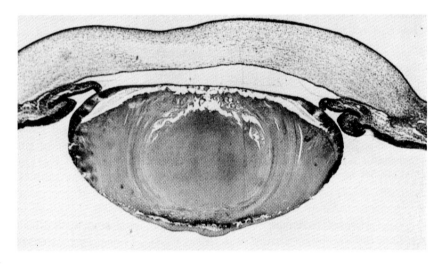

FIG. 115. Turkey embryo 18 days old. Degeneration of the lens immediately beneath the capsule and a large area in the cornea where cells are absent. (Haematoxylin and eosin, × 32.) From Ferguson *et al.* (1956).

change was in the lens and consisted of degeneration and proliferation of the lens epithelium with extensive liquefaction of the lens fibres (Fig. 115).

H. Iron, Copper and Manganese

It was reported that skeletal and eye defects resulted in the young of rats fed on one of four dried wholemilk diets from weaning (O'Dell *et al.*, 1961). These diets were deficient in either iron, manganese, or copper. No account is given of the precise nature of the eye defects. They occurred with a 3.3% incidence in the control group but the incidence rose in the young of those animals receiving the deficient diets as follows: iron-deficient 7.4%, manganese-deficient 10.0%, and copper-deficient 4.2%.

I. Zinc

Microphthalmos was among the many deformities produced in chick embryos of hens fed on a ration deficient in zinc (Blamberg et al., 1960). Small or missing eyes occurred in about one-third of the progeny of zinc-deficient rats; defects in other organs were even more common (Hurley and Swenerton, 1966). Duncan and Hurley (1978) have shown that deficiency of both zinc and vitamin A increased the incidence of malformations of all kinds to 100%.

J. Selenium

Mention has already been made of the possible implications of necrosis in the embryo in the causation of congenital defects above. This work was carried out by feeding selenium compounds to chickens. Necrosis occurred in certain areas of the brain, spinal cord, eyes, and limb buds after $2\frac{1}{2}$ to 3 days of incubation. In 4- and 5-day-old embryos the optic cups were abnormal and the lenses affected by necrosis (Gruenwald, 1958).

K. Strontium

Fujino et al. (1959) reported ocular malformations in newborn rats of mothers receiving a diet containing 200 mg of non-radioactive strontium carbonate per 100 g body weight for an unspecified period. In 93 malformed rats 29 had central cataract and 44 folding of the retina.

L. Protein and Amino Acids

No macroscopic abnormalities were found in any of the young of rats put onto protein-free or protein-deficient diets on the day of mating (Nelson and Evans, 1953). They confirmed earlier work (Guilbert and Goss, 1932; Pearson et al., 1937) that had shown that a dietary level of protein below about 5% is usually insufficient for ovulation and reproduction in the rat. Lepkovsky and Borson (1955) discussed the effects of protein deficiency on pregnancy but did not mention malformations. Another study used female rats fed after mating on an experimental diet containing either 5 or 3% casein (Curtiss, 1953). In all, 52% did not complete their pregnancy, and the fetuses of those that did weighed less than normal and were often eaten by their mothers within the first 24 hours. Reference is made to one malformed fetus, but details are not given as to the nature of the defects or as to the diet of the mother.

The view that a general deficiency of protein is not so harmful to the embryo as absence of specific amino acids has been referred to above. These results would seem to confirm the innocence of protein deficiency in this regard. It was observed by Waddington and Perry (1958) that amino acid and purine antagonists brought about embryological defects in chick embryos developing in culture. In view of the partial origin of the eye from the nervous system it is of interest that the vesicles of the brain were particularly sensitive to these effects.

In this connection some experiments of a preliminary nature are of considerable interest, e.g. feeding to mother rats a diet (Diet 1: see Chapter 6, Section I) containing 4% protein with methionine as the limiting amino acid. These animals had been reared on this same diet since weaning. They were mated with stock male rats but out of a considerable number of them kept in this way for more than 1 year only one female conceived, illustrating the difficulty known to occur in obtaining litters from rats fed on low protein diets. The account which follows is of the subsequent history of this single rat and her litters.

Twenty-one days after conception, identified by the finding of three "mating plugs", a litter of four pups (litter I) was produced weighing only 4 g each in contrast to the usual 5 g or more. The dam had already begun to eat the tails of her offspring when they were discovered and as it was evident that they could not be reared it was decided to kill them. Macroscopic examination revealed no abnormalities. On sectioning the heads the following changes were found in each eye of all the pups. (1) The eye was much smaller than normal. (2) The most marked changes were in the lens (Fig. 116a and b); this showed almost complete absence of normal fibre formation and the epithelium consisted of a disorderly mass of irregular cells extending far into the anterior part of the lens. The lens bow was barely recognizable. The capsule stained poorly and irregularly with periodic acid-Schiff (PAS) stain, whereas it is normally strongly positive. The lens fibres normally stain very strongly with Bennett's reagent for sulphydryl groups. Compared with lenses from control newborn rats there was a pronounced reduction in the intensity of staining. Staining with toluidine blue revealed metachromatic material scattered throughout the disorganized lens substance, whereas controls did not show any metachromasia in the lens. (3) The lids of newborn rats have not separated but a zone of future separation is clearly visible. This zone in the normal newborn rat is packed full of strongly PAS-positive material and it extends for some distance in either direction on the inner aspect of the lids (Fig. 117a). In the deficient rats there was complete absence of this material from both the zone of separation and the inner surface of the

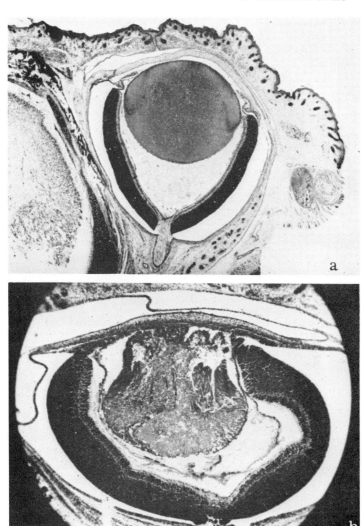

FIG. 116. (a) Eye of newborn rat from control dam. (Haematoxylin and eosin, × 9.) (b) Eye of newborn rat from protein-deficient dam. The eye is small and the lens grossly disorganized. (Haematoxylin and eosin, ×45.) From D. S. McLaren (1960).

lids (Fig. 117b). (4) Poor development of the iris and ciliary body. (5) The stroma of the cornea in the control was uniformly PAS-positive at birth. In the deficient animals only the deeper layers stained. This suggests immaturity of development because the same localization of the stain is seen in the

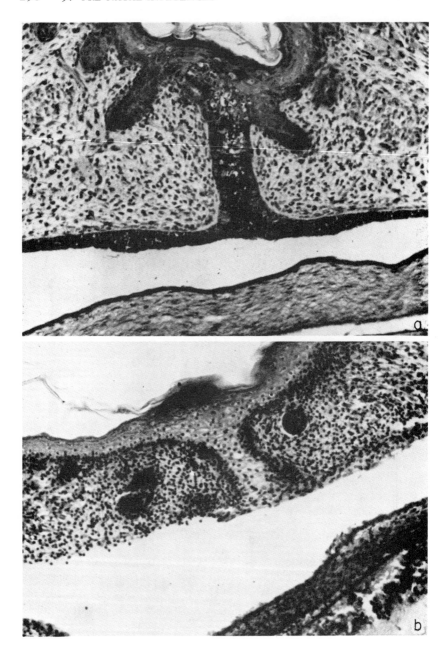

cornea of the normal fetus some days before birth. The metachromatic staining properties of the cornea were, however, not affected.

The following changes were also seen, but in only some of the eyes: absence of the anterior chamber; presence of a retrolental membrane; in one eye the retina was much folded, the outer nuclear layer was very thick in places with thinning out of the inner nuclear layer and persistence of part of

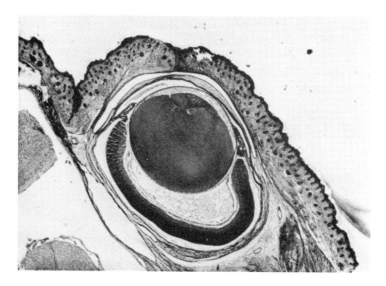

FIG. 118. Eye of rat of litter II. (×9). Compare with Fig. 116.

the hyaloid system. In this eye there was also material, homogeneous in structure and staining with eosin, deep to the capsule of the lens anteriorly.

In this experiment both parent rats were from stock with no history of eye defects. In order to rule out causal genetic influences as far as possible, breeding was continued after transfer of both animals to the stock diet. After 42 days of this diet a second litter (litter II) of six pups was born, four were found alive and two recently dead. After a further 47 days on the stock diet a third litter (litter III) of six was produced.

Histological examination of the eyes of all the newborn rats of these two litters showed the following appearances. The eyes were larger than those of litter I rats, but not quite as large as normal. In the lens there was a marked improvement in the orderliness of lens fibre formation, regularity of the

FIG. 117. (a) Lids of normal newborn rat. There is heavy staining in the zone of separation of the lids and for some way along the posterior surface. (b) Lids of newborn rat from protein-deficient dam. Note lack of PAS-positive material in these areas. (Both PAS stain, × 145.) From D. S. McLaren (1960).

epithelial bow, and a normal intensity of staining by Bennett's method. The lens was not normal, however, for some fibres were degenerate, with globules of material scattered between the fibres (Figs. 118 and 119). A consistent finding was the presence of eosinophilic material with a granular appearance under the anterior part of the epithelium. The PAS-positive material in the zone of separation of the lids and on their inner aspect was consistently present as in the control.

Only 21 days after the birth of litter III another litter (litter IV) was born to the same pair of rats still fed on stock diet. Four pups were born and all of these were reared by a stock dam as the experimental dam failed to lactate. The eyes opened normally on the 15th day and slit lamp examination revealed no cataract or any other abnormality. At 21 days of age three of the

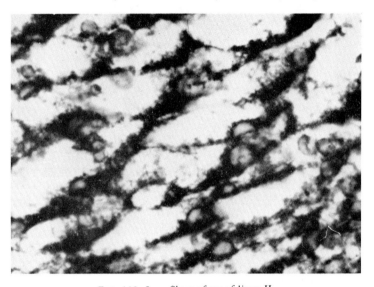

Fig. 119. Lens fibres of rat of litter II.

rats were weaned on to stock diet and the other was killed and the eyes taken for sectioning. At 75 days of age the three rats had grown normally and showed no eye changes and they were then killed. The eyes were found to be normal in weight and with those of the rat killed at 21 days old showed no abnormalities histologically.

A fifth and final litter (litter V) was born only 23 days after the birth of litter IV. Pregnancy was discovered 2 days before birth took place and it was decided to see what the effect of a low protein diet acting during late pregnancy and lactation might be. A diet providing 4% protein from arachin was fed the pregnant dam for the last 2 days of pregnancy. At the same time a lactating stock rat was given the same diet and the four pups that were born were transferred to this rat for suckling. Lid opening was delayed until the 17th or 18th day in each instance. Body growth was much retarded, the four rats together at 20 days old weighed only 42 g, less than half the normal weight for this age. No abnormalities in any of the eyes of these rats were detected with the slit lamp up to 21 days of age, when two of them died, and 28 days, when the other two were eaten by the foster dam. Histologically the only change was that in the posterior subcapsular portion of the lens the lens fibres ended short of the capsule and the interval contained some foam-like material.

These results have been presented in some detail because, although they need to be extended, they do provide some evidence for the view that maternal supplies of protein, and of the sulphur-containing amino acids in particular, are of importance in intrauterine development of the eye. That the gross changes were confined to animals in litter I, and present in all of them, and that the subsequent litters born while the dam was on the stock diet showed marked and progressive regression of ocular defects seems to rule out the likelihood of solely genetic influences being responsible.

Diet 1 was particularly deficient in the amino acids methionine and cystine, containing less than one tenth of these than the amount present in the stock diet. A deficiency of these might well have been responsible for the poor staining with Bennett's compound for sulphydryl groups. There is some evidence that these amino acids, as well as the general level of protein, may be important also in the production of the lid changes. Reference was made earlier (see Chapter 6, Section IC) to the role of methionine and cystine in wound healing and the accumulation of mucopolysaccharide in protein deficiency. Several reports link increased cellular activity in certain tissues with depolymerization and increased PAS positivity—in the lens following radiation injury (Permutt and Johnson, 1953), in the development of the chick eye (Elchlepp, 1956), in connective tissue invaded by tumour cells (Gersh and Catchpole, 1949), and in regeneration of liver (Aterman, 1952). The zone of separation of the lids would seem to be another such area of marked cellular activity. It is discernible at least a week before birth, and even at this time there is much PAS-positive material present there in the fetuses of control rats.

Reference has already been made (see Chapter 1, Section IA2) to the delay in opening of the lids associated with deficiency states. There was a similar delay in this phenomenon in the rats of litter V, but those of litter IV opened at the normal time. Rats of litters II and III all had a normal amount of mucopolysaccharide in the zone at birth. Furthermore in the normal rat this material begins to disappear from the zone soon after birth and has all gone by about 1 week before the lids open.

The collagen of the cornea differs from most other collagens in its ability to stain with both the periodic acid-Schiff stain and with toluidine blue. In fetal life the cornea shows metachromatic substance first nearest the anterior chamber, and not over the entire thickness until the time of lid opening. This also was true in the deficient animals. On the other hand, the cornea of the newborn rat normally stains uniformly by the periodic acid-Schiff method, but in the deficient animals stained only in the part nearest to the anterior chamber. This suggests some delay in development, for the same localization of stain is seen in the corneae of normal fetuses some days before birth.

Grau *et al.* (1965) reported arrest of retinal pigmentation and degeneration of the neural retina in tyrosine-deficient chick embryos.

The amino acid monosodium glutamate in only 0.3 mM concentration caused severe damage to the 12-day chick embryo retina in culture after only a few hours of exposure. Glutamyl transferase induction was shown to be inhibited (Reif-Lehrer *et al.*, 1975).

M. Carbohydrates

The importance of carbohydrates in metabolism is well known and there is considerable evidence now for the vital part they play *in utero* (Giroud, 1959). The central nervous system appears to be especially exacting in its nutrient requirements as far as sugars are concerned. The brain and spinal cord and optic vesicles, for example, will not develop in concentrations of sugar substrate that are quite adequate for the formation and pulsation of the heart. Very little is known about the part played by certain sugars. Fructose, for instance, is present in many embryos but its function is not understood. It occurs in the rat lens (Kuck, 1961).

Two pieces of evidence suggest that both deficiency and excess of sugars may have deleterious effects on the eye. Brinsmade (1957) produced insulin shock in pregnant rabbits on two successive days between the 6th and 11th day of pregnancy. The surviving embryos on the 15th day showed severe malformations of the central nervous system as a result of incomplete closure of the neural tube. In a further experiment insulin was given between the 6th and 12th days but only in amounts sufficient to lower the blood sugar without producing shock. Many embryos on the 15th day showed vacuolar changes in the lens and certain signs of brain and spinal cord damage. Although in the first group circulatory disturbance accompanying the condition of shock might be held partly responsible for the defects this could not be said of the second, in which a glucose deficiency would seem to have been the cause.

Young rats fed on diets with a high content of galactose readily develop cataract (Chapter 7, Section IA). Identical lens damage has been observed in the embryos of mother rats fed on a diet containing 25% galactose during pregnancy, the lenses remaining normal until the 16th day (Bannon *et al.*, 1945). In addition to various degrees of vacuolization and necrosis of the lens, de Meyer (1959) noted defective or even absent migration of the optic fibres toward the diencephalon.

Rats maintained exclusively on yoghurt grew normally and gave birth to normal litters but all the young developed cataract (Richter and Duke, 1970). The high galactose content was blamed; nearly 25% of the energy content in commercial yoghurt compared with only 14% when made from whole milk.

N. Ethanol

There is considerable interest at present in the possible production of congenital malformations by maternal ingestion of alcohol (Section IIE). Chernoff (1975) reported embryo resorption, low birth weight, skeletal, eye ("open eyes"), cardiovascular and nervous system lesions in the offspring of mice given ethanol during gestation.

O. Cyclamate and Saccharin

These artificial sweeteners are under attack for their carcinogenic properties in very large doses in experimental animals. A negative study has recently been reported by Luckhaus and Machemer (1978). Female Wistar rats received 5% sodium cyclamate or 0.4% sodium saccharin in their food for 20 days after mating. The ingested dose of sweetener amounted on average to 1495 mg sodium cyclamate, or 98.8 mg sodium saccharin, per animal per day. The fetuses delivered by caesarian section on day 20 of pregnancy and the young killed 3 weeks after parturition showed no treatment-related anomalies. There were no histological changes in the lens, vitreous, insertion of the optic nerve or other parts of the eye.

II. Human Studies

A. Low Birth Weight

Body weight at birth of 2.5 kg or less constitutes low birth weight. About 7% of all babies born in the UK and USA have a low birth weight and the figure is about three to five times greater in many developing countries. Perinatal and neonatal mortality rates are considerably raised in this group.

Low birth weight may result from a shorter than normal gestational period (preterm). These infants are physiologically immature, but with a diet designed to promote catch-up growth they are usually not materially handicapped. Another group of babies are of low birth weight because they have not grown normally during the gestation period that may be normal or shorter than normal in duration ("light for dates"). It is especially among this latter group that serious defects are to be expected.

During the period when high levels of oxygen were administered to low birth weight babies at birth a high incidence of retrolental fibroplasia occurred. With the recognition that this treatment was responsible for most cases of this condition the incidence has been greatly reduced. There is, however, some not very convincing evidence that vitamin E may be beneficial (Chapter 4, Sections IC and IIC). However, many reports of eye changes are unrelated to oxygen therapy.

1. Cataract

Cataract was found in 1% of 1128 children aged 6–8 years who had a birth weight less than 1.8 kg (McDonald, 1962, 1964). Mental retardation of all degrees and a history of fits were more common among those with cataract. In a study of 553 children legally blind born in New York State over a 12-year period Goldberg et al. (1967) found a greater proportion of cases

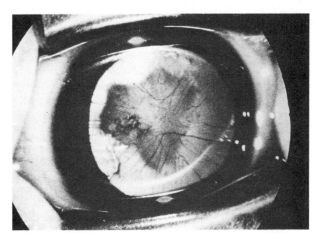

FIG. 120. Left eye of infant with well-developed transient cataracts. Radial strands are remnants of the tunica vasculosa lentis. From Alden et al. (1973).

than expected among non-whites, those born to mothers aged less than 20 years or more than 35 years, and mothers with pre-eclampsia. Congenital cataract was the most notable defect and the proportion of blind who were twins was greater than expected. Dann *et al.* (1964) reported a 2% incidence of cataracts in 100 infants of birth weight less than 1 kg.

Transient cataracts were reported in seven of 17 low birth weight infants (McCormick, 1968). A 2.7% incidence (Alden *et al.,* 1973) was reported in 692 infants. These are symmetrical, bilateral, and consist of clear fluid vacuole formation just anterior to the posterior lens capsule (Fig. 120). The onset is usually about 16 days after birth and they disappear within a further 25–30 days (Gerhard, 1974). They are reversible at any stage and resolution is opposite to their formation. The aetiology is unknown but respiratory distress, periods of apnoea, acidosis and sepsis are frequently present.

2. *Refractive Errors*

Refractive errors have frequently been reported in low birth weight infants. Myopia in marasmic infants was discussed in Chapter 6, Section IIA. In 1955 Fletcher and Brandon studied 462 low birth weight infants at 6 months of age. They found myopia more marked in the smaller infants and closely associated with retrolental fibroplasia, present in 136. A high incidence of a low degree of myopia is the commonly reported finding (Graham and Gray, 1963; Hosaka, 1963; Eames, 1964; Tabuchi and Yamamoto, 1974; Šeba, 1974). In 500 infants with high myopia at birth Rivara and Gemme (1966) described a diminution in the refractive error to 3 months of age, with the higher degrees of myopia remaining in those of especially low birth weight. Grignolo and Rivara (1968) found a marked increase in axial length of the eye during the first year of life, particularly in the first 3 months in low birth weight and in normal infants. The axial length, smaller in those of low birth weight, increased more rapidly as did hypermetropic refraction. However, the total refractive power, as well as corneal and lens power, decreased progressively. After 4 months of age none of these differences was found between the two groups. These workers explained the transient myopia by an increase in total dioptric strength, especially in the lens, due to incomplete development of the peripheral part of the lens (Rivara and Gemme, 1965).

Fledelius (1976) examined 539 children at about 10 years of age. 302 had a birth weight of 2 kg or less and the rest a normal birth weight. The low birth weight group had a mean refraction of +0.75 with myopia in 13.3%. The normal birth weight group had a mean refraction of +1.07 and 9.3% respectively. Eyes of the low birth weight group were 0.3 mm shorter on average and the radius of the cornea 0.18 mm shorter. Mean height, head circumference, interpupillary distance and corneal diameter were all shorter in the low birth weight group. In this group 1% were blind; two cases of retrolental fibroplasia and one case of cataract occurred. Heterotropia was 29.5% in those of low birth weight and 5.9% in the control. Hosaka (1963) reported astigmatism in 31% of 60 low birth weight babies, but only 3% had astigmatism in the 100 very low birth weight (less than 1 kg) studied by Dann *et al*. (1964).

3. Other Ocular Findings

Other ocular abnormalities have been much less commonly reported. Dann *et al*. (1964) reported 37% incidence of strabismus. Hosaka (1963) noted frequent attenuation of the fundus vessels and a pale optic disc was more common than in mature infants. In the series of Fledelius (1976) 5% of the low birth weight group had ocular malformations compared with 2% in those of normal birth weight. In a very large series of 138 281 newborns Pilman and Weinbaum (1974) found congenital ocular defects no more numerous in premature than in full-term infants.

B. Vitamin A

There is no strong evidence of a human counterpart to the lesions described in vitamin A deficient animals (Section IA). Sarma (1959) reported an infant with microcephaly and microphthalmos born to a mother in India who was totally blind, reputedly from severe vitamin A deficiency. It is not known whether the "deficiency" was active during the organogenetic period of the fetus and no biochemical evidence is presented. The only other possible case known is that of a blind and mentally retarded girl with bilateral microphthalmos, coloboma of iris and choroid and retinal aplasia. The only evidence of vitamin A deficiency in the mother was a history of night blindness during pregnancy (Lambda and Sood, 1968).

There is no evidence for ocular damage in the human fetus resulting from large doses during pregnancy.

C. Folic Acid

Folic acid deficiency is not uncommon in pregnancy and it is customary to supplement the diet at this time. Anticonvulsants may accentuate a deficiency and there is evidence that their efficacy is dependent upon this effect. Congenital malformations, especially neural tube defects, have been reported in offspring of mothers receiving anticonvulsants during pregnancy and although eye malformations have not been reported (Warkany *et al.*, 1959; Smithells, 1976) they might be expected to occur, in the light of animal work (Section IC).

D. Iodine

Eye defects have been among the malformations of which there is reported to be an increased incidence in goitrous areas (Giroud, 1959).

E. Ethanol

Jones *et al.* (1973) reported a fetal alcohol syndrome in babies born to mothers who were chronic alcoholics. Microcephaly, mental retardation, short palpebral fissures and small eyes have been commonly reported and some have had strabismus and asymmetric ptosis (see Section IN).

Chapter 10

Dietary Toxins

A large number of toxic substances that have an adverse effect on the eye are ingested. Some may be taken in, voluntarily or involuntarily, as poisons, and many drugs used in treatment have ocular side effects.

In this chapter attention is limited to those toxins which are found in certain items of food and to ethanol which acts as a source of energy in the body; and to their effects on the eyes. The toxic consequences of some vitamins and some essential elements when consumed in excessive amounts are dealt with in their respective chapters. The role of cyanide from tobacco smoke and untreated cassava in the aetiology of optic neuropathy is discussed in Chapter 3, Section B*1*.

I. Animal Studies

A. Ethanol

Degenerative changes in the ganglion cells of the retina were found in rabbits chronically poisoned with ethyl alcohol, but a monkey kept in a state of constant inebriation for 6 months appeared to suffer no ocular effects (Duke-Elder, 1954).

B. Lathyrism

This is a human disease occurring in parts of India and a few other places as the result of consumption of lathyrus peas (Section IIB). A possible toxin in the peas is β,β'-iminodiproprionitrile. Ocular lesions have not been described in the human disease and it is unclear why Yamashita (1972, 1973) applied this substance to the cornea of rats, resulting in non-specific epithelial damage. The neurotoxin isolated from lathyrus seeds is β-N-oxalyl-amino-L-alanine (BOAA).

C. Argemone Oil, Sanguinarine, and Citral

Interest in the causation of the raised intraocular tension that has been reported as one of the clinical features of the human disease known as epidemic dropsy justifies a joint consideration of these substances. The ocular aspects of the disease in man are dealt with later (Section IIB).

Argemone oil is derived from the seeds of *Argemone mexicana*, a member of the poppy family, and sanguinarine is an alkaloid of the isoquinoline group found in this oil. Citral is an unsaturated aldehyde found in citrus fruits and in the oil of lemon grass *(Cymbopogon flexuosus)*. Contamination of cooking oil with argemone oil has been shown quite conclusively to be responsible for outbreaks of epidemic dropsy. Several workers have reported that sanguinarine is the toxic agent, producing among other features of the condition the glaucoma. Subconjunctival injection of argemone oil or sanguinarine in rabbits and monkeys (Hakim, 1954), intravenous injections of sanguinarine and related alkaloids in rabbits (Lieb and Scherf, 1956), injection of sanguinarine into the lateral ventricles in the cat (Hakim, 1957), and prolonged feeding by mouth of sanguinarine to monkeys (Leach and Lloyd, 1956) have all been claimed to result in marked rise in the intraocular tension, in some cases for prolonged periods.

A careful reinvestigation of the whole subject carried out by Dobbie and Langham (1961) raised doubts concerning the activity of sanguinarine in epidemic dropsy and the ability of either this alkaloid or the parent oil to cause glaucoma. Only transient rises in intraocular tension resulted from intravenous and intraventricular injections of sanguinarine in both cats and rabbits. Adult rabbits fed approximately 175 mg sanguinarine or 1 ml argemone oil daily for a period of 3 weeks appeared in normal health at the termination of the experiment, showed no rise in intraocular pressure at any time, and the eyes on histological examination were all normal. Similar results were obtained in hens. Argemone oil also had negative results as far as the eyes were concerned in rabbits and hens but in the latter animal the finding of Hart (1941) that the wattles and combs become oedematous was confirmed.

Conflicting results have also been reported concerning the toxic effects of citral. It was during the course of a study of sanguinarine poisoning that Leach (1955) found that the eyes of some of their control monkeys showed histological changes in the trabecular meshwork of the anterior chamber angle similar to those observed in animals receiving sanguinarine. Eyes of control monkeys receiving a synthetic diet were normal but those of monkeys eating an orange twice a week with a stock diet were not. They claimed that orange oil prepared from orange peel when fed by mouth or injected subcutaneously raised the intraocular pressure of rabbits (Leach and Lloyd, 1956). It was postulated that citral acted as a vitamin A antagonist and they claimed that vitamin A dosing could prevent or reverse its poisonous action.

Other workers have failed to confirm both the reported rise in intraocular tension and the structural changes in the trabeculum using rabbits (Berggren, 1957; Rodger *et al.*, 1960a) and monkeys (Rodger *et al.*, 1960b) nor did vitamin A-deficient animals show any differences from those receiving citral alone.

D. Ergot

Poisoning with the parasitic fungus *Claviceps purpurea* of grain cereals has been, and occasionally still is, responsible for outbreaks of convulsive ergotism in man in which cataract and retinal changes have been reported (Section IIC). This type of cataract has never been recorded in the experimental animal and the only account known in which damage to the eye occurred is that of Peters (1902). He stated that there were degenerative changes in the ganglion cells of the retina and the retinal vessel walls. Ergothioneine was found in high concentration in the lens of several species (D. S. McLaren, unpublished observations).

E. Bracken Fern *(Pteris aquilina)*

This fern is a potent source of thiaminase (see also Chapter 3, Section IE). Many species, from rat to horse, fed on bracken fern die from acute thiamine deficiency within 30 days. Blindness and extensive brain lesions do not occur. Ruminants such as sheep and cattle have been thought to obtain thiamine from microbial synthesis in the rumen. Cattle fed bracken fern have been reported to die of haematologic changes not responding to thiamine. There have, however, been reports from the USA and the UK of young sheep and cattle fed on bracken fern developing "central" blindness and extreme cerebrocortical necrosis, with presumed damage to optic nerves or tracts. It is not clear whether reported cure with thiamine may not have been influenced by a change of diet (Anon, 1969).

More recently "bright blindness" has been produced experimentally in sheep by feeding bracken nuts (Barnett and Watson, 1970) or a ration of 50% dried bracken (Watson *et al.*, 1972). In both studies retinal degeneration was observed but the changes do not appear to have been described in detail yet and the toxin remains obscure.

F. Male Fern *(Felix mas)*

In 1967 two outbreaks of a blinding disease in cattle occurred in Kirkcudbright, Scotland (Rosen *et al.*, 1969). Among 68 animals which became ill,

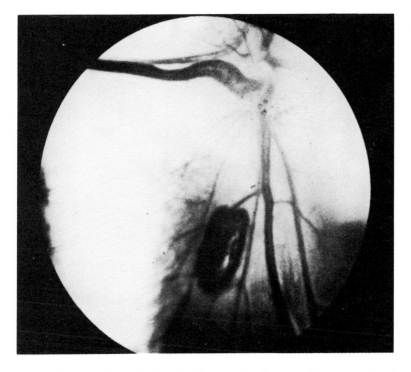

Fig. 121. Left fundus of acutely affected calf two weeks after onset of symptoms, showing a discrete ovoid haemorrhage adjacent to the disc. From Rosen *et al.* (1969).

61 were judged to have visual impairment. Within a week 53 animals appeared fully recovered but four cows and four calves remained permanently blind. In the acute stage haemorrhages around the optic discs and papilloedema were noted. Optic atrophy was evident 9 months after the incidents in those permanently affected (Figs. 121 and 122). Consumption of the

apical buds of rhizomes of male fern was suspected as the cause. The authors state that extract of male fern is known to cause poisoning, which has

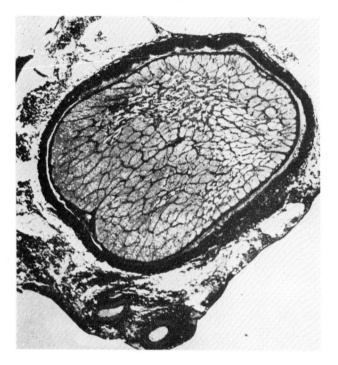

FIG. 122. Left optic nerve 3 mm behind lamina. Pale paracentral zone of nervous tissue destruction with area of septal collapse. From Rosen *et al.* (1969).

included blurring or loss of vision. *Felix mas* has been used as a vermifuge in man and occasionally resulted in similar changes.

G. Locoweed

This term is applied to many plants of oxytropis and astragulus genera of the family leguminosae. Neurological complications are common ("loco" means crazy in Spanish) in cattle, sheep and horses that graze on this weed. Van Kampen and James (1971) reported damage to the ganglion layer of the retina and epithelium of the ciliary body in these species. The toxic factor is probably selenium (see Chapter 5, Section IE).

H. Ocular Cancer

In a 20-year study of 435 range beef cows it was reported that those on a "high level feed" had increased incidence and earlier development of ocular squamous-cell carcinoma (Anderson *et al.*, 1970). This appears to be a special instance of the general effect of high energy diets increasing the incidence of tumours (Ross and Bras, 1965).

II. Human Studies

A. Ethanol

Two important conditions affecting the eyes in which chronic ethanol ingestion is involved are dealt with elsewhere. The Wernicke-Korsakoff syndrome is due mainly to thiamine deficiency and is discussed in Chapter 3, Section B2. Retrobulbar neuropathy in chronic alcoholism is recognized as being a secondary nutritional deficiency and is considered in Chapter 3, B1*g*.

1. Acute Alcoholism

Visual acuity and visual fields are almost normal and in the few authenticated cases of total blindness the fundi have been normal and the vision has invariably returned to normal within a few days. The common term "blind drunk" is therefore a misnomer.

Disturbances of higher visual functions are very well known and, apart from the diplopia, are usually denied by the subject. Sensitivity to light is lowered and the brightness difference threshold is increased. Complex judgments such as depth perception and reaction time are considerably impaired. Ocular movements are affected at an early stage (Newman and Fletcher, 1941). Levett and Karras (1977) found in three volunteers that accommodation times were increased by 10–30% over those of controls when blood alcohol was 50–100 mg/100 ml.

2. Chronic Alcoholism

Apart from the conditions mentioned in the introduction, reports of eye involvement in chronic alcoholism have related to liver cirrhosis. Most of these have been concerned with disordered rod and cone function. In some patients this may be attributed to vitamin A deficiency (Chapter 2, Section

IIIB) but there is increasing evidence that a deficiency of zinc is involved in some (Chapter 5, Section IIC).

Summerskill and Molnar (1962) reported a 12% incidence of lid retraction and lag, sometimes with apparent ptosis, compared with 1% and no proptosis in non-cirrhotic controls. Of 20 cases reported from Yugoslavia (Čavka, 1963) 19 had yellowish sclerae and telangiectasia with small aneurysms on arterioles and venular varices of palpebral and bulbar conjunctivae. Eleven had powdery opacification of the vitreous and all had abnormal retinae, with 14 showing degenerative changes in the pigmented layer. Chronic uveitis has been reported (Rapidis et al., 1975). Baron (1972) found temporal pallor with central or central-focal scotomata in 30% of 220 male cases examined.

Visual fields in white light are usually normal, but constriction was found in red and green light, the degree being related to the clinical stage of alcoholism, as were colour vision defects (Travinskaya and Shtilman, 1973). Cruz-Coke (1965) claimed that X-linked genes for defective colour vision predispose either to alcoholism or cirrhosis. Fialkow et al. (1966) were unable to confirm this. In 46 patients with alcoholic cirrhosis, one had the very rare blue-yellow defect and 19 had red-green defects. Most of these latter defects cleared up during convalescence. In another study (Rothstein et al., 1973) 14 out of 16 patients with proven alcoholic cirrhosis had significant dyschromatopsia (colour vision defects) on the Farnsworth–Munsell 100-hue test. There was no relation to serum B_{12} levels but 10 had low serum folate levels. Results of treatment are not discussed and the significance of the findings is doubtful as serum folate is indicative of recent intake rather than folate status.

The chronic consumption of large amounts of alcohol during gestation has resulted in malformations in the offspring, including the periocular tissues (Chapter 9, Sections IN and IIE).

B. Epidemic Dropsy

It is necessary at the outset of the discussion of the ocular features of this disease to point out that the disease known as epidemic dropsy has no connection with beriberi, in the acute form of which disease dropsy is a prominent sign. Some of the early writers suggested such an association before the aetiology of epidemic dropsy had been discovered and this may account for the persistence of this wrong impression in some quarters. Clinical descriptions include bullous eruptions on the skin and glaucoma.

The disease was first described in India in the nineteenth century, since when it has occurred in epidemic form not only in India but also in Indian communities in other parts of the world such as Mauritius, Fiji, and South Africa. It was shown by Lal and Roy (1937) and Lal *et al.* (1940) that the cause was the ingestion of argemone oil. This oil is obtained from the seeds of the poppy *Argemone mexicana* which is a common contaminant of the mustard plant, the oil from which is used for cooking by many Indian communities. Typical signs of the disease have been produced in human volunteers by feeding 40–50 oz of argemone oil over a period of about 30 days (Chopra *et al.*, 1939; Lal *et al.*, 1941).

In neither of these experimental studies in man was glaucoma produced, although in one instance two out of five volunteers complained of dimness of vision. There was also no rise in intraocular tension in the eyes of hens, rabbits, or cats fed argemone oil by Dobbie and Langham (1961), contrary to the results of other workers (Section IC) Maynard (1909) in Calcutta appears to have been the first to report glaucoma in association with an epidemic of the condition, and Kirwan (1934, 1936) and Dutt (1950) have also stated that glaucoma is common in those with epidemic dropsy. As Dobbie and Langham (1961) pointed out there is really no convincing clinical evidence for a causal relationship. One piece of evidence in favour of the existence of such a relationship is, however, that the histological appearance of the eye in epidemic dropsy is quite different from that of ordinary open-angle glaucoma. Kirwan (1935) reported that there was a dilatation of the capillaries of the whole of the uveal tract, especially marked in the ciliary processes and the choroid. It was postulated that this led to an increased permeability of the endothelial walls and a consequently raised output of aqueous humour into the anterior chamber. It is evident, however, that there is now some doubt as to whether or not the eye is really affected in epidemic dropsy.

Sanguinarine has been isolated from nearly 50 species of poppy-fumiraria weeds. Hakim (1957) showed that the ingestion of these plants by cattle, goats and sheep led to the secretion of sanguinarine in their milk. He suggested that consumption of contaminated milk was responsible for widespread glaucoma, but this has never been substantiated.

C. Ergotism

The widespread consumption of rye contaminated with ergot fungus led to many devastating epidemics of the disease in Europe during the Middle Ages (Barger, 1931). The two main groups of symptoms, the gangrenous and the nervous, had been described for centuries but it was not until the middle of the nineteenth century that cataract was included in the symptomatology. Meier (1862) found that 23 out of 283 affected people of Siebenburgen, in

Transylvania, months after an epidemic in 1857 due to eating contaminated rye, developed cataract, young people being more affected than old. Several subsequent reports (Bellows, 1944; Duke-Elder, 1954) largely from Russia in the later years of the nineteenth and earlier part of the twentieth century confirmed the occurrence of cataract usually a matter of months or a year or two after recovery from the acute systemic effects. The latent period is reported to be shorter in children than in older people and in the aged the lens changes are described as being indistinguishable from those of senile cataract.

Retinal changes occur during the acute illness and consist of vasoconstriction and oedema with an amblyopia in which there is peripheral contraction of the fields and a central scotoma. These symptoms are all transitory and optic atrophy does not occur (Kaunitz, 1932).

There seems little doubt from their nature that the retinal signs are caused by the alkaloids of ergot. The nature of the lens damage is less certain, although many theories have been devised to explain it, such as spasm of the ciliary vessels, alteration of the composition of the aqueous, damage to the lens epithelium, and so on.

Scott (1962) pointed out that no instance of cataract has been reported following the medical use of ergot or its alkaloids. He suggested that ergotism of the convulsive type might have been confused with tetany, with which cataract is not infrequently associated (Chapter 4, Section IIB).

D. Favism

Choremis et al. (1960) described severe impairment of vision in two boys aged 3 and 6 years who had eaten broad beans. Retinal haemorrhages in one appeared to be part of a general haemorrhagic state and in the other papilloedema and constriction of retinal vessels were present. They reviewed the few case reports in the literature and noted that visual symptoms usually appear 3 to 7 days after the onset of haemorrhages elsewhere. Complete blindness may ensue within a few hours and the ultimate prognosis is poor; half showing no improvement and only 10% recovering full vision.

E. Oxalosis

Toxicity may result from excessive intake, increased intestinal absorption, increased endogenous synthesis, or retention due to renal dysfunction. Rhubarb and spinach are especially rich sources. Deposits may occasionally occur in the retina, optic nerve, uvea and oculomotor muscles (Timm,

1963). Garner (1974) described a case with oxalate deposits in the outer layers of a detached and degenerate retina.

F. Finger Cherry Tree Poisoning

The fruit of the finger cherry tree (Australian horror tree, *Rhodomyrtus macrocarpa*) native to Queensland and New Guinea, may give rise to blindness when eaten (Flecker, 1944). The local people rub off the skin before eating it and are unaffected. The toxin is unknown.

Chapter 11

Miscellaneous Human Eye Conditions

There are some human eye conditions that are in some way or another related to nutrition but which do not fit into any of the previous categories as they are not directly due to nutritional deficiency nor do they respond to dietary treatment. In some instances they are discussed here in order to dispel the suggestion of a role for nutrition that has been made on inadequate evidence.

A. Refractive Errors

An account has already been given of the common occurrence of myopia in low birth weight babies (Chapter 9, Section IIA) and of a similar, reversible, change in severely malnourished infants (Chapter 6, Section IIA). The question may now be considered as to whether communities in different parts of the world, who might be subject to chronic undernutrition of an unspecified nature, might have refraction distributions that differ from those found in well nourished communities.

Consideration may first be given to the way in which the growth of the eye as a whole and its component parts affects the refractive state.

During early intrauterine life the optic vesicle is the "organizer" of a normal eye. Sorsby *et al.* (1957) postulated, with supporting data, that the retina takes over this function as an "organizer" of emmetropia. The size of the retina will determine the size of the overlying sclera, which in turn will control the curvature of the cornea. That is to say, a large eye with a long axial length will have a flat cornea, and a short eye a highly curved one. Furthermore, the lens will be highly curved in a short eye, and flatter in a long eye. Thus the retina would seem to continue the function of the optic vesicle of determining and moulding the lens.

In a subsequent study of 408 ametropic eyes Sorsby *et al.* (1962a) showed that most refractive errors are correlation ametropias, that is to say there is failure of correlation of ocular components that are not in themselves abnormal. Component ametropia is seen in less than 3% of subjects and is generally due to an axial length that is outside the range seen in emmetropia. Axial length was shown to be the essential factor in 68 cases of anisometropia (Sorsby *et al.*, 1962b).

The study of twins by Sorsby *et al.* (1957) has demonstrated the overriding importance of heredity in the correlation of the optical components of refraction in the absence of adverse environmental influences acting early in life. However, that these influences may produce refractive errors when acting *in utero* (Chapter 9, Section IIA) or in infancy (Chapter 6, Section IIA) has also been shown.

There is also considerable, although less direct, evidence that differences in refraction of population groups may be related to environmental, most like nutritional, influences.

An early and almost constant feature of any nutritional deficiency state is retardation of body growth. It has been shown however in the experimental animal that, at least as far as general inanition (Chapter 1, Section IA) and protein deficiency (Chapter 6, Section IA) are concerned, the eye is one of the most resistant organs to such adverse influences. The question naturally arises, to which no complete answer can be given, as to whether malnutrition operating during the organogenetic period of the eye could influence the growth of the retina. In this way there would be a lasting effect on the scleral size, the axial length, the corneal and lens curvatures, and consequently on the overall refraction of the eye. If malnutrition could exert such an influence, and it is difficult to see how it could be actually demonstrated in man, then it would be not an isolated influence but would act in conjunction with genetic factors which are known to be of primary importance.

There has been a great deal of speculation concerning the possibility of influencing high refractive errors, particularly the serious condition of high myopia, by dietary treatment. It hardly seems profitable to give an account of the various ill-founded theories and treatment trials that have been reported in this connection. The subjects of these experiments have not been shown to be deficient in any nutrient, and it is not surprising that the various claims of response have not been confirmed by others.

The claims of Gardiner (1956, 1958) that London schoolchildren with advancing myopia eat less first class protein than do those whose eyesight is not deteriorating, and that the progress of myopia may be retarded by dietary means, are of this nature. His work has been criticized from both the nutritional and the ophthalmological points of view (Anon, 1959).

As was pointed out earlier, the eye receives preferential treatment for nutrients over most other organs when these are in short supply. Only in the organogenetic period of intrauterine life, when differentiation is taking place, is it at all likely that nutritional deficiency might have an effect. Once myopia, or any other refractive error has become established, it is unlikely that it will be influenced by dietary or any other means.

Many studies of refraction in populations have been carried out, mostly in Caucasians. They indicate that about 70% of all eyes fall into the refraction

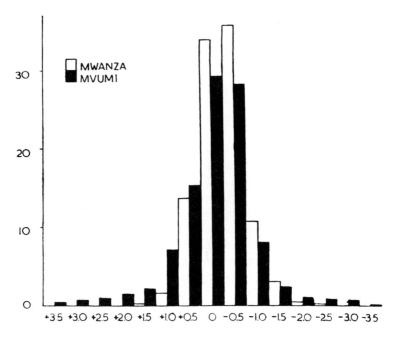

FIG. 123. Percentage distribution of mean refraction within the limits ± 4.0 D. Beyond these limits the differences were even more marked; 23 high myopes and five high hypermetropes at Mvumi compared with one high hypermetrope at Mwanza. From McLaren (1960a).

class 0 to plus 1.0 D, and that refractions close to emmetropia are more frequent than would be expected on a curve of normal distribution (e.g. Hyams *et al.*, 1977). Similar results have been reported for Negroes, aged 20–40, numbering 2147 eyes, in Gabon in Africa (Holm, 1937), Eskimos (Skeller, 1954), and high caste Indian children in Poona, India (Pendse, 1954) and Mwanza, Tanganyika (McLaren, 1961). While children of the Sukuma tribe in Mwanza gave normal values, a marked scatter with a high incidence of myopia in excess of 4.0 D was found in children of another tribe, the Gogo, in Mvumi, Tanganyika (McLaren, 1960a) (Fig. 123). A similar, but much smaller, skewness on the myopic side was found among "untouch-ables" by Pendse (1954) in India.

All the Gogo children were survivors of a severe famine in 1953–54, varying in age at that time from about 1 or 2 years to 7 or 8 years. The Sukuma children had known no food shortage. In addition there is continuing vitamin A deficiency in Ugogo affecting mainly infants, but no such problem in Sukumaland. Patterns of marriage are identical in the two areas; cousin marriages are forbidden by both tribes. Two other Tanganyika tribal groups have also been examined, in non-famine areas, and their refraction follows the usual pattern. It is tempting to suppose that among the Gogo famine or possibly vitamin A deficiency in early life has acted to exaggerate innate genetic influences. If similar results were obtained in other areas of chronic food shortage considerable weight would be added to this argument.

Johnstone and McLaren (1963) extended these studies to six areas of Tanzania, including a resurvey of the prior famine area. The incidence of myopia was about 1.3 % in the five areas unaffected by famine, comparable with figures for Europe and North America. The incidence in the famine area was 4.4 %. A high incidence of myopia and anisometropia was also found in relatives of the children in the famine area.

One thing is clear: the marked difference in incidence of refractive errors between these two closely related tribes, the Gogo and the Sukuma, should discourage sweeping statements which have been made in the past to the effect that myopia does not occur in Africa. Similarly these results invalidate the conclusion Holm (1937) draws from the lack of refractive errors in his Gabon Negroes that inheritance plays an all-important part. It probably does, but it cannot be argued on the grounds that primitive people always show lack of variation of characteristics, one being refraction, which they have inherited from their primordial ancestors. On this argument the highly myopic Gogo should be very sophisticated, but are if anything less so even than the Sukuma.

It may, conversely, be asked whether there is any evidence that malnutrition has played any part among racial groups that are known to have a high incidence of refractive errors. Certain groups are notoriously myopic, for instance the Chinese, Japanese, Arabs, and Jews (Duke-Elder, 1954). One wonders if, in view of the marked differences found in Tanzania, such generalizations can be justified. If the results of a survey among schoolchildren in Japan (Majima et al., 1960) are compared with those for Gogo schoolchildren of the same age (McLaren, 1960a) it will be seen that axial myopia (i.e. errors greater than minus 4.0 D) was three times as common among the Gogo as in the Japanese during the same period.

Several studies provide further evidence for the role of environmental factors. Wangspa and Limpaphayom (1965) refracted 5733 Thai schoolchildren between 6 and 15 years of age and found that the incidence of myopia among those in urban areas was more than double that in the rural areas. Young *et al.* (1969) found that there was no correlation between the refractive state of Eskimo parents and their children, but a high correlation between siblings. There was virtually no myopia in grandparents or parents but a 58% incidence in their offspring. Sato (1965) reported a 50–70% decrease in the incidence of myopia among Japanese in recent years. This was attributed to measures taken against continual accommodation for near work, but it must be remembered that the nutritional status has remarkably improved, as evidenced by considerably greater mean height, over the same period. However, among 3511 Danish conscripts myopes were found to be on average 1.6 cm taller than emmetropes, and myopia was most frequent among grammar-school pupils and undergraduates, who were tallest, and myopia was least in labourers and seamen, who were shortest (Goldschmidt, 1966, 1968). Similar results were obtained in a study of 403 myopic children in Britain who were taller, had a higher birth rank, and tended to come from smaller, non-manual labouring families as compared with a normal nationally representative sample (Peckham *et al.*, 1977).

Among the ocular changes reported from prisoners-of-war camps refractive errors have figured from time to time, although never having the prominence attained by nutritional amblyopia. Several authors mention the development of myopia or the deterioration of an existing myopia (Livingston and Ridley, 1946; Balcet, 1948; Rich, 1946; Reed, 1947; Smith and Woodruff, 1951). The latter state that 22 adults, whose sight was known to be normal previously, developed myopia, the mean extent of which was 1.9 D in the worse eye and 0.8 D in the better. Among 44 patients known to have been myopic before the war, exactly half showed an increase of myopia far greater than would normally have been expected. On the other hand, premature onset and unusually rapid progress of presbyopia was also reported (Ridley, 1945; Smith and Woodruff, 1951). Myopia and presbyopia tend to act in opposition and it is difficult to understand how the two could arise under the same conditions, albeit in different individuals, if malnutrition was causative.

Finally the same children who were examined for lens damage as a result of infant malnutrition (see Section B, below) were also refracted. All were within normal limits.

B. Cataract

In some earlier chapters evidence for the nutritional aetiology of cataract involving several different nutrients was brought forward, and this in a number of animal species. Despite all this suggestive evidence from animal studies and the widespread occurrence of cataract in man, there is at the present time nothing to show conclusively that the human lens may also be damaged by malnutrition. Such suggestions have frequently been made, for example in association with riboflavin deficiency (Torokhova, 1947; Falcone, 1952) and pellagra (Spillane, 1947) but without any real foundation.

The term cataract implies opacification of the lens, this being almost without exception the only pathological change which the lens can undergo. There are, however, many causes of cataract formation and an equally great variety of anatomical forms and sites in the lens of the opacities. Cataractous change may be manifest at birth as a result of damage to the fetal lens, or may show itself at any age thereafter (Chapter 9, Section IIA1). We are ignorant of the fundamental changes in the physical and chemical nature of the lens which are responsible for all the different types of cataract, although this is not for lack of research.

The adjective "senile" has become attached to the most common of all forms of cataract, about the precise aetiology of which nothing is known. Although usually occurring in its mature form in elderly individuals it is not uncommonly seen in relatively young subjects, in their 40s or 50s, who would not be regarded as being senile in any other respect. On the other hand many truly senile individuals of a great age do not have cataract, at least not a degree giving rise to visual impairment. Acknowledgment of the unsatisfactory state of the terminology is evinced by the use of "presenile" by some when the cataract occurs in younger people. It would seem that the best course to adopt is to retain the expression senile cataract for what is a well recognized and clearly understood entity, but to place the word "senile" in quotation marks to remind the reader that the association of this kind of cataract with an advanced stage of the ageing process is by no means constant and not necessarily aetiological.

One other kind of cataract, developmental cataract, has long been suspected of arising sometimes as a result of maternal or early infantile malnutrition. The frequent association of zonular cataract with the hypocal-caemia of tetany and other stigmata of calcium deficiency, such as rickets and hypoplasia of dental enamel, has been noted elsewhere (Chapter 5, Section IIAa). While it is considered most unlikely that lens damage could arise in this way as a dietary deficiency of calcium and vitamin D alone, the possibility of lack of other essential nutrients at this stage has never been investigated as a cause of cataract. This relatively uncommon form of cataract will not be considered further here, but attention will now be turned to the evidence that has from time to time been brought forward suggesting that malnutrition may sometimes play a part in the causation of "senile" cataract.

The various deficiency diseases and undernutrition in general are not evenly distributed throughout the world but are virtually absent from some countries while still rife in others. The demonstration of a similar distribution of "senile" cataract would certainly suggest, although it could do no more, that the two were in some way associated. If it were thought that the considerable volume of writing on this subject provided a factual basis for the belief that "senile" cataract is more common in some parts of the world than in others, then it would be recorded here in some detail, but this is not so. Compilations of the data of many authors have been made and the interested reader is referred in particular to Bellows (1944), Sorsby (1950), and Fuchs (1960).

In countries where registration of the blind is in force, statistics on "senile" cataract are made from this registry. In many countries, however, there is no such registration and the only sources of data have been eye department records including cataract extraction figures. Eye surgery is highly specialized work wherever it is performed. In the underdoctored countries of the world the dearth of ophthalmologists is, of course, even greater than that of general duty physicians and surgeons. Blindness being the incapacitating thing it is, help for its alleviation will be sought from afar by those who can afford it. The chronic, painless nature of "senile" cataract, and the usual lack of urgency for surgery contribute to the accumulation of large numbers of cases in certain centres where a reputation has been established. All hospital statistics are notoriously unreliable as indications of the disease situation in the area around the hospital. Especially will they be so for such a condition as "senile" cataract under the conditions prevailing in most countries of the world. They may suggest the fame of an eye surgeon or the state of communications, but they cannot reflect the incidence of the condition in a population at large.

Although satisfactory statistics are lacking, the general consensus of opinion of numerous ophthalmologists with many years of experience of cataract in both temperate and tropical areas is that in the latter "senile" cataract is more common and occurs at an earlier age than in the former (Vanneste, 1956—Congo; Pi, 1934—China; D'Haussy et al., 1958—Sudan; Budden, 1956—Nigeria; Wright, 1936; Rambo, cited in Fuchs, 1960—India; and many others).

Chatterjee (1973) commented that eye camps for cataract surgery are required especially in North West India, but not at all in Kerela, in the South. Surveys suggest a high incidence and earlier onset in hot and dry parts of the country. The wet parts of Bengal have a lower incidence than the dry. There is a higher reported incidence among Indians in South Africa than among other racial groups in that country.

In view of the paucity of data on this subject the results of surveys in three large villages in the Khond Hills, India (McLaren, 1960c) in the early 1950s may be of interest. Among 2126 people of all ages there were eight with mature cataract of the "senile" type. All of these had sufficient impairment of vision for them to have been included on the register of the blind if they had been in England and Wales. According to Sorsby (1950) the number of registered blind in England and Wales in 1948 was 77 390 of whom 24.6%, or 19 347, were blind due to cataract. This was roughly 1/44 400 of the total population. It is obvious that the incidence of cataract was much higher in the Khond Hills villages than in England and Wales, even without taking into account the fact that the proportion of people over the age of 45 was nearly three times greater in England and Wales than in the Indian villages surveyed. A similarly high incidence was found among the approximately 2000 people examined at Mvumi (McLaren, 1960a).

In Table XIV a tentative comparison has been made on an age basis between the same data for England and Wales and a series of 517 patients operated upon for "senile" cataract in the Khond Hills by my former colleague Dr S. F. Thomas of the Moorshead Memorial Hospital, to whom I am indebted for the data. Although the two groups of data are rather different in nature the differences in age distribution are striking.

Several workers have reported that the type of cataract observed in the tropics is different from that most commonly seen outside the tropics. Mingelen (1933) in Indonesia found that of 135 patients (260 eyes) with cataract, 72% had the nuclear type compared with 29% in the United States (Kirby, 1936) and 22% for England (Foster and Benson, 1935). Cooper (in Fuchs, 1960) finds a high incidence of black cataract and nuclear sclerosis in Bombay, and Murray and Asregadoo (1959) stated that in the West Indies most senile and presenile cataracts begin centrally. In Western Australia, Mann (1959) found that cataract was nearly always due to nuclear sclerosis, in contrast to New Guinea where more of the soft water-cleft type was found. She suggested a correlation with atmospheric humidity although not with temperature.

An important difficulty in assessing the incidence of "senile" cataract is connected with its very nature. The process of cataract formation is an extremely chronic one. The condition as it is recorded in hospital data consists largely of the end stages when the cataract is mature and causing impairment of vision, if not actual blindness. To take into account only such cases in determining the incidence of "senile" cataract is to miss the majority.

The appearance of water-clefts in the cortical portion of the lens is one of the commonest manifestations of incipient cataract of the "senile" type. These clefts lead gradually to spoke-like opacities, which are merely water-clefts with a cloudy medium. The conversion of clear water-clefts into opaque spokes may take several years and more usually pass before these, together with lamellar separations which give rise to cuneiform opacities,

TABLE XIV. *A Comparison of the Incidence of Cataract in the Khond Hills, India, and in England and Wales*[a]

1	2	3	4	5	6	7	8	9	10
Age (years)	No. of cataracts in Khond Hills series	Percentage in each group	Distri-bution of Khond Hills population	Relative incidence of cataract (i.e. 3:4 as %)	No. of cataracts in Sorsby's data	Percentage in each group	Distri-bution of England and Wales population	Relative incidence of cataract (i.e. 7:8 as %)	Relative percentage incidences compared (i.e. 5:9[b])
Under 30	7	1.4	67.5	0.14	—	—	41.0	—	—
30–39	16	3.1	14.2	1.14	4	0.1	14.6	0.10	11.4
40–49	73	14.1	8.2	8.95	51	1.2	14.8	1.32	6.8
50–59	193	37.3	3.6	54.26	218	5.2	13.1	6.44	8.4
60 and over	228	44.1	6.5	35.51	3931	93.5	16.5	92.14	0.4
Total	517	100	100	100	4204	100	100	100	100

[a]From D. S. McLaren (1960c).
[b]There is a much higher proportion of cataract in the Khond Hills in the three 10-year periods, leaving relatively few in the 60 and over group as compared with England and Wales.

lead to the immature stage of "senile" cataract (Bellows, 1944). These changes are exceptional in the earlier decades of life. Pfeiffer (1921) found that in 111 subjects, 28% of those aged about 50 years and 37% of those older showed water-clefts.

Retinoscopy carried out on the eyes of Bantu children of several tribes and of Indian children in Tanganyika (McLaren, 1960a, 1961) under full hyoscine cycloplegia revealed the presence in a high proportion of radially situated dark areas in the lens. These were referred to originally as opacities but it would be more correct to call them "sectorial alterations in the refractive indices of the lense fibres" (Duke-Elder, 1959). They precede actual opacification and may be regarded as being the earliest indication of the development of cataract of the "senile" type. The significance of these lens changes at such an early age in African and Indian children, but not in European children who have lived most of their lives in the tropics, is not known. Whether due to malnutrition or not, they would seem to be the very beginning of cataract formation.

A special group of subjects who might be thought to provide evidence of lens damage from infantile malnutrition, if such occurs, are children who are known to have had kwashiorkor or marasmus in the past. The writer examined five such children in Kampala under the care of Dr H. Welbourn and six more in Guatemala City being followed up by INCAP. None showed signs of such damage.

From Indonesia, Zuidema (1955, 1959) has reported calcification and fibrosis of the pancreas in young adults presenting with severe, and often insulin-resistant, diabetes. In 45 such cases there was also advanced cataract in 43. In a personal communication to the writer Zuidema confirms that these were of the "senile" and not diabetic type. It is thought that the pancreatic changes may be a late effect of kwashiorkor and if so would provide evidence for the ultimate damage of the lens by protein deficiency.

Prchal et al. (1978) studied 22 patients aged under 50 with cataract in Alabama. Five were heterozygous for galactokinase deficiency and two for galactose-1-phosphate uridyl transferase deficiency. Eight had erythrocyte glutathione reductase activity suggestive of riboflavin deficiency (see also Chapter 7, Section IIA).

In India, Bhat and Gopalan (1974a, b) in a small series of cataract patients found a high incidence of riboflavin deficiency and abnormal galactose tolerance. The results suggest that while galactose metabolism is not affected by riboflavin deficiency the latter might facilitate the reduction of galactose and lead to accumulation of galactitol in the lens, if galactose were to accumulate in tissues as a result of a metabolic error or extensive feeding of sugar (Anon, 1976).

Cotlier and Sharma (1980) report the finding, of doubtful significance, of raised plasma total, bound and free tryptophan in senile cataract and aphakia.

C. Measles Keratoconjunctivitis

This was a not-infrequent complication of morbilli in Europe during the nineteenth century and until the second world war (Duke-Elder, 1965). Most of the patients were described as being malnourished. It is now a rare occurrence and measles appears to be in every way a milder condition, although the rare involvement of the cornea and most other ocular tissues is occasionally still reported (see Sauter, 1976).

In many developing countries, and especially those in Africa, however, measles keratoconjunctivitis is considered to be one of the most important causes of blindness in children (Pratt-Johnson, 1959: Armengaud *et al.,* 1961; Quéré, 1964; Morales *et al.,* 1965; Lagraulet and Bard, 1967; Oomen, 1971; Franken, 1974; Sauter, 1976; and others). The serious eye complications almost invariably occur in severely malnourished chldren. It is significant that the active process and the resulting scars resemble those described in xerophthalmia (Chapter 2, Section IIIA3g).

A contributory role for vitamin A deficiency must always be considered under these circumstances. One example of misdiagnosis comes from Haiti, where xerophthalmia is known to be endemic (Chapter 2, Section IIIA9e). An epidemic of rubeola (measles) was blamed for 25 cases of corneal ulceration, 14 with perforation (Frederique *et al.,* 1969). Although the patients were malnourished, vitamin A deficiency was wrongly ruled out because Bitot's spots and xerosis of the conjunctiva were not present (McLaren, 1970).

A very mild keratoconjunctivitis is an almost constant finding in measles, presumably responsible for the characteristic photophobia (Thygeson, 1959). In the series of Azizi and Krakovsky (1965) it also occurred in two of five subjects given gammaglobulin, but was absent in all 20 cases of other exanthematous diseases.

Well-nourished children may develop a marked ocular reaction, with severe photophobia, irritation, increased lacrimation, blepharospasm, chemosis and diffuse micropunctate corneal staining with 1% fluorescein. There is a discharge, mainly purulent with very little mucus, due to deficiency of goblet cells in the conjunctiva, as was demonstrated in the respiratory and digestive tracts (Scheifele and Forbes, 1973). The pre-ocular tear film is deficient and the BUT (break-up time) is shortened. Tiny particles in the pre-ocular film consist of degenerating and dead epithelial cells. There is giant cell formation in the conjunctival and corneal epithelium, as elsewhere (Scheifele and Forbes, 1973). These cells contain measles virus (Sauter, 1976) as do similar cells from the nasopharynx (Suringa *et al.,* 1970). Sauter (1976) suggests that profuse tear production

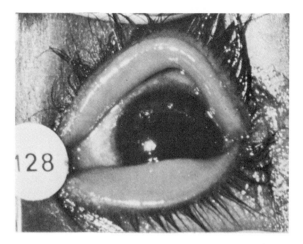

FIG. 124. Xerophthalmia and measles keratoconjunctivitis. Corneal erosions stained with 1% fluorescein, conjunctival xerosis stained by 1% rose Bengal. From Sauter (1976).

under these circumstances probably provides considerable protection against secondary infection.

In children with measles keratoconjunctivitis accompanied by xerophthalmia Sauter (1976) described a strikingly mild degree of inflammatory response; presumably related to the known impairment of cell-mediated immunity in vitamin A deficiency (Figs. 124 to 130). Apart from general

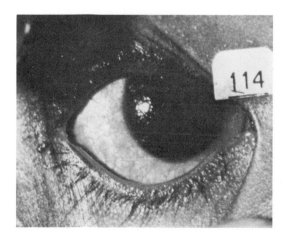

FIG. 125. Xerophthalmia and measles keratoconjunctivitis. Corneal reflex is distorted and pre-ocular tear film lacking. From Sauter (1976).

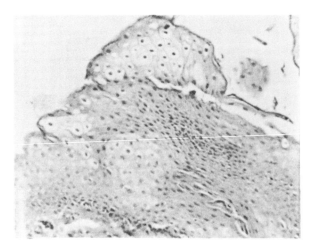

FIG. 126. Histology of measles keratoconjunctivitis. (Haematoxylin and eosin, × 100). Thickened hyperplastic epithelium, goblet cells lacking. From Sauter (1976).

supportive and local treatment of the eye in severe measles it is clearly important to institute therapy with vitamin A (see Chapter 2, Section IIIA10). A recent study (Whittle et al., 1978) in Nigeria of children with measles, many of whom were malnourished, showed that herpes simplex virus could be cultivated from corneal and mouth ulcers, suggesting that

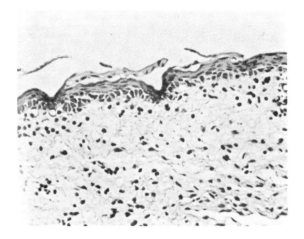

FIG. 127. Conjunctival xerosis (XIA) of vitamin A deficiency. (Haematoxylin and eosin, × 100.) Very thin desquamating epithelium. Keratinized cell layers with flattened nuclei on degenerating basal cells. From Sauter (1976).

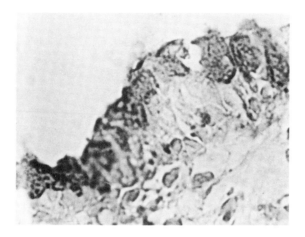

FIG. 128. Healing conjunctival xerosis (XIA). (PAS and alanine blue, × 400.) Epithelium still very thin, numerous mucus-secreting goblet cells. From Sauter (1976).

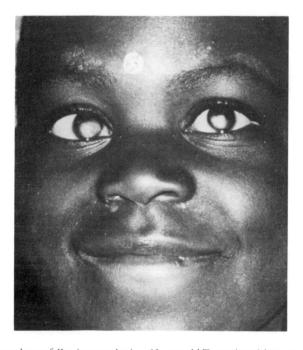

FIG. 129. Corneal scars following measles in a 13-year-old Tanzanian girl (courtesy of Dr J. J. M. Sauter). They resemble those following xerophthalmia, and where both conditions are common and occur in association it is impossible at this stage to identify the role played by each disease.

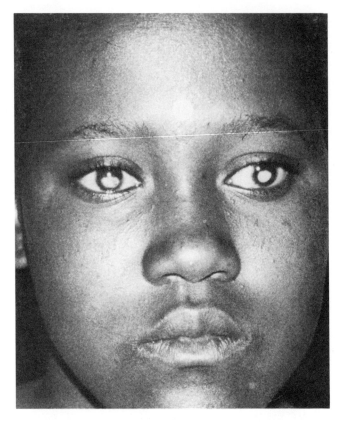

FIG. 130. Another example of corneal scars following measles in a 17-year-old Tanzanian girl (courtesy of Dr J. J. M. Sauter).

these may have resulted from immunosuppression and that this might explain the poor response of some cases to vitamin A therapy.

D. Trachoma

It may be categorically stated at the outset that the role of malnutrition in trachoma has never been properly investigated. The Expert Committee on Trachoma (1956) of WHO concluded that diet was one of the factors that did not "directly and appreciably affect the development of trachoma". The reasons given for this view were that it "occurs equally in vegetarian populations, in meat eaters, in persons living on a mixed diet, in well-nourished persons, and in persons showing a certain amount of protein, calorie, and vitamin deficiencies". It is not clear what the Committee meant to imply by the word "equally". If they meant that trachoma occurs in all these groups then the statement is acceptable, although it cannot be assumed from this that nutrition plays no part. If on the other hand they meant that the incidence and severity of the disease is uniform throughout these groups then the statement is not acceptable, for such is not the case.

One of the members of this WHO Committee, Bietti (1955, 1956), noted a predilection of the disease for ill-nourished communities from his experience in Sardinia, the Middle East, East Africa, and Indonesia. He excludes any association with vitamin A deficiency, and regards deficiency of calories, protein, and fat of importance. It has been stated that the aboriginals living in the Central Desert area of Australia, who are heavily infected with trachoma, are exceptional in that they are exclusively meat eaters. Mann (1959) confirmed that they have a high incidence of trachoma but when game is not available they live on berries, wild fruits, leaves, and yams, living on a "feast and famine" basis. As Bietti points out, it may be supposed that malnutrition of the host organism might hinder the establishment of the disease by rendering the cells deficient in enzyme systems which the virus needs for multiplication. In support of this he quotes the finding of Wilson that while trachoma is almost universal in the Egyptian population, cachectic children did not have the disease.

It is not difficult to find many records of strongly expressed views both for and against the existence of a role for nutrition in the aetiology of trachoma. There is little point in referring to these in detail here for a question like this cannot be answered by clinical impressions alone. On the one hand nutritional deficiencies are complex, usually multiple and long-lasting processes, and on the other trachoma is an exceedingly chronic disease. In the amount of damage it does trachoma appears to be influenced greatly by the presence of other infections of the conjunctiva and cornea, and in practice this may be almost impossible to separate from any influence nutrition may have.

This is not the place to consider in detail the clinical features and evolution of trachoma, but an outline of some studies in Tanzania may serve to indicate some of the problems and how they may be approached, although it will not provide the answer. This work was carried out in village primary schools near Mwanza, Bukoba, and Mvumi, the headquarters towns of East Lake, West Lake, and Central Provinces, respectively. In the first two places the annual rainfall is adequate and there has not been any serious food shortage in modern times. The country becomes much drier and dustier the further one goes from Lake Victoria, and Mvumi has suffered numerous famines of which that in 1919–20 was perhaps the most disastrous and that of 1953–54 the most recent (Johnstone and McLaren, 1963).

The typical disease pattern of trachoma with early lesions in young children was observed in all places, but in the dry, famine area of Mvumi the general incidence of the disease was highest and the stage tended to be more advanced. In Mwanza and Bukoba about 10% of nearly 800 schoolchildren had trachoma. At Mvumi nearly 60% of 450 children had the disease. In addition to the recurrence of famine at Mvumi there is also a continuing vitamin A deficiency problem as evidenced by a high incidence of xerophthalmia in infants (Chapter 2, Section III9c). The drier climatic conditions at Mvumi are, of course, not only responsible for food shortage, especially of fruit and vegetables, but also for poorer standards of hygiene and a greater fly problem than in the other areas, all of which factors may be expected to play a part.

Johnstone and McLaren (1963) considered the possibility of trachoma affecting the upper limbal area causing astigmatism. Both conditions were common among the schoolchildren examined in the famine area of Tanzania. There was, however, no such association found.

E. Discrete Colliquative Keratopathy (DCK)

This is the name that has been applied (McLaren, 1960c) to a condition of the cornea, first described by Blumenthal (1950) as "malnutritional keratoconjunctivitis" in the Bantu of South Africa. In this and a subsequent paper (1954), Blumenthal outlined the essential features of this disease as he had observed it over a number of years in the Eastern Cape Province. His statement that this was "numerically the only important cause of preventable blindness in the Union" brought much criticism from workers in other parts of South Africa. They claimed to see such cases only rarely and maintained that much of what Blumenthal had included was due to trachoma, healed injuries, and purulent infections. Although these criticisms appear valid there still emerges a separate entity characterized by localized softening of the cornea frequently with prolapse of the iris. If there is no secondary infection this heals with varying degrees of corneal scarring and with leucoma adherens if the iris has been involved. In the presence of infection total leucoma with ectasia, anterior staphyloma, phthisis bulbi, and all the consequences of panophthalmitis may result, obscuring the underlying condition and producing an end result indistinguishable from that due to many other causes.

Typically this condition affects the Bantu toddler in the postweaning period and is especially common in the chubby child rather than in the marasmic. It is just this age group and this very type of child that should be suspected of suffering from early protein-energy malnutrition or prekwashiorkor. It is therefore disconcerting to find that Blumenthal (1961) denied that his cases had kwashiorkor, although their basic diet of mealie-meal with little else causes many cases of kwashiorkor every year in South Africa as a whole.

Outside South Africa the condition has been seen in East Africa (McLaren, 1960b) in its acute form, and in a personal communication to Dr W. J. Darby of Vanderbilt University, Dr M. F. Gelfand of Salisbury mentioned

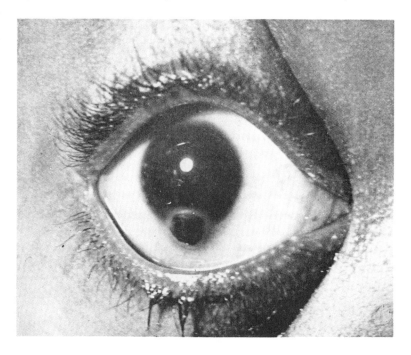

FIG. 131. Clean iris prolapse in DCK. From Blumenthal (1950).

that he had seen painless dissolution of the cornea in Bantu adolescents in Southern Rhodesia. This disease has not been reported so far other than in the Bantu race, although malnutrition is of course rife in many other parts of the world. The writer has had the opportunity during many years of examining the eyes of malnourished children in many of these countries and of discussing this condition with many ophthalmologists, paediatricians, and other interested medical personnel. Without exception, outside Africa, they have failed to recognize this condition from their own experience. Dr Ida Mann, the eminent and widely travelled ophthalmologist, in a personal communication to the writer, said that she had discussed the condition with Blumenthal in South Africa and had not seen anything comparable anywhere else in the world.

In the typical case a small area of cornea of the middle zone between limbus and central area, usually in the lower half, either down and in or down and out, in either one or both eyes, softens and when seen for the first time frequently has an associated prolapsed knuckle of iris (Fig. 131). More often than not the eye is "quiet" with no accompanying photophobia, increased lacrimation, or injection. The first indication to the mother that there is anything wrong with her child's eye may be the prolapse of the iris and she may ask the physician to "wipe off the black thing from the eye!"

The softening of the cornea takes place from within outward, and is in no sense of the term an ulceration. The early stage of the condition before perforation has occurred is not common, but in one case seen by the writer with a typical prolapse in one eye there was an earlier stage without corneal perforation in the other. Under the slit lamp a small area of endothelium contained bleb-like areas resembling those in that structure that accompany Fuch's epithelial dystrophy. The overlying deep stroma was infiltrated with cells, invaded by small blood vessels, and there was migration of a little pigment.

It cannot be too strongly emphasized that this condition is totally different in nature from keratomalacia, although they have been confused by some. Blumenthal (1954) stressed the differences, although he had to rely on textbook descriptions of keratomalacia as he had not encountered this condition. The writer is in the fortunate position of being one of the few who have had experience with both; a table contrasting their characteristics may prove of value (Table XV).

Pratt-Johnson (1959) suggested that DCK is nothing but measles keratitis. In the latter there is much more reaction in the eye, but the main reason against this view is simply that the vast majority of cases have not had measles. The aetiology remains, about 30 years after the first description of the condition, a complete mystery. Apart from the common occurrence in malnourished subjects there is no real evidence that it is nutritional in nature and for this reason the original name is best avoided. The term "spontaneous iris prolapse" has also been used. Although it describes one feature of the most typical phase it is quite insuitable for the condition as a whole for the iris does not always prolapse and the lesion is primarily of the cornea. Vitamin therapy has been without effect and healing by scar formation takes place eventually (Fig. 132).

There was a marked seasonal and annual fluctuation in the incidence of the disease as seen at Mwanza from 1958 to 1962. All cases were confined to the rainy season (October–May), and no case was seen at all in 1960 and 1961, although about 10 were seen by Dr R. Smith (personal communication) in Dodoma, Central Province between December 1960 and February 1961.

Blumenthal was impressed by the rarity of the stigmata of this condition in the older age groups of Bantu people in East London. This would seem to indicate one of two things. Either the disease is new in the area, or else

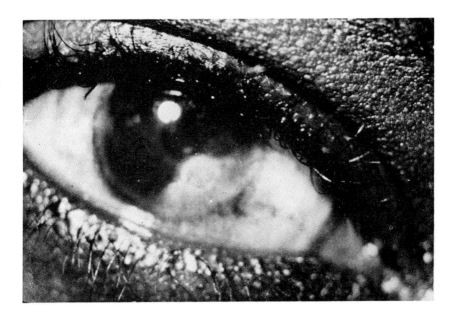

FIG. 132. Healed case of DCK with leucoma adherens.

childhood cases do not survive into later life, possibly because the corneal softening is symptomatic of a generalized defect in connective tissue.

Further accounts of DCK do not appear to have been reported and the aetiology and present status are unclear. Duke-Elder (1965) summarized the work under this name in his System of Ophthalmology.

F. Onchocerciasis

Rodger (1957, 1960) claimed that there were two distinct types of posterior segment lesions in onchocerciasis, an atrophic type with no evidence of inflammation and absence of microfilariae, and an inflammatory type with

TABLE XV. *Keratomalacia and Discrete Colliquative Keratopathy (DCK) Compared and Contrasted*

Feature	Keratomalacia	DCK
Age	Main incidence in pre-school child, especially ages 3 and 4	Pre-school child
Sex	Sexes equally affected in first year of life. Pre-school child, 1.4 male to 1.0 female. Ten years and over, 6.0 male to 1.0 female.	Sexes equally affected
Global occurrence at present time	Major problem in certain parts of Southeast Asia, Central and South Amercia, Middle East, and Africa.	South and East Africa
Race	No influence directly.	Reported only in Bantu.
Periodicity	Usually endemic. Occasionally in special circumstances of privation.	Possible relationship to wet season.
General condition of patient	Usually kwashiorkor or marasmus. Frequent with infectious disease, e.g. measles. Ill child, high mortality.	Often malnourished, especially prekwashiorkor, less serious.
Clinical appearance of eye in acute stage	Usually xerosis conjunctivae. Frequently Bitot's spot. Always xerosis corneae.	No xerosis. Quiet eye. Typical myencephalon (4 or 8 o'clock)
Late result	Central scarring of cornea, ectasia, phthisis bulbi.	Leucoma adherens
Pathology	Keratinizing metaplasia of corneal epithelium proceeding to colliquative necrosis discrete or total.	Ill-defined process commencing in deep corneal stroma
Treatment	Rapid response to vitamin A	No response

abundant microfilariae. He suggested that vitamin A deficiency played a part in the first type.

A very thorough study of 244 cases with posterior segment lesions attributable to onchocerciasis was made by Bird *et al.* (1976). Other retinopathies were carefully excluded and fluorescence angiography of the fundus was employed. No evidence of vitamin A deficiency was found. Specific biochemical tests of vitamin A status and vitamin A therapy were not carried out, so conclusive evidence for lack of a role for vitamin A deficiency has not been obtained, but it seems to be most unlikely.

G. Retinitis Pigmentosa

Serum vitamin A levels were reported to be lower than normal in this condition (Campbell and Tonks, 1962), but this has not been confirmed (Massoud *et al.*, 1975). Retinol-binding protein was reported to be low in 82% of 51 patients (Rahi, 1972), but others have found normal levels and unaltered fluorescent properties (Maraini, 1974; Futterman *et al.*, 1974; Maraini *et al.*, 1975). 11-*cis*-Vitamin A is quite ineffective (Chatzinoff *et al.*, 1968). Of considerable importance is the demonstration by Bergsma *et al.* (1977) that in one case of retinitis pigmentosa only 2S receptors for retinol were present, while in normal human retina both 2S and 8S receptors for retinol were demonstrated.

Recently Airaksinen *et al.* (1979) have described defective uptake of the amino acid taurine by the platelets of 12 patients with retinitis pigmentosa compared with that in healthy controls (see also Chapter 6, Section IE).

H. Food Allergy

Liu *et al.* (1973) studied a group of children with growth failure, bouts of malabsorption with rapid weight loss, induced by cow's milk protein. Some cases had eyelid oedema, conjunctival injection, increased lacrimation and a high concentration of glucose in tears. Potter and Duncan (1976) reported allergy to various foods as a common cause of mild chronic conjunctivitis. There was lasting relief when the food responsible was eliminated.

I. Gout

Ocular manifestations are uncommon but may include tophi in the conjunctiva, subconjunctival haemorrhage, crystalline deposits of urate in the conjunctiva and lens, and rarely sclerosing keratitis. In acute attacks of ocular gout there is conjunctival congestion, episcleritis and anterior granulomatous uveitis (Heinz *et al.*, 1971).

A purine-free diet and reduced alcohol intake are especially indicated in acute attacks.

References

Chapter 1

Addis, T., Poo, L. J. and Lew, W. (1936). Quantities of protein lost by various organs and tissues of body during fast. *J. biol. Chem.* 115, 111–116.

Barry, L. W. (1920). The effects of inanition in the pregnant albino rat with special reference to changes in the relative weights of the various parts, systems and organs of the offspring. *Carnegie Inst. Wash. Publ.* (*Contribution to Embryology*) No. 53, 91–136.

Barry, L. W. (1921). *Pap. Mayo Fdn med. Educ.* 1, 590.

Bich, I. A. (1895). "Changes in the Retina of Dogs During Hunger (With or Without Water)." Med. Dissertation, St Petersburg. Cited by C. M. Jackson (1925).

Bourgeois, L. (1870). Étude de physiologie expérimentale. De la mort par inanition. *Thèse* No. 186, Paris. Cited by C. M. Jackson (1925).

Carville and Bochefontaine (1874). Notes sur quelques lésions anatomo-pathologiques consécutive à l'inanition observées chez duex chiens. *Gaz. méd. Paris* 3, 549–551.

Carville and Bochefontaine (1875). Notes sur quelques lésions anatomo-pathologiques consécutive à l'inanition observées chez duex chiens. *C. r. Séanc. Soc. Biol.* 26, 314–322.

Derrien, E. and Turchini, J. (1924). Sur l'accummulation d'une porphyrine dans la glande de Harder des rongeurs du genre Mus et sur son mode d'excrétion. *C. r. Séanc. Soc. Biol.* 91, 637–639.

Djacos, C. (1949). Les altérations oculaires dans les oedèmes de carence. *Archs Ophthal. Paris* 9, 421–426.

Durig, A. (1901). Wassergehalt und Organfunction. *Pflügers Arch. ges. Physiol.* 85, 401–504.

Edge, J. R. (1945). Partial starvation in prisoners-of-war. *Lancet* ii, 317–318.

Eleftheriou, D. S. and Djacos, C. (1950). Lésions anatomo-pathologiques de la cornée dans les oedèmes de carence. *Archs Ophthal. Paris* 10, 217–227.

Fajgenblat, S. (1946). "Maladie de Famine." Apfelbaum, Warsaw.

Falck, F. A. (1875). *Beitr. Physiol. Hyg. Pharmakol. Toxikol.* 1, 128.

Falck, F. A. and Scheffer, T. (1854). *Arch. Physiol. Heilk.* 13, 508.

Figge, F. H. J. and Atkinson, W. B. (1941). Relation of water metabolism to porphyria incrustations in pantothenic acid-deficient rats. *Proc. Soc. exp. Biol. Med.* 48, 112–114.

Heinsius, E. (1950). Die Beteiligung des Augenhintergrundes bei Mangelernährung. *Dt. med. Wschr.* 75, 419–421.

Helleström, B. E. (1956). Experimental approach to the pathogenesis of retrolental fibroplasia. V. The influence of the state of nutrition on oxygen-induced changes in the mouse eye. *Acta paediat.* 45, 43.

Jackson, C. M. (1915). Changes in the relative weights of the various parts, systems and organs of young albino rats held at constant body-weight by underfeeding for various periods. *J. exp. Zool.* 19, 99–156.

Jackson, C. M. (1925). "The Effects of Inanition and Malnutrition upon Growth and Structure." Blakiston, Philadelphia.

Jackson, C. M. (1932). Structural changes when growth is suppressed by undernourishment in the albino rat. *Am. J. Anat.* 51, 347–379.

Jackson, C. M. (1936). Recovery in rats upon refeeding after prolonged suppression of growth by dietary deficiency of protein. *Am. J. Anat.* 58, 179–193.

Jackson, C. M. (1937). Recovery of rats upon refeeding after prolonged suppression of growth by underfeeding. *Anat. Rec.* 68, 371–381.

Jess, A. (1930). *In* "Kurzes Handbuch der Ophthalmologie" (Eds F. Schieck and A. Brückner), Vol. 3, 170. Springer, Berlin.

Kammerer, P. (1912). Experimente über Fortpflanzung, Farbe, Augen und Körperreduction bei Proteus anguinis Laur. *Arch. Entw Mech. Org.* 33, 349–461.

Kauffman, R. C., Norton, H. W., Harmon, B. G. and Breidenstein, B. C. (1967). Growth of the porcine eye lens as an index to chronological age. *J. Anim. Sci.* 26, 31–5.

Keys, A., Brozek, J., Henschel, A., Mickelsen, O. and Taylor, H. L. (1950). "The Biology of Human Starvation," Vol. 1, 675. University of Minnesota Press, Minneapolis.

Kornfeld, W. (1922). Uber den Zellteilungsrhythmus und seine Regelung. *Arch. EntwMech. Org.* 50, 526–592.

Kudo, T. (1921a). Studies on the effects of thirst. I. Effects of thirst on the weights of the various organs and systems of adult albino rats. *Am. J. Anat.* 28, 399.

Kudo, T. (1921b). Studies on the effects of thirst. II Effects of thirst upon the growth of the body and of the various organs in young albino rats. *J. exp. Zool.* 33, 435–461.

Lamy, M., Lamotte, M. and Lamotte-Barillon, S. (1948). "La Dénutrition." Doin, Paris.

Lee, Y., Kauffman, R. G. and de Venicia, G. (1974). Effects of fasting and refeeding on morphological and biochemical properties of the porcine lens. *Invest. Ophthal.* 13, 308–310.

Leyton, G. B. (1946). Effects of slow starvation. *Lancet* ii, 73–79.

Lodato, G. (1898a). Sulle alterazione oculari nella inanizione. *Arch. Ottal.* 5, 285–298. Cited by C. M. Jackson (1925).

Lodato, G. (1898b). *Accad. Med. clin., Palermo* 3 Aprile. Cited by C. M. Jackson (1925).

Lowrey, L. G. (1913). The growth of the dry substance in the albino rat. *Anat. Rec.* 7, 143–168.

Lucas, D. R. and Newhouse, J. P. (1957). The toxic effect of sodium L-glutamate on the inner layers of the retina. *A.M.A. Archs Ophthal.* 58, 193–201.

McLaren, D. S. (1958). Growth and water content of the eyeball of the albino rat in protein deficiency. *Br. J. Nutr.* 12, 254–9.

McMeekan, C. P. (1940). Growth and development of the pig. I With special reference to carcase quality characters. Development II Influence of the plane of nutrition on growth and development. Growth III Effect of the plane of nutrition on the form and composition of the bacon pig. *J. agric. Sci., Camb.* 30, 276–343, 387–427, 511–569.

Manassein, V. (1869). Materijalidlja voprosa o golodanii. "Materials on the Question of Starvation." Russian Med. dissertation, St Petersburg. Cited by C. M. Jackson (1925).

Miller, D. (1958). A case of anorexia nervosa in a young woman with development of subcapsular cataracts. *Trans. ophthal. Soc. U.K.* 78, 217–222.

Obal, A. (1950). Makulaschäden bei Inanition, Schneeblindheit und Sonnenblendung. Probleme der Ernährung der Netyhaut. *Klin. Mbl. Augenheilk.* 117, 28–45.

Palich-Szántó, O. (1924). Schnell reifende Katarakt nach Encephalitis lethargica. *Klin. Mbl. Augenheilk.* 72, 657–660.

Patterson, J. W. (1954). Effect of partial starvation on development of diabetic cataracts. *Proc. Soc. exp. Biol. Med.* 87, 395–6.

Petzetakis, M. (1950). Les tròubles oculaires pendant la trophopénie (maladie oedémateuse) et l'épidemie de pellagre (1941–4). La kératite superficielle trophopénique (kératopathie épithéliale). *Presse méd.* 58, 1082–4.

Scholtyssek, H. (1950). Beobachtungen über tiefe Augenveränderungen nach Mangelernährung. *Klin. Mbl. Augenheilk.* 117, 1–18.

Schuchardt, B. (1847). Inaugural Dissertation, Marburgi, Hesse. Cited by C. M. Jackson.

Siegert, P. (1956). Über Augenerkrankugen bei mangelernährten Spätheimkehrern. *Klin. Mbl. augenheilk.* 129, 3–13.

Smith, S. G. (1932). A new symptom complex in vitamin-G deficiency in rats. *Proc. Soc. exp. Biol. Med.* 30, 198–200.

Spyratos, S. (1949). Héméralopie et altérations oculaires par carence en Grèce pendant les années 1941–45. *Annls Oculist, Paris* 182, 672–685.

Stewart, C. A. (1918). Changes in the relative weights of the various parts, systems and organs of young albino rats underfed for various periods. *J. exp. Zool.* 25, 301–353.

Stewart, C. A. (1919). Changes in the weight of the various parts, systems and organs in albino rats kept at birth weight by underfeeding for various periods. *Am. J. Physiol.* 48, 67–78.

Stigmar, G. (1965). Anorexia nervosa associated with cataracts (report of a case). *Acta Ophthal.* 43, 787–789.

Tashiro, S., Smith, C. C., Badger, E. and Kezur, E. (1940). Chromodacryorrhea, a new criterion for biological assay of acetylcholine. *Proc. Soc. esp. Biol. Med.* 44, 658–661.

von Bechterew, W. (1895). Uber den Einfluss des Hungers auf die neugeborenen Thiere insbesondere auf das Gewicht und die Entwickelung des Gehirns. *Zentbl. Neurol.* 14, 810–817.

Widdowson, E. M. and McCance, R. A. (1960). Some effects of accelerating growth. I. General somatic development. *Proc. R. Soc. B* 152, 188–206.

Winkler, G. (1948). Über Augenhintergrundsveränderungen (Degeneration der Makula) bei Hungerkranken. *Klin. Mbl. Augenheilk.* 113, 231–234.

Živkov, E. and Teoharov, B. (1958). Clinical and pathological aspects of retinal oedema in alimentary dystrophy. *Archs Path.* 2, 71–76.

Chapter 2

Abrahamson, I. A. Sr and Abrahamson, I. A. Jr (1962). Hypercarotenemia. *Archs Ophthal.* 68, 4–7.

Achar, S. T. (1950) Nutritional dystrophy among children in Madras. *Br. med. J.* i, 701–703.

Achar, S. T. and Benjamin, V. (1953). Observations on nutritional dystrophy. *Indian J. child Hlth* 2, 1.

Adams, J. F., Johnstone, J. M. and Hunter, R. D. (1960). Vitamin A deficiency following total gastrectomy. *Lancet* i, 415–417.

Agarwal, L. P. and Adhaulia, H. N. (1954). Role of Vitamin A in healing corneal ulcers. *Ophthalmologica* 128, 6–14.

Aguilar, J. R., Arroyave, G. and Gallardo, C. (1977). Manual de supervisión y control de programs de fortificaciôn de azúcar con vitamina A. *I.N.C.A.P. Publ.* E-913.

Appelmans, M., Lebas, P. and Missotten, L. (1957). Vitamin A deficiency and its ocular manifestations. *Scalpel, Liege* 110, 217–234.

Arlt, F. (1851). *Die Krankheiten des Auges, Prague* 1, 211.

Arroyave, G., Wilson, D., Méndez, J., Béhar, M. and Scrimshaw, N. S. (1961). Serum and liver vitamin A and lipids in children with severe protein malnutrition. *Am. J. clin. Nutr.* 9, 180–185.

Ascher, K. W. (1954). Study of 22 malnourished patients with Bitot's spots. *Am. J. Opthal.* 38, 367–373.

Autret, M. and Béhar, M. (1954). Sindrome policarencial infantil (kwashiorkor) and its prevention in Central America. *FAO Nutr. Stud.* No. 13, v and 81.

Aykroyd, W. R. (1928). Vitamin A deficiency in Newfoundland. *Ir. J. med. Sci.* 6th Series, 161–165.

Aykroyd, W. R. (1930). Beriberi and other food-deficiency diseases in Newfoundland and Labrador. *J. Hyg. Camb.* 30, 357–386.

Baas, K. L. (1894). Uber eine Ophthalmia hepatitica nebst Beiträgen zur Kenntniss der Xerosis conjunctivae und zur Pathologie der Augenmuskelerkrankungen. *Albrecht v. Graefes Arch. Ophthal.* 40, 212–246.

Bagchi, K., Halder, K. and Chowdhury, S. R. (1959). Study of Bitot's spot with special reference to protein malnutrition. *J. Indian med. Ass.* 33, 401–407.

Balletto, G. M. (1954). Nutritional survey in central province of Tanganyika. *E. Afr. med. J.* 31, 459–464.

Bampfield (1814). *Med.-Chir. Trans.* 5, 32.

Bashor, M. M., Toft, D. O. and Chytil, F. (1973). In vitro binding of retinol to rat-tissue components. *Proc. natn. Acad. Sci. USA.* 70, 3483–3487.

Basu, N. M. and De, N. K. (1941). Assessment of vitamin A deficiency among Bengalees and determination of minimal and optimal requirements of vitamin A by simplified method for measuring visual adaptation in dark. *Indian J. med. Res.* 39, 591–612.

Beaver, D. L. (1961). Vitamin A deficiency in the germ-free rat. *Am. J. Path.* 38, 335–357.

Beitch, I. (1970). The induction of keratinization in the corneal epithelium. A comparison of the "dry" and vitamin A deficient eye. *Invest. Ophthal.* 9, 827–843.

Ben Sira, I., Ticho, V. and Yassur, Y. (1972). Surgical treatment of active keratomalacia by "covering graft". *Israel J. Med. Sci.* 8, 1209–1211.

Bergen, C. A. à and Weise, J. C. (1754). "De nyctalopia seu caecitate nocturna."

Berson, E. L. (1973). Experimental and therapeutic aspects of photopic damage to the retina. *Invest. Ophthal.* 12, 35–44.

Bessey, O. A. and Wolbach, S. B. (1938). Vitamin A: physiology and pathology. *J. Am. med. Ass.* 110, 2072–2080.

Bhattachayya, A. K. and Chatterjee, S. (1964). Karatomalacia in kwashiorkor and marasmus. *Calcutta Bull. Med.* 12, 152–154.

Bicknell, F. and Prescott, F. (1953). "The Vitamins in Medicine," 3rd edn, p.1. Heinemann, London.

Bietti, G. B. (1940). "Le Vitamine in Oftalmologia." Cappelli, Bologna.

Birnbacher, T. (1928). Zur Physiologie des fettlöslicher vitamines A. *Münchner med. W schr.* 75, 1114–5.

Bitot, C. (1863). Sur une lesion conjonctivale non encore décrite, coincidant avec l'héméralopie. *Gas. hebd. Med. Chir.* 10, 284.

Blackfan, K. D. and Wolbach, S. B. (1933). Vitamin A deficiency in infants: clinical and pathological study. *J. Pediat.* 3, 679–706.

Blakemore, F., Ottaway, C. W., Sellers, K. C., Eden, E. and Moore, T. (1957). The effects of a diet deficient in vitamin A on the development of the skull, optic nerves and brain of cattle. *J. comp. Path. Ther.* 67, 277–288.

Blegvad, O. (1924). Xerophthalmia, keratomalacia and xerosis conjunctivae. *Am. J. Ophthal.* 7, 89–117.

Blessig (1866). *Petersburger med. Z.* Cited by Blegvad, O. (1924).

Bloch, C. E. (1917). Diseases of infancy caused by preponderantly carbohydrate diet for protracted period: atrophy, dystrophy and amylogenic colitis. *Ugeskr. Laeg.* 79, 279–292.

Bloch, C. E. (1919). Klinische Untersunchungen über Dystrophie and Xerophthalmie bei jungen Kindern. *Jb. Kinderheilk.* **89**, 405–441.

Bloch, C. E. (1921). Clinical investigation of xerophthalmia and dystrophy in infants and young children. *J. Hyg., Camb.* **19**, 283–304.

Bloch, C. E. (1924a). Blindness and other diseases in children arising from deficient nutrition (lack of fat-soluble A factor). *Am. J. Dis. Child.* **27**, 139–148.

Bloch, C. E. (1924b). Further clinical investigation into the diseases arising in consequence of a deficiency in the fat-soluble A factor. *Am. J. Dis. Child.* **28**, 659–667.

Boëthius, J., Carlson, S. D., Höglund, G. and Struwe, G. (1972). Light sensitivity of the compound eye of a moth (*mànduca sexta*) reared on a retinol-deficient diet. *Acta Physiol. scand.* **84**, 289–294.

Bors, F. and Fells, P. (1971). Reversal of the complications of self-induced vitamin A deficiency. *Br. J. Ophthal.* **55**, 210–214.

Bouman, H. D., and van Creveld, S. (1940). Fetal keratomalacia. *Z. Vitaminforsch.* **10**, 192–197.

Bouzas, A. (1959). Significance of Bitot's spots. *Bull. Soc. ophthal. Fr.* **72**, 185–191.

Bowles, L. L., Allen, L., Sydenstricker, V. P., Hock, C. W. and Hall, W. K. (1946). The development and demonstration of corneal vascularization in rats deficient in vitamin A and in riboflavin. *J. Nutr.* **32**, 19–35.

Brammer, J. D. and White, R. H. (1969). Vitamin A deficiency: effect on mosquito eye ultrastructure. *Science, N.Y.* **163**, 821–823.

Brandenburger, J. L., Reed, C. T. and Eakin, R. M. (1975). Freeze fracture study of photoreceptors of dark and light adapted snails. *Ann. Zool.* **15**, 782.

Brëslau, R. C. (1957). Hypervitaminosis A. *Archs Pediat.* **74**, 139–152, 178–197.

Bridges, C. D. (1975). Storage, distribution and utilization of vitamins A in the eyes of adult amphibians and their tadpoles. *Vision Res.* **15**, 1311–1323.

Bridges, C. D. (1977). The visual pigment and vitamin A of *Xenopus laevis* embryos, larvae and adults. *Expl Eye Res.* **24**, 7–13.

Brink, E. W., Davey, W., Perera, A., Broske, S. P., Cash, R. A., Smith, J. L., Sauberlich, H. E. and Bashor, M. M. (1979). Vitamin A status of children in Sri Lanka. *Am. J. clin. Nutr.* **32**, 84–91.

Brock, J. F. and Autret, M. (1952). Kwashiorkor in Africa. *Monograph. Ser. W.H.O.* No. 8.

Bronte-Stewart, J. and Foulds, W. S. (1972). Acquired dyschromatopsia in vitamin A deficiency. *Mod. Probl. Ophthal.* **11**, 168–173.

Brown, J. (1827). Case of ulcerated cornea, from inanition. *Edin. J. med. Sci.* **3**, 218.

Brown, K. T. and Wiesel, T. N. (1958). Intraretinal recording in the unopened cat eye. *Am. J. Ophthal.* **46**, 91–96; discussion 96–98.

Brown, S. I., Weller, C. A. and Shinobu Akiya. (1970). Pathogenisis of ulcers of the alkali-burned cornea. *Archs Ophthal.* **83**, 205–208.

Bruce, G. M., Denning, C. R. and Spalter, H. F. (1960). Ocular findings in cystic fibrosis of the pancreas. *A.M.A. Archs Ophthal.* **63**, 391–401.

Buchanan, W. J. (1900). *Indian med. Gaz.* **35**, 424.

Carlos Negro, R. and Gentile Ramos, I. (1957). More frequent deficiencies in the children of Montevideo. *Archs Pediat. Uruguay* **28**, 633–652.

Carlson, S. D., Steeves, H. R. III, Vandeberg, J. S. and Robbins, W. E. (1967). Vitamin A deficiency: effect on the retinal structure of the moth *Manduca sexta*. *Science, N.Y.* 158, 268–270.

Carr, R. E., Margolis, S. and Siegel, I. M. (1976). Fluorescein angiography and vitamin A and oxalate levels in fundus. *Am. J. Ophthal.* 82, 549–558.

Carvalho, M. (1946). *Medna Cirurg. Farm.* 122, 303.

Carvalho, M. (1947). *Hospital, Rio de Janeiro* 32, 307.

Castellanos, A. (1935). Contribucion al estudio clinico de las avitaminosos B en Cusa; el sindrome pelagroide-ber-berico. *Boln Soc. cub. Pediat.* 7, 5–54.

Castellanos, A. (1937). El sindrome pelagroide-beri-berico. *Vida nueva* 40, 199–216.

Chandra, H., Venkatachalam, P. S., Belavadi, B., Reddy, V. and Gopalan, C. (1960). Some observations on vitamin A deficiency in Indian children. *Indian J. child Hlth* 9, 589–595.

Charpentier, G. (1936). Das Elektroretinogramm normaler und hemeraloper Raten. *Acta ophthal.* Suppl. No. 9, 1–85.

Chen, J. (1942). Nutritional œdema in children. *Am. J. Dis. Child.* 63, 552–580.

Chen, P. C. (1972). Sociocultural influences on vitamin A deficiency in a rural Malay community. *J. trop. Med. Hyg.* 75, 231–236.

Chevallier, A. (1946). *VII Congr. int. chimie Biol.*

Cobb, B. and Awdry, P. N. (1968). Xerophthalmia. *Trans. ophthal. Soc. U.K.* 88, 579–585.

Collins, E. T. (1930). Harderian gland; xerophthalmia; vitamin A deficiency; keratomalacia. *Trans. ophthal. Soc. U.K.* 50, 201–230.

Committee on Nutrition in the Colonial Empire (1939). First Report, Part 2. H.M.S.O., London.

Coward, K. H. (1942). The relative needs of young male and female rats for vitamin A. *Br. med. J.* i, 435–436.

Czerny, A. and Keller, A. (1906). "Des Kindes Ernährung, Ernährungsstörungen und Ernährungstherapie." Deutlicke, Leipzig.

Dansey-Browning, G. C. (1958). Ophthalmic disease in Hong Kong. *Br. J. Ophthal.* 42, 394–401.

Darby, W. J., McGanity, W. J., McLaren, D. S., Paton, D., Alemu, Z. and Medhen, M. G. (1960). Bitot's spots and vitamin A deficiency. *Publ. Hlth Rep., Wash.* 75, 738–743.

Darby, W. J. and McLaren, D. S. (1957). *W.H.O. Document* SEA/NUT/4.

De Gouvêa, H. (1883). Beiträge zur Kenntnis der Hemeralopie und Xerophthalmie aus Ernährungsstörungen. *Albrecht v. Graefes Arch. Ophthal.* 29, 167–200.

De Haas, J. H., Posthuma, J. H. and Meulemans, O. (1940). Xerophthalmia among children in Batavia. *Geneesk. Tijdschr. Ned.-Indië* 80, 928–950.

Dehority, B. A., Hazzard, D. G., Eaton, H. D., Grifo, A. P., jun., Rousseau, J. E., jun., Helmboldt, D. F., Jungherr, E. L. and Gosslee, D. G. (1960). Some biochemical constituents in serum cerebrospinal fluid, and aqueous humour of vitamin A deficient Holstein calves. *J. Dairy Sci.* 43, 630–644.

De Leonibus, F. (1939). *Annal Ottal. Clin. ocul.* 67, 512.

Delmelle, M., Noell, W. K. and Organisciak, D. T. (1975). Herditary retinal dystrophy in the rat: rhodopsin, retinol, vitamin A deficiency. *Expl Eye Res.* 21, 369–380.

348   NUTRITIONAL OPHTHALMOLOGY

De Ocampo, G. (1956). Changing concepts and patterns of approach in blinding diseases. *J. Philippine med. Ass.* 32, 1–6.

Dhanda, R. P. (1955). Electroretinography in night blindness and other vitamin A deficiencies. *A.M.A. Archs Ophthal.* 54, 841–849.

Dhanda, R. P. (1956). Clinical application of electroretinography with special reference to clinical manifestations of vitamin A deficiency, cataract and glaucoma. *Indian J. med. Res.* 44, 295–303.

Dixit, D. T. (1966). Night blindness in third trimester of pregnancy. *Indian J. med. Res.* 54, 971–975.

Donath, W. F. and Gorter, F. J. (1938). Determination of vitamins A and C and of carotenoids in blood of Dessa population in regions around Grisse, Segalaherang and Tjlandjoer. *Geneesk. Tijdschr. Ned.-Indië* 78, 2235–2274.

Dowling, J. E. (1960). Night blindness, dark adaptation, and the electroretinogram. *Am. J. Ophthal.* 50, 875–889.

Dowling, J. E. and Gibbons, I. R. (1961). The effect of vitamin A deficiency on the fine structure of the retina. *In* "The Structure of the Eye" (Ed. G. K. Smelser), 85–99. Academic Press, London and New York.

Dowling, J. E. and Wald, G. (1958). Vitamin A deficiency and night blindness. *Proc. natn. Acad. Sci. U.S.A.* 44, 648–661.

Drummond J. C. and Wilbraham, A. (1939). "The Englishman's Food," 95. Cape, London.

Ebbell, B. (1924). Die ägyptischen krankheitsnamen. *Z. ägyptische Sprache* 59, 57.

Ehrengut, W. (1955). Akuter benigner Hydrocephalus durch Hypervitaminosis-A (Syndrom Marie-Sée) bei Keratomalacie. *Z. Kinderheilk.* 77, 468–482.

Elkan, E. and Zwart, P. (1967). The ocular disease of young terrapins caused by vitamin A deficiency. *Path. vet.* 4, 201–222.

Elliot, R. H. (1920). "Tropical Ophthalmology", 80. Frowde, London.

Emran, N. and Sommer, A. (1979). Lissamine green staining in the clinical diagnosis of xerophthalmia. *Archs Ophthal.* 97, 2332–2335.

Etzine, S. (1968). The blindness of Tobit. *Med. Proc.* 14, 106–107.

Evetzki, A. (1890). *Archs ophthal. Paris* 10, 377.

Falta, W. and Noeggerath, C. T. (1905). Fütterwigsversuche mit künstlicher Nahrung. *Beitr. chem. Physiol. Path.* 7, 313–322.

Fedden, R. and Thomson, J. (1950). "Crusader Castles", p. 60. John Murray, London.

Fell, H. B. and Mellanby, E. (1953). Metaplasia produced in cultures of chick ectoderm by high vitamin A. *J. Physiol., Lond.* 119, 470–488.

Fells, P. and Bors, F. (1969). Ocular complications of self-induced vitamin A deficiency. *Trans. ophthal. Soc. U.K.* 89, 221–228.

Field, J. W. (1931). Some observations on vitamin A starvation among immigrant Indians in Malaya. *Malay. med. J.* 6, 46–53.

Findlay, G. M. (1925). A contribution to the aetiology of experimental keratomalacia. *Br. J. exp. Path.* 6, 16–21.

Fischer, J. N. (1843). Keratomalacie nach Masern. *In* "Lehrbuch de gesamt Entzündungen." Cited by Oomen, H.A.P.C. (1961).

Frape, D. L., Allen, R. S., Speer, V. C., Hays, V. W. and Catron, D. V. (1959).

Relationship of vitamin A to ^{35}S metabolism in the baby pig. *J. Nutr.* **68**, 189–201.

Frazier, C. N. and Hu, C. K. (1936). Nature and distribution according to age of cutaneous manifestations of vitamin A deficiency. *Arch Derm. Syph.* **33**, 825–852.

Freise, E., Goldschmidt, M. and Frank, A. (1915). Experimentelle Beiträge zur Aetiologie der Keratomalazie. *Mschr. Kinderheilk.* **13**, 424–430.

Friderichsen, C., and Edmund, C. (1937). Studies of hypervitaminosis A. II. A new method for costing the resorption of vitamin A from medicaments. *Am. J. Dis. Child.* **53**, 89–109.

Fridericia, L. S. and Holm, E. (1925). Experimental contribution to the study of the relation between night blindness and malnutrition. *Am. J. Physiol.* **73**, 63–78.

Friedenwald, J. S., Buschke, W. and Morris, M. E. (1945). Mitotic activity and wound healing in the corneal epithelium of vitamin A deficient rats. *J. Nutr.* **29**, 299–308.

Friis-Hansen, B. and McCullough, F. S. (1962). Vitamin A deficiency in African children in Northern Rhodesia. *J. Pediat.* **60**, 114–121.

Frontali, G. (1948). *Pediat. int.* **1**, 1.

Fuchs, A. (1947). Influence of general metabolic and nutritional disturbances upon resistance of cornea. *Am. J. Ophthal.* **30**, 721–727.

Fuchs, A. (1959). White spots of the fundus combined with night blindness and xerosis (Uyemura's syndrome). *Am. J. Ophthal.* **48**, 101–103.

Gama Lobo. (1866). Ophthalmia brasiliana. *Klin. Mbl. Augenheilk.* **4**, 65.

Genest, A. A., Sarwono, D. and Gyorgy, P. (1967). Vitamin A blood serum levels and electroretinogram in 5- to 14-years age group in Indonesia and Thailand. *Am. J. clin. Nutr.* **20**, 1275–1279.

Gershoff, S. N., Andrus, S. B., Hegsted, D. M. and Lentini, E. A. (1957). Vitamin A deficiency in cats. *Lab. Invest.* **6**, 227–240.

Gil, A. C. (1934). *Rev. méd. Yucatán* **17**, 467.

Giorgio, A. J., Cartwright, G. E. and Wintrobe, M. M. (1964). Pseudo-Kayser-Fleischer rings. *Archs intern. Med.* **113**, 817–818.

Goldschmidt, M. (1915). Experimenteller Beitrag zur Aetiologie der Keratomalacie. *Albrecht v. Graefes Arch. Ophthal.* **90**, 354–366.

Goldsmith, T. H., Barker, R. J. and Cohen, C. F. (1964). Sensitivity of visual receptors of carotene-depleted flies: a vitamin A deficiency in an invertebrate. *Science, N.Y.* **146**, 65–67.

Gorduren, S. and Ören, C. (1958). Bitot's spots not related to vitamin insufficiency. *XVIII Concilium Ophthalmologicum Belgica Acta* **2**, 1080.

Gorman, J. J., Cogan, D. G. and Gellis, S. S. (1957). An apparatus for grading the visual acuity in infants on the basis of opticokinetic nystagmus. *Pediatrics* **19**, 1088–1100.

Gow, W. H. (1934). Some clinical observations on cases of keratomalacia in Manchuria. *Chin. med. J.* **48**, 885–889.

Griffiths, A. W. and Behrman, J. (1967). Dark adaptation in mongols. *J. ment. Defic. Res.* **11**, 25–30.

Guerrero, L. E. and Conception, I. (1920). Xerophthalmia in fowls fed on polished rice and its clinical importance. *Philipp. J. Sci.* **17**, 99–103.

Guillemeau, J. (1585). "Traité des Maladies de l'oeil."

Haigh, L. D., Moulton, C. R. and Trowbridge, P. F. (1920). *Univ. Missouri Coll. Agric. Expl. Sta. Res. Bull.* **38**, 47.

Harris, W. A., Ready, D. F., Lipson, E. D. and Hudspeth, A. J. (1977). Vitamin A deprivation and Drosophila photopigments. *Nature, Lond.* **266**, 648–650.

Hartmann, E. and Saraux, H. (1957). Vitamin A and ocular tension. 200 000 "units" daily reduced ocular tension in man and the rabbit, probably owing to action against ascorbic acid. *Annls Oculist Paris* **190**, 508–523.

Hayes, K. C. (1974). Retinal degeneration in monkeys induced by deficiency of vitamin E or A. *Invest. Ophthal.* **13**, 499–510.

Hecht, S., Hendley, C. D., Ross, S. and Richmond, P. N. (1948). Effect of exposure to sunlight on night vision. *Am. J. Ophthal.* **31**, 1573–1580.

Hecht, S. and Mandelbaum, J. (1938). Rod-cone dark adaptation and vitamin A. *Science, N.Y.* **88**, 219–221.

Hecht, S. and Mandelbaum, J. (1939). The relation between vitamin A and dark adaptation. *J. Am. med. Ass.* **112**, 1910–1916.

Hecht, S. and Mandelbaum, J. (1940). Dark adaptation and experimental human vitamin A deficiency. *Am. J. Physiol.* **130**, 651–664.

Helgebostad, A. (1955). Experimental excess of vitamin A in fur animals. *Nord. VetMed.* **7**, 297–308.

Heller, J. (1975). Interactions of plasma retinol-binding protein with its receptor. *J. biol. Chem.* **250**, 3613–3619.

Heller, J. and Bok, D. (1976). Specific receptor for retinol binding-protein as detected by binding of human and bovine retinol-binding protein to pigment epithelial cells. *Am. J. Ophthal.* **81**, 93–97.

Herbert, H. (1897). Epithelial xerosis in natives of India. *Indian med. Gaz.* **32**, 130–134.

Herlinger, H. (1950). Nutritional dystrophy. *Br. med. J.* i, 1199–1200.

Herron, W. L., Riegel, B. W., Myers, O. E. and Rubin, M. L. (1969). Retinal dystrophy in the rat—a pigment epithelial disease. *Invest. Ophthal.* **8**, 595–604.

Hess, C. (1907). Uber Dunkeladaptation und Sehpurpur bei Hühnern und Tauben. *Archs Augenheilk.* **57**, 298–317.

Hess, C. (1909). Untersuchungen über Hemeralopie. *Archs Augenheilk.* **62**, 50–70.

Hetler, R. A. (1934). The development of xerophthalmia and the keratinization of epithelial tissue on withdrawal of vitamin A from the diet of the monkey (*Macacus rhesus*), guinea pig, rabbit and adult albino rat. *J. Nutr.* **8**, 75–103.

Hicks, R. J. (1867). *Richmond med. J.* **3**, 34.

Hime, J. M. (1972). Eye disease in terrapins. *Vet. Rec.* **91**, 493.

Hodges, R. E., Sauberlich, H. E., Canham, J. E., Wallace, D. L., Rucker, R. B., Mejia, L. A. and Mohanram, M. (1978). Hematopoietic studies in vitamin A deficiency. *Am. J. clin. Nutr.* **31**, 876–885.

Holm, E. (1925). Demonstration of hemeralopia in rats nourished on food devoid of fat-soluble A-vitamin. *Am. J. Physiol.* **73**, 79–84.

Holm, E. (1929). Demonstration of vitamin A in retinal tissue and comparison with vitamin content of brain tissue. *Acta Ophthal.* **7**, 146–161.

Holm, K. and Kessing, S. V. (1975). Conjunctival goblet cells in patients with cystic fibrosis. *Acta ophthal.* **53**, 167–172.

Hong, K. and Hubbell, W. L. (1972). Preparation and properties of phospholipid bilayers containing rhodopsin. *Proc. natn. Acad. Sci. U.S.A.* **69**, 2617–2621.

Hoogenkamp, P. A. (1956). "Ontwikkeling, Voeding en Voedingstoestand van zuigelingen en kleuters bij de Ngadju-Dajak op Kalimantan-Selatan (Zuid-Borneo), Indonesië." Thesis, University of Amsterdam.

Houet, R. and Lecomte-Ramioul, S. (1950). Répercussions sur l'enfant des avitaminosis de la mère pendant la grossesse. Un cas de bec-de-lièvre et xérophtalmie néonatale chez un enfant dont la mere présente une carance en vitamines A et B_2. *Ann. Pediat.* **175**, 378–388.

Hsu, K. L. (1927). Nutritional keratomalacia; report of cases. *Chin. med. J.* **41**, 825–836.

Hubbenet, M. (1860). *Annls Oculist. Paris* **44**, 293.

Huenemann, R. L., Collazos, C. C., Hegsted, D. M., Bravo De Rueda, Y., Castellanos, A., Dieseldorff, A., Escobar, M., Moscoso, I., White, P. L. and White, H. S. (1955). Nutrition and care of young children in Peru; Chacan and Vicos, rural communities in Andes. *J. Am. diet. Ass.* **31**, 1121–1133.

Hughes, J. S., Lienhardt, H. F. and Aubel, C. E. (1929). Nerve degeneration resulting from avitaminosis A. *J. Nutr.* **2**, 183–186.

Hume, E. M. and Krebs, H. A. (1949). Vitamin A requirement of human adults: an experimental study of vitamin A deprivation in man. A report of the vitamin A Sub-Committee of the Accessory Food Factors Committee. *Spec. Rep. Ser. med. Res. Coun.* No. 264.

Imai, R. (1930). *Acta Soc. Ophthal. Japan* **24**, 771.

Ishihara, S. (1913). Zur Aetiologie der idiopathischen Hemeralopie bzw. Xerosis conjunctivae. *Klin. Mbl. Augenheilk.* **15**, 596–603.

Ishikawa (1921). Cited by Sugita (1926).

Jan, L. Y. and Revel, J-P. (1974). Ultrastructural localization of rhodopsin in the vertebrate retina. *J. Cell Biol.* **62**, 257–273.

Jayle, G. E. and Ourgaud, A. G. (1950). "La vision nocturne et ses troubles." Masson, Paris.

Jelliffe, D. B. (1955). Infant nutrition in the subtropics and tropics. *Monograph. Ser. W.H.O.* No. 29.

Jensen, E. (1903). Xerophthalmia in small children. *Hospitalstidende* xi, 749–758.

Jensen, O. A. (1968). Necrotizing keratitis (keratomalacia) with corneal perforation and expulsive uveal haemorrhage in a newborn. *Acta Ophthal.* **46**, 215–7.

Jess, A. (1921). Die Nachtblindheit mit besunderer Berücksichtgung der während des Krieges gesammelten Erfahrungen. *Zentbl. ges. Ophthal.* **6**, 113.

John, I. (1931). The disturbances of sensibility of the cornea and conjunctiva in xerosis and keratomalacia of adults. *Archs Ophthal.* **5**, 374–391.

Johnson, M. L. (1939). The effect of vitamin A deficiency on the retina of the cat. *J. exp. Zool.* **81**, 67–89.

Johnson, M. L. (1943). Degeneration and repair of rat retina in avitaminosis A. *Archs Ophthal.* **29**, 793–810.

Jones, B. R., Darougar, S., Mohsenine, H. and Poirer, R. H. (1976). Communicable ophthalmia; the blinding scourge of the Middle East. Yesterday, today and ? tomorrow. *Br. J. Ophthal.* **60**, 492–498.

Jones, J. H. (1927). The relation of the inorganic constituents of A ration to the production of ophthalmia in rats. *J. biol. Chem.* 75, 139–146.

Josephs, H. W. (1944). Hypervitaminosis A and carotenaemia. *Am. J. Dis. Child* 67, 33–43.

Juzwa, J. (1958). Decreased corneal sensitivity in infants with xerophthalmia and keratomalacia. *Klin. Oczna* 28, 129–138.

Kanai, M., Raz, A. and Goodman, D. S. (1968). Retinol-binding protein: the transport protein for vitamin A in human plasma. *J. clin. Invest.* 47, 2025–2044.

Katznelson, A. B. (1947). Vitamin insufficiency in the pathology of the cornea. *Vest. Oftalmol.* 26, 3–7.

Keefer, C. S. and Yang, C. S. (1929). *Nat. med. J. China* 15, 701.

Kessler, E., Mondino, B. J. and Brown, S. I. (1977). The corneal response to *Pseudomonas aeruginosa*: histopathological and enzymatic characterization. *Invest. Ophthal. Vision Sic.* 16, 116–125.

Keys, A., Brozek, J., Hanschel, A., Mickelson, O. and Taylor, H. L. (1950). *"The Biology of Human Starvation,"* Vols 1 and 2. University of Minnesota Press, Minneapolis.

Khalap, N. V. (1956). Observations on "kwashiorkor" or nutritional dystrophy in Poona. *Indian J. child Hth* 5, 306–313.

Kirwan E. O'G., Sen, K. and Bose, N. (1943). Nutrition and its bearing on preventable blindness and eye diseases in Bengal. *Indian J. med. Res.* 31, 49–62.

Knapp, P. (1908). Experimenteller Beitrag zur Ernährung von Ratten mit Künstlicher. Nahrung und zum Zusammerhang von Ernährungs-störungen mit Erkrankungen der Conjunctiva. *Z. expl. Path. Ther.* 5, 147–169.

Ko Lay (1968). Causes of blindness in Burma. *Union Burma J. Life Sci.* 1, 85–87.

Kollock, C. W. (1890). A form of xerosis. *Ophthal. Rev.* 9, 249–251.

Konno, T., Hansen, J. D. and Truswell, A. S. (1968). Vitamin A deficiency and protein-calorie malnutrition in Cape Town. *S. Afr. med. J.* 42, 950–955.

Kreger, A. S. and Griffin, O. K. (1975). Cornea-damaging proteases of *Serratia marcescens. Invest. Ophthal.* 14, 190–198.

Kreiker, A. (1930). Zur Klinik und Histologie der epithelialen Bindehautxerose. *Albrecht v. Graefes Arch. Ophthal.* 124, 191–205.

Kubli, T. (1887). Zur Lehre von der epidemischen Hemeralopie. *Archs Augenheilk.* 17, 409–411.

Kuming, B. S. and Politzer, W. M. (1967). Xerophthalmia and protein malnutrition in Bantu children. *Br. J. Ophthal.* 51, 649–666.

Kusin, J. A., Soewando, W. and Parlindungan Dinaga, H. S. R. (1979). Rose Bengal and lissamine green vital stains: useful diagnostic aids for early stages of xerophthalmia? *Am. J. clin. Nutr.* 32, 1559–1561.

Kuwahara, Y. (1935). *Acta Soc. Ophthal. Japan* 39, 143.

Lahiri, L. M. (1938). Night blindness and cataract in bullocks. (A deficiency disease?) *Indian vet. J.* 15, 58.

Lambert, R. A. and Yudkin, A. M. (1923). Changes in the paraocular glands accompanying the ocular lesions which result from a deficiency in vitamin A. *J. exp. Med.* 38, 25–32.

Leber, T. (1883). Ueber die Xerosis der Bindehaut und die infantile Hornhaut-verschwärung; neben Bemerkungen über die Entstehung des Xerophthalmus.

Albrecht v. Graefes Arch. Ophthal. 29, 225–290.

Lechat, M. F., Bouche, R., Ville De Goyet, C. de. and Boucquey, C. (1976). Epidemiologie de l'avitaminose A au Niger. *Annls Soc. belg. Méd. trop.* 56, 333–343.

Lee, O. S. Jr and Hart, W. M. (1944). Metabolism of cornea; studies on oxygen consumption of corneas of riboflavin- and Vitamin A-deficient rats. *Am. J. Ophthal.* 27, 488–500.

Leitner, Z. A., Moore, T. and Sharman, I. M. (1960). Vitamin A and vitamin E in human blood. I. Levels of vitamin A and carotenoids in British men and women, 1948–57. *Br. J. Nutr.* 14, 157–169.

Lemp, M. A. (1973). The mucin-deficient dry eye. *Invest. Ophthal.* 13, 185–189.

Lemp, M. A., Holly, F. J., Iwata, S. and Dohlman, C. H. (1970). The pre-corneal tear film. I. Factors in spreading and maintaining a continuous tear film over the corneal surface. *Archs Ophthal.* 83, 89–94.

Levine, R. A. and Rabb, M. F. (1971). Bitot's spot overlying a pinguecula. *Archs Ophthal.* 86, 525–528.

Levy, N. S. and Toskes, P. P. (1974). Fundus albi punctatus and vitamin A deficiency. *Am. J. Ophthal.* 78, 926–929.

Lietman, P. S., di'Sant'Agnese, P. A. and Wong, V. (1964). Optic neuritis in cystic fibrosis of the pancreas. *J. Am. med. Ass.* 189, 924–927.

Lim, K. H. (1975). Causes of blindness in Singapore. *Med. J. Malay.* 29, 263–269.

Livingston, P. C. (1944). Visual problems of aerial warfare. *Lancet* ii, 33–38.

Loewenthal, L. J. A. (1935). An enquiry into vitamin A deficiency among the population of Teso, Uganda, with special reference to schoolchildren. *Ann. trop. Med. Parasit.* 29, 349–360.

Loh, R. C. K. (1967). Xerophthalmia (keratomalacia) in Singapore—a study. *Singapore med. J.* 8, 128–133.

Lund, C. J. and Kimble, M. S. (1943). Plasma vitamin A and carotene of the newborn infant: with consideration of fetal–maternal relationships. *Am. J. Obstet. Gynec.* 46, 207–221.

McCarrison, R. (1923). On the occurrence of ophthalmia in pigeons fed exclusively on parboiled rice and on its prevention by the addition of soil to the food. *Indian J. med. Res.* 11, 323–335.

McCollum, E. V. (1957). Pioneer studies of vitamin A. *In* "A History of Nutrition," 229–243. Mifflin, Boston.

McCollum, E. V. and Davis, M. (1913). The necessity of certain lipins in the diet during growth. *J. biol. Chem.* 15, 167–175.

McCollum, E. V., Simmonds, N. and Becker, J. E. (1922). On a type of ophthalmia caused by unsatisfactory relations in the inorganic portion of the diet. An ophthalmia not due to starvation for fat-soluble A, and not curable by its administration. *J. biol. Chem.* 53, 313–321.

McCollum, E. V., Simmonds, N. and Becker, J. E. (1926–27). Studies on "salt ophthalmia" III. *Proc. Soc. exp. Biol. Med.* 24, 952.

McKenzie, A. (1939). An examination of vitamin A deficiency among African natives by the dysadaptation test. *Trans. R. Soc. trop. Med. Hyg.* 32, 717–728.

Mackenzie, W. (1830). "A Practical Treatise on the Diseases of the Eye," 88, 199. Longman, Ree, Orme, Brown and Green, London.

McLaren, D. S. (1956). A study of the factors underlying the special incidence of keratomalacia in Oriya children in the Phulbani and Ganjam districts of Orissa, India. *J. trop. Pediat.* 2, 135–140.

McLaren, D. S. (1958). Involvement of the eye in protein malnutrition. *Bull. Wld Hlth Org.* 19, 303–314.

McLaren, D. S. (1959). Influence of protein deficiency and sex on the development of ocular lesions and survival time of the vitamin A-deficient rat. *Br. J. Ophthal.* 43, 234–241.

McLaren, D. S. (1960a). The effects of malnutrition on the eye: with special reference to work with experimental animals. *Wld Rev. Nutr. Dietet.* 2, 25–51.

McLaren, D. S. (1960b). Nutrition and eye disease in East Africa: experience in Lake and Central Provinces, Tanganyika. *J. trop. Med. Hyg.* 63, 101–122.

McLaren, D. S., Shaw, M. J. and Dalley, K. R. (1961). Eye disease in leprosy patients. A study in central Tanganyika. *Int. J. Leprosy.* 29, 20–28.

McLaren, D. S. (1963). "Malnutrition and the Eye." Academic Press, London and New York.

McLaren, D. S. (1966). Present knowledge of the role of vitamin A in health and disease. *Trans. R. Soc. trop. Med. Hyg.* 60, 436–462.

McLaren, D. S. (1976). "Nutrition and Its Disorders," 2nd edn. Churchill Livingston, Edinburgh.

McLaren, D. S., Shirajian, E., Tchalian, M. and Khoury, G. (1965a). Xerophthalmia in Jordan. *Am. J. clin. Nutr.* 17, 117–130.

McLaren, D. S., Tchalian, M. and Ajans, Z. A. (1965b). Biochemical and hematologic changes in the vitamin A-deficient rat. *Am. J. clin. Nutr.* 17, 131–138.

McLaren, D. S., Oomen, H. A. P. C. and Escapini, H. (1966a). Ocular manifestations of vitamin A deficiency in man. *Bull. Wld Hlth Org.* 34, 357–361.

McLaren, D. S., Read, W. W. C. and Tchalian, M. (1966b). Extent of human vitamin A deficiency. *Proc. Nutr. Soc.* 25, xxviii.

McLaren, D. S. and Zekian, B. (1971). Failure of enzymic cleavage of beta-carotene: the cause of vitamin A deficiency in a child. *Am. J. Dis. Child.* 121, 278–280.

MacManus, E. P. (1968). Xerophthalmia in Matabeleland. *Cent. Afr. J. Med.* 14, 166–170.

MacPhail, N. P. (1929). *United Fruit Co. Med. Dept., 18th Ann. Rep.* p. 172.

McPherson, H. J. (1956). "Investigation of ophthalmological conditions and the need for ophthalmological services in Kelantan." *Serv. Rep. Min. Health, Malaya* 1955–56.

Magendie, F. (1816). *Ann. Chim. Phys.* 3, 66.

Majima, A., Nakajima, A., Ichikawa, H. and Watanabe, M. (1960). Prevalence of ocular anomalies among schoolchildren. *Am. J. Ophthal.* 50, 139–146.

Manchanda, S. S. and Gupta, H. L. (1958). Malnutrition in the Punjab—with particular reference to protein deficiency (a review of 200 cases). *Indian J. child Hlth* 7, 386–395.

Mann, I. (1959). Researches into the regional distribution of eye disease. *Am. J. Ophthal.* 47, 134–144.

Mann, I., Pirie, A., Tansley, K. and Wood, C. (1946). Some effects of vitamin A deficiency on eye of rabbit. *Am. J. Ophthal.* 29, 801–815.

Manson-Bahr, P. E. C. (1951). Malignant malnutrition in Fiji. *Trans. R. Soc. trop. Med. Hyg.* 44, 555–8.

Mar, P. G. and Read, B. E. (1936). Chemical examination of Chinese remedies for night blindness. *Chin. J. Physiol.* 10, 273–283.

Marie, J. and Sée, G. (1951). Hydrocéphalie aiguë bénigne du nourrisson après l'ingestion d'une dose massive et unique de vitamines A et D. *Seamaine Hôp.* 27, 1744–1746.

Marie, J. and Sée, G. (1954). Acute hypervitaminosis A of the infant: its clinical manifestation with benign acute hydrocephalus and pronounced bulge of the fontanel; a clinical and biologic study. *Am. J. Dis. Child.* 87, 731–6.

Marmor, M. F. (1977). Fundus albi punctatus: a clinical study of the fundus lesions, the physiologic deficit and the vitamin A metabolism. *Doc. Ophthal.* 43, 277–302.

Martin, P. H. (1930). *Malay. med. J.* 4, 103.

Maxwell, J. P. (1932). Vitamin deficiency in the antenatal period, its effects on the mother and the infant. *J. Obstet. Gynaec. Br. Emp.* 39, 764–776.

Mayer, J. and Krehl, W. A. (1935). Influence of vitamin A deficiency on the gross efficiency of growth of rats. Yale J. Biol. Med. 20, 403–405.

Mayou, M. S. (1904). The pathological anatomy of plaques in epithelial xerosis. *Trans. ophthal. Soc. U.K.* 24, 9–16.

Mekki el Sheikh (1960). Vitamin deficiencies in relation to the eye. *Br. J. Ophthal.* 44, 406–414.

Mellanby, E. (1934). Xerophthalmia, trigeminal degeneration and vitamin A deficiency. *J. Path. Bact.* 38, 391–407.

Mellanby, E. (1943). The effect of bone dysplasia (overgrowth) on cranial nerves in vitamin A deficient animals. *J. Physiol., Lond.* 101, 408–431.

Mellanby, E. (1944). Nutrition in relation to bone growth and the nervous system. *Proc. R. Soc. B* 132, 28–46.

Mellanby, E. (1947). Vitamin A and bone growth: the reversibility of vitamin A-deficiency changes. *J. Physiol., Lond.* 105, 382–399.

Meneghello, J., Espinosa, J. and Coronel, L. (1949). Value of biopsy of the liver in nutritional dystrophy: evaluation of treatment with choline and dried stomach. *Am. J. Dis. Child.* 78, 141–152.

Meneghello, J., Niemeyer, H. and Espinosa, J. (1950). Liver steatosis in undernourished Chilean children. I. Its evolution as followed by serial puncture biopsies. *Am. J. Dis. Child.* 80, 889–897.

Métivier, V. M. (1941). Bitot spots in Trinidad. *Am. J. Ophthal.* 24, 1029–1034.

Meulemans, O. and De Haas, J. H. (1936). Over het gehalte aan carotine en vitamine A van moedermelk in Batavia. *Geneesk. Tijdschr. Ned.-Indië* 76, 1538–1571.

Meyerhof, M. (1916). Nightblindness as a war disease. *Am. J. Ophthal.* 33, 139–143.

Mikkelsen, B., Ehler, S. N. and Thomsen, H. G. (1974). Vitamin A intoxication causing papilloedema and simulating acute encephalitis. *Acta neurol.* 50, 642–650.

Milano, A. (1936). Incidence of eye diseases due to vitamin deficiency in the Naples Eye Clinic from 1930 to 1935. *Quad. Nutri., Roma* 3, 82–92.

Millen, J. W., Woollam, D. H. M. and Lamming, G. E. (1953). Hydrocephalus associated with deficiency of vitamin A. *Lancet* ii, 1234–1236.

Millen, J. W., Woollam, D. H. M. and Lamming, G. E. (1954). Congenital hydrocephalus due to experimental hypervitaminosis A. *Lancet* ii, 679–683.

Miś, M. (1958). A simplified instrument for making the darkness adaptation curve by means of an objective method based on the optokinetic nystagmus symptom. *Klin. Oczna* 28, 95–100.

Moore, L. A. (1939). Relationship between carotene, blindness due to constriction of the optic nerve, papillary œdema and nyctalopia in calves. *J. Nutr.* 17, 443–459.

Moore, L. A. (1941). Some ocular changes and deficiency manifestations in mature cows fed a ration deficient in vitamin A. *J. Diary Sci.* 24, 895.

Moore, L. A. and Sykes, J. F. (1941). Terminal cerebrospinal fluid pressure values in vitamin A deficiency. *Am. J. Physiol.* 134, 436–439.

Moore, L. A., Huffman, C. F. and Duncan, C. W. (1935). Blindness in cattle associated with a constriction of the optic nerve and probably of nutritional origin. *J. Nutr.* 9, 533–551.

Moore, T. (1957a). "Vitamin A," p. 239. Elsevier, Amsterdam.

Moore, T. (1957b). "Vitamin A," p. 326. Elsevier, Amsterdam.

Moore, T. (1957c). "Vitamin A," p. 425. Elsevier, Amsterdam.

Moore, T. (1957d). "Vitamin A", p. 432. Elsevier, Amsterdam.

Moore, T. and Wang, Y. L. (1945). Hypervitaminosis A. *Biochem. J.* 39, 222–228.

Mori, M. (1904). Ueber den sogenanten Hekam (Xerosis conjunctivae infantum eventuell Keratomalacie). *Jb. Kinderheilk.* 59, 175–195.

Mori, S. (1922a). Primary changes in eyes of rats which result from a deficiency of fat-soluble A in diet. *J. Am. med. Ass.* 79, 197–200.

Mori, S. (1922b). The changes in the paraocular glands which follow the administration of diets low in fat-soluble A. *Johns Hopkins Hosp. Bull.* 33, 357–359.

Mori, S. (1923). The pathological anatomy of ophthalmia produced by diets containing fat-soluble A, but unfavourable contents of certain inorganic elements. *Am. J. Hyg.* 3, 99–102.

Morrice, G., Havener, W. H. and Kapetansky, F. (1970). Vitamin A intoxication as a cause of pseudotumor cerebri. J. Am. med. Ass. 173, 1802–1803.

Mouriquand, G., Rollet, J. and Edel, V. (1949). Sur l'avitaminose A du pigeon. *C. r. Seanc. Soc. Biol.* 142, 980–981.

Mouriquand, G., Rollet, J., Edel, V. and Chighizola, R. (1955). Avitaminose et hypervitaminose A du pigeon. Identité de leur séméiologie oculair. *C. r. hebd. Séanc. Acad. Sci., Paris* 241, 348–350.

Mullins, M. M. (1960). Keratomalacia associated with adrenal hypoplasia in a defective. *Br. J. Ophthal.* 44, 300–5.

Mulock Houwer, A. W. (1956). "Kouwenaar's Leerboek der trop. Gen," p. 539. Schletema and Holkema, Amsterdam.

Mutch, J. R. and Richards, M. B. (1939). Keratoconus experimentally produced in rat by vitamin A deficiency. *Br. J. Ophthal.* 23, 381–387.

Neave, M. (1968). Protein and calorie malnutrition of early childhood in Western Samoa. *Trop. geogr. Med.* 20, 191–201.

Nelson, V. E. and Lamb, A. R. (1920). The effect of vitamin deficiency on various species of animals. I. The production of xerophthalmia in the rabbit. *Am. J. Physiol.* 51, 530–535.

Netrasiri, A. and Netrasiri, C. (1955). Kwashiorkor in Bangkok (analytical study of 54 cases). *J. trop. Pediat.* 1, 148–155.

Netter (1870). *C. r. hebd. Séanc Acad. Sci., Paris* 70, 577.

Nguyen Dinh Cat (1958). *XVIII Conc. Ophthal. Belg. Acta* 2, 1127.

Nicholls, L. (1933). Phrynoderma: condition due to vitamin deficiency. *Indian med. Gaz.* **68**, 681–686.

Nicholls, L. and Nimalasuriya, A. (1939). Bitot's spots in Ceylon. *Lancet* i, 1432–1434.

Nicotra, C., Livrea, M. A. and Cacioppa, F. (1976). Retinol and retinyl esters in pigment epithelia of rats with inherent retinal degeneration. *Experientia* **32**, 147–8.

Noell, W. K. (1958). Differentiation, metabolic organization and viability of the visual cell. *A.M.A. Archs Ophthal.* **60**, 702–733.

Noell, W. K. and Albrecht, R. (1971). Irreversible effects of visible light on the retina: role of vitamin A. *Science, N.Y.* **172**, 76–79.

Noell, W. K., Delmelle, M. C. and Albrecht, R. (1971). Vitamin A deficiency effect on retina: dependence on light. *Science, N.Y.* **172**, 72–75.

Norden, A. and Stigmar, G. (1969). Measurement of dark adaptation in vitamin A deficiency by a new quantitative technique. *Acta Ophthal.* **47**, 716–722.

Norn, M. S. (1974). Alizarin red. Vital staining of cornea and conjunctiva. *Acta ophthal.* **52**, 468–476.

Oliver, T. K. and Havener, W. H. (1958). Eye manifestations of chronic vitamin A intoxication. *A.M.A. Archs Ophthal.* **60**, 19–22.

Ong, D. E. and Chytil, F. (1975). Retinoic acid-binding protein in rat tissue. Partial purification and comparison to rat tissue retinol-binding protein. *J. biol. Chem.* **250**, 6113–6117.

Oomen, H. A. P. C. (1953). Infant malnutrition in Indonesia. *Bull. Wld Hlth Org.* **9**, 371–384.

Oomen, H. A. P. C. (1954). Xerophthalmia in the presence of kwashiorkor. *Br. J. Nutr.* **8**, 307–318.

Oomen, H. A. P. C. (1955). The external pattern of malnutrition in Djakarta toddlers. *Documenta Med. geogr. trop.* **7**, 1–9.

Oomen, H. A. P. C. (1957). The incidence of xerophthalmia in Java in relation to age and sex. *Documenta Med. geogr. trop.* **9**, 357–368.

Oomen, H. A. P. C. (1958). Hypovitaminosis A. III. Clinical experience of Hypovitaminosis A. *Fedn Proc. Fedn Am. Socs exp. Biol.* **17**, Suppl. No. 2, 111–128.

Oomen, H. A. P. C. (1960). *W.H.O. Document* Malaya 12.

Oomen, H. A. P. C. (1961). An outline of xerophthalmia. *Int. Rev. trop. Med.* **1**, 131–213.

Oomen, H. A. P. C. and Grubben, G. J. H. (1977). "Tropical Leafy Vegetables in Human Nutrition." Royal Institute for the Tropics, Amsterdam.

Oomen, H. A. P. C., McLaren, D. S. and Escapini, H. (1964). Epidemiology and public health aspects of hypovitaminosis A. A global survey on xerophthalmia. *Trop. geogr. Med.* **16**, 271–315.

Oomen, J. M. V. (1971). Xerophthalmia in northern Nigeria. *Trop. geogr. Med.* **23**, 246–249.

Oropeza, P. (1946). Los estados distróficos en la segunda infancia (sindromes policarenciales). *Archos venez. puericult. Pediat.* **8**, 1570–1782.

Ouwehand, C. D. (1900). Over "Rondar Manok." *Geneesk. Tijdschr. Ned.-Indië* **40**, 227–229.

358 NUTRITIONAL OPHTHALMOLOGY

Pagola, J. G. (1948). Los estados cerenciales en Mexico. *Acta Paediat.* 36, 329–332.

Parinaud (1881). Des modifications pathologiques de la perception de la lumière, des couleurs et des formes, et des differéntes espèces de sensibilité oculaire. *Gaz. méd. Paris* 3, 411–413.

Patek, A. J. and Haig, C. (1939). The occurrence of abnormal dark adaptation and its relation to vitamin A metabolism in patients with cirrhosis of the liver. *J. clin. Invest.* 18, 609–616.

Paton, D. and McLaren, D. S. (1960). Bitot spots. *Am. J. Ophthal.* 50, 568–574.

Patwardhan, V. N. (1969). Hypovitaminosis A and epidemiology of xerophthalmia. *Am. J. clin. Nutr.* 22, 1106–1118.

Pernetta, C. and de Martino, H. (1945). Pelagra na la infância. *Hospital, Rio de Janeiro* 27, 211–230.

Petersen, R. A., Petersen, V. S. and Robb, R. M. (1968). Vitamin A deficiency with xerophthalmia and night blindness in cystic fibrosis. *Am. J. Dis. Child.* 116, 662–665.

Pfister, R. R. and Renner, M. E. (1978). Corneal and conjunctival surface in vitamin A deficiency—a scanning electron microscope study. *Invest. Ophthal. Vision. Sci.* 17, 874–883.

Pillat, A. (1929). Does keratomalacia exist in adults? *A.M.A. Archs Ophthal.* 2, 256–287.

Pillat, A. (1930). Ueber Praexerosis und Xerosis corneae als selbständige Krankheitsbilder der Mangelerkrankung des Auges beim Erwachsenen. *Albrecht v. Graefes Arch. Ophthal.* 124, 486–506.

Pillat, A. (1931). Ueber eine eigenartige Pigmentierung der Bindehaut bei den verschiedenen Formen des Vitamin-A Manglerkrankung d. Erwachsenen. *Albrecht v. Graefes Arch. Ophthal.* 127, 575–597.

Pillat, A. (1932). Uber Mumifizierung des Hornkautepithels bei Vitamin-A-Mangel. *Z. Augenheilk.* 79, 200–208.

Pillat, A. (1933). Production of pigment in conjunctiva in night blindness, prexerosis, xerosis and keratomalacia of adults. *A.M.A. Archs Ophthal.* 9, 25–47.

Pillat, A. (1939). Mangel an Vitamin A. *In* "Ernahrungslehre" (Ed. W. Stepp), 283–330. Springer, Berlin.

Pillat, A. (1940). Die klassischen Symptome des Vitamin A-Mangels und der Vitamin A-Mangel als Gesamterkrankung des Körpers. *Wien. klin. Wschr.* 53, 779–783.

Pirie, A. (1977). Effect of locally applied retinoic acid on corneal xerophthalmia in the rat. *Expl. Eye Res.* 25, 297–302.

Pirie, A. and Overall, M. (1972). Effect of vitamin A deficiency on the lens epithelium of the rat. *Expl Eye Res.* 13, 105–109.

Pirie, A., Werb, Z. and Burleigh, M. C. (1975). Collagenase and other proteinases in cornea of retinol-deficient rat. *Br. J. Nutr.* 34, 297–309.

Platt, B. S. (1958). Hypovitaminosis A. *Fedn Proc. Fedn Am. Socs exp. Biol.* 17, Suppl. No. 2, 109.

Pohlman, M. E. and Ritter, E. F. (1952). Observations on vitamin deficiencies in eye, ear, nose and throat clinic of Japanese prison hospital. *Am. J. Ophthal.* 35, 228–230.

Postmus, S. (1956). *Voeding* 17, 403.

Prasad, L. N., and Upadhaya, M. P. (1967). Blindness as observed in Katmandu. *J. Nepal med. Ass.* 5, 92–101.

Protein-Calorie Advisory Group (1976). *Prot. Adv. Group Bull.* 6, No. 4.

Puretić, B., Raić, F. and Sarajlić-Vrsalović, M. (1967). Těski oblici avitaminoze A dojenčadi. Osvrt na 19 bolesnika. *Jugoslav. Pedijat.* 10, 3–10.

Quéré, M. A., Satgé, P., Graveline, J., Charnay, C., Diallo, J., and Blatt, C. (1967). Les kératopathies infantiles dans les kwashiorkors et les dénutrirons graves en Afrique tropicale. *Bull. Soc. ophthal. Fr.* 80, 69–77.

Raica, N. Jr., Scott, J., Lowry, L. and Sauberlich, H. E. (1972). Vitamin A concentration in human tissues collected from five areas in the United States. *Am. J. clin. Nutr.* 25, 291–296.

Ramalingaswami, V. (1948). Nutritional diarrhoea due to vitamin A deficiency. *Indian J. med. Sci.* 2, 665.

Ramalingaswami, V., Leach, E. H. and Sriramachari, S. (1955). Ocular structure in vitamin A deficiency in the monkey. *Q. Jl exp. Physiol.* 40, 337–347.

Rambo, V. C. (1958). *XVIII Conc. Ophthal. Belg. Acta* 2, 1850.

Rao, M. V. R. (1936). Studies on vitamin A deficiency. I. Xerophthalmia and trigeminal nerve degeneration. *Indian J. med. Res.* 24, 439–457.

Reddy, V. and Vijayalaxmi (1977). Colour vision in vitamin A deficiency. *Br. med. J.* i, 81.

Reichel, H. and Bleichert, A. (1958). Der einfluss von Vitamin A auf die Zapfenadaptation des Menschen. *Klin. Wschr.* 36, 225–227.

Remé, C. E. and Young, R. W. (1977). The effect of hibernation on cone visual cells in the grey squirrel. *Invest. Ophthal. Vision Sci.* 16, 813–840.

Rezgallah, A., Tcherevco, S. and Zaghdane, M. (1967). Atteinte de l'oeil dans la malnutrition protéique chez le nourisson. *Tunis. Med.* 45, 35–39.

Rodger, F. C., Saiduzzafar, H., Grover, A. D. and Fazal, A. (1963). A reappraisal of the ocular lesions known as Bitot's spot. *Br. J. Nutr.* 17, 475–485.

Rogers, N. E. Jr, Bieri, J. G. and McDaniel, E. G. (1971). Vitamin A deficiency in the germ-free rat. *Fedn Proc. Fedn Am. Socs exp. Biol.* 30, 1773–1778.

Roels, O. A., Debeir, O. and Trout, M. (1958a). Vitamin A deficiency in Ruanda-Urundi. *Trop. geogr. Med.* 10, 77–92.

Roels, O. A., Trout, M. and Dujacquier, R. (1958b). Carotene balances in boys in Ruanda where vitamin A deficiency is prevalent. *J. Nutr.* 65, 115–127.

Rumbaur, W. (1922). Augenerkrankungen bei Enten infolge von Avitaminose. *Klin. Mbl. Augenheilk.* 68, 744–9.

Russell, B. M., Smith, V. C., Multrack, R., Krill, A. E. and Rosenberg, I. H. (1973). Dark adaptation testing for diagnosis of subclinical vitamin A deficiency and evaluation of therapy. *Lancet* ii, 1161–1164.

Russell, R. M., Morrison, S. A., Smith, F. R., Oaks, E. V. and Carney, E. A. (1978). Vitamin A reversal of abnormal dark adaptation in cirrhosis. Study of effects on the plasma retinol transport system. *Ann. int. Med.* 88, 622–626.

Sabella, J. D., Bern, H. A., and Kahn, R. H. (1951). Effect of locally applied Vitamin A and oestrogen on rat epidermis. *Proc. Soc. exp. Biol. Med.* 76, 499–503.

Saemisch, T. (1876). *Handb. Augenheilk.* 4, 128.

Said, M. (1955). Kwashiorkor in Negri Sembilan. *Med. J. Malaya* 10, 20–47.

Salley, J. J. and Bryson, W. F. (1957). Vitamin A deficiency in the hamster. *J. dent. Res.* 36, 935–944.

Salus, R. (1957). Ophthalmology in a concentration camp. *Am. J. Ophthal.* 44, 12–17.

Sandberg, M. A., Rosen, J. B. and Berson, E. L. (1977). Cone and rod functions in vitamin A deficiency with chronic alcoholism and in retinitis pigmentosa. *Am. J. Ophthal.* 84, 658–665.

Sarin, B. P. (1957). Clinical observations on "kwashiorkor" or protein undernutrition in Rangoon. *Indian J. child Hlth* 6, 300–307.

Sauberlich, H. E., Hodges, R. E., Wallace, D. L., Kolder, H., Canham, J. E., Hood, J., Raica, N. Jr. and Lowry, L. K. (1974). Vitamin A metabolism and requirements in the human studied with the use of labelled retinol. *Vitams Horm.* 32, 251–275.

Sauer, M. E. (1939). A demonstration of nerve fibres in the metaplastic epithelium of vitamin A deficient rats. *Anat. Rec.* 74, 223–230.

Sauter, J. J. M. (1976). "Xerophthalmia and Measles in Kenya." Thesis, Univ. Groningen. Drukkeru van Denderen Bv, Groningen.

Schmidt, H. (1941). Vitamin A deficiencies in ruminants. *Am. J. vet. Res.* 2, 373–389.

Schneider, B., Hood, D. C., Cohen, H. and Stamper, M. (1977). Behavioural threshold and rhodopsin content as a function of vitamin A deprivation in the rat. *Vision Res.* 17, 799–806.

Scott, P. P. and Greaves, J. P. (1964). Retinal degeneration and other signs of vitamin A deficiency in the cat. *Proc. Nutr. Soc.* 23, xxxiv.

Scragg, J. and Rubidge, C. (1960). Kwashiorkor in African children in Durban. *Br. med. J.* ii, 1759–1766.

Scrimshaw, N. S., Béhar, M., Arroyave, G., Viteri, F. and Tejade, C. (1956). Characteristics of kwashiorkor (syndrome pluricarencial de la infancia). *Fedn. Proc. Fedn Am. Socs exp. Biol.* 15, 977–985.

Scullica, F. and Fulchignoni, E. (1937). Comportamento del fondo oculare per deficienza della Vitamina A nel coniglio. Osservazioni sul metabolismo della porposa retinica. *Annali Ottal. Clin. ocul.* 65, 427–445.

Shah, P. M. (1978). Strategies for prevention of malnutritional blindness in India: operational methodology, management, monitoring and cost/benefit. *Rep. R. Commonw. Soc. Blind.*

Sheldon, H. and Zetterqvist, H. (1956a). An electron microscope study of the corneal epithelium in the vitamin A deficient mouse. *Johns Hopkins Hosp. Bull.* 98, 372–405.

Sheldon, H. and Zetterqvist, H. (1956b). Experimentally induced changes in mitochondrial morphology: vitamin A deficiency. *Expl Cell Res.* 10, 225–228.

Sheorey, U. B. (1976). Clinical assessment of rhodopsin in the eye: using a standard fundus camera and a photographic technique. *Br. J. Ophthal.* 60, 135–141.

Sie Boen Lian. (1938). Over vlekken van Bitot niet behorend tot het ziektebeeld der xerophthalmie. *Geneesk. Tijdschr. Ned.-Indië* 78, 665–670.

Sie Boen Lian. (1960). *Adv. Ophthal.* 10, 49.

Simmonds, N., Becker, J. E. and McCollum, E. V. (1927a). The relation of vitamin E to iron assimilation. *J. biol. Chem.* 74, lxviii–lxix.

Simmonds, N., Becker, J. E. and McCollum, E. V. (1927b). The relation of vitamin E to iron assimilation. *J. Am. med. Ass.* 88, 1047–1050.

Singh Gurbak and Malik, A. R. K. (1973). Therapeutic penetrating keratoplasty in keratomalacia. *Br. J. Ophthal.* 57, 638–640.

Sinha, D. P. and Bang, F. B. (1973). Seasonal variation in signs of vitamin A deficiency in rural West Bengal children. *Lancet* ii, 228–230.

Sivasubramaniam, P. (1958). Keratomalacia. *Trans. Ophthal. Soc., Ceylon* 1, 21–7.

Sloan, L. L. (1947). Rate of dark adaptation and regional threshold gradient of dark-adapted eye: physiologic and clinical studies. *Am. J. Ophthal.* 30, 705–720.

Smith, F. R., Goodman D. S., Zaklama, M. S., Gabt, M. K., El Marashi, S. and Patwardhan, V. N. (1973). Serum vitamin A, retinol-binding protein and prealbumin concentration in protein and calorie malnutrition. *Am. J. clin. Nutr.* 26, 973–981.

Smith, F. R., Suskind, R., Thanangkul, O., Leitzmann, C., Goodman, D. S. and Olson, R. E. (1975). Plasma vitamin A, retinol-binding protein and prealbumin concentration in protein and calorie malnutrition. III. Response to varying dietary treatments. *Am. J. clin. Nutr.* 28, 732–738.

Smolin, G., Okumoto, M., Friedlaender, M. and Kwok, S. (1979). Herpes simplex keratitis treatment with vitamin A. *Archs Ophthal.* 97, 2181–2183.

Snell, S. (1881). On nyctalopia with peculiar appearances on the conjunctiva. *Trans. ophthal. Soc. U.K.* 1, 207–215.

Sobel, A. E., Besman, L. and Kramer, B. (1949). Vitamin A absorption in the newborn. *Am. J. Dis. Child.* 77, 576–591.

Solon, F. S., Popkin, B. M., Fernandez, T. L. and Latham, M. C. (1978). Vitamin A deficiency in the Philippines: a study of xerophthalmia in Cebu. *Am. J. clin. Nutr.* 31, 360–368.

Someswara Rao, K., De, N. K. and Subba Rao, D. (1953). Investigation of an outbreak of nightblindness in a village near Madras. *Indian J. med. Res.* 41, 349–357.

Sommer, A. (1978). "Field Guide to the Detection and Control of Xerophthalmia." W.H.O., Geneva.

Sommer, A. and Emran, N. (1978). Topical retinoic acid in the treatment of corneal xerophthalmia. *Am. J. Ophthal.* 86, 615–617.

Sommer, A., Emran, N. and Tamba, T. (1979). Vitamin A responsive punctate keratopathy in xerophthalmia. *Am. J. Ophthal.* 87, 330–333.

Sommer, A., Faich, G. and Quesada, J. (1975a). Mass distribution of vitamin A and the prevention of keratomalacia. *Am. J. Ophthal.* 80, 1073–1080.

Sommer, A., Hussaini, G., Muhilal, Tarwotjo, I., Susanto, D. and Saroso, J. S. (1980). Night blindness: a simple tool for xerophthalmia screening. *Am. J. clin. Nutr.* in press.

Sommer, A., Muhilal, Tarwotjo, I., Djunaedi, E. and Glover, J. (1980). Oral versus intramuscular vitamin A in the treatment of xerophthalmia. *Lancet* i, 557–559.

Sommer, A., Quesada, J., Doty, M. and Faich, G. (1975b). Xerophthalmia and anterior segment blindness among preschool-age children in El Salvador. *Am. J. Ophthal.* 80, 1066–1072.

Sommer, A., Tjakrasdjatma, S., Djunaldi, E. and Green, R. (1978). Vitamin A-responsive panocular xerophthalmia in a healthy adult. *Archs Ophthal.* 96, 1630–1634.

Sorsby, A., Reading, H. W. and Bunyan, J. (1966). Effect of vitamin A deficiency on the retina of the experimental rabbit. *Nature, Lond.* 210, 1011–1015.

Squires, B. T. (1956). Nutrition in the Bechuanaland Protectorate. *Centr. Afr. J. Med.* 2, 112–118.

Stark, W. S. and Zitzmann, W. G. (1976). Isolation of adaptation mechanisms and photopigment spectra by vitamin A deprivation in drosophila. *J. comp. Physiol.* Part A, 105, 15–27.

Steadman, B. St J. (1942). Investigation of night vision among personnel of A.A-Unit. *Jl Roy. Army Med. Corps* 78, 14–24.

Steenbock, H., Nelson, E. M. and Hart, E. B. (1921). Fat-soluble vitamin. IX. The incidence of an ophthalmic reaction in dogs fed a fat-soluble vitamin deficient diet. *Am. J. Physiol.* **58**, 14–19.

Stephenson, M. and Clark, A. B. (1920). A contribution to the study of keratomalacia among rats. *Biochem. J.* **14**, 502–521.

Stephenson, S. (1898). *Trans. ophthalmol. Soc. U.K.* **18**, 55.

Steven, D. and Wald, G. (1941). Vitamin A deficiency: a field study in Newfoundland and Labrador. *J. Nutr.* **21**, 461–476.

Stock, F. E. (1946). Blindness in an urban centre in Nigeria. *Br. med. J.* **1**, 525–526.

Stransky, E. (1950). Nutritional dystrophy. *Br. med. J.* **1**, 1370–1371.

Stransky, E., Dauis-Lawas, D. F. and Lawas, I. (1951). On hypoproteinaemia due to malnutrition in tropics. *J. trop. Med. Hyg.* **54**, 53–60.

Suthutvoravoot, S. and Olson, J. A. (1974). Plasma and liver concentration of vitamin A in a normal population of urban Thai. *Am. J. clin. Nutr.* **27**, 883–891.

Studer, A. and Frey, J. R. (1949). Ueber Hautveränderungen der Ratte nach Groben oralen Dosen von Vitamin A. *Schweiz. med. Wschr.* **79**, 382–384.

Sugita, Y. (1926). Experimentelle Untersuchungen über die Wirkung der Galle und ihre Bestandteile auf das Auge, speziell auf den Lichtsinn und den Sehpurpur, nebst Bemerkungen über meine Sehpurpur-Lösungsmethode. *Albrecht v. Graefes Arch. Ophthal.* **116**, 653–666.

Sullivan, W. R., McCully, J. P. and Dohlman, C. H. (1973). Return of goblet cells after vitamin A therapy in xerosis of the conjunctiva. *Am. J. Ophthal.* **75**, 720–725.

Sweet, L. K. and K'ang, H. J. (1935). Clinical and anatomic study of avitaminosis A among the Chinese. *Am. J. Dis. Child.* **50**, 699–734.

Tansley, K. (1931). Regeneration of visual purple; its relation to dark adaptation and night blindness. *J. Physiol., Lond.* **71**, 442–458.

Tansley, K. (1934). Factors affecting the development and regeneration of visual purple in the mammalian retina. *Proc. R. Soc. B* **114**, 79–103.

Tarwotjo, I., Gunawan, S., Reedy, S., ten Doesschate, J., House, E. and Pettiss, S. T. (1975). An Evaluation of the Vitamin A Deficiency Prevention Pilot Project in Indonesia 1973–1975." American Foundation for Overseas Blind, New York.

Taylor, F. S. (1944). St Jerome and vitamin A. *Nature, Lond.* **154**, 802.

Ten Doesschate, J. (1968). "Causes of Blindness in and around Surabaja, East Java, Indonesia." Thesis, University of Indonesia, Jacarta.

Teng Khoen Hing (1959). Fundus changes in hypovitaminosis A. *Ophthalmologica* **137**, 81–85.

Teng Khoen Hing. (1965). Serum vitamin A and protein levels in fundus xerophthalmicus. *Trop. geogr. Med.* **17**, 273–281.

Teuscher, O. (1867). *Jena, Z. Med. Naturw.* **3**, 103.

Thaler, A., Helig, P. and Zehetbauer, G. (1976). The influence of deficiency of vitamin A on the electro-oculogram. *Albrecht v. Graefes Arch. Ophthal.* **199**, 187–190.

Thomson, F. A. (1949). Dietary deficiencies in children in island of Viti Levu, Fiji. *Trans. R. Soc. trop. Med. Hyg.* **42**, 487–492.

Thonnard-Neumann, E. (1957). Clinical notes on the climate and nutrition in Colombia. *Z. Tropenmed. Parasit.* **8**, 367–376.

Tijssen, J. (1936). De avitaminose van het oog en hare oorzaken. *Geneesk. Tijdschr. Ned.-Indië* **76**, 2891–2898.

Timmer, M. (1961). "Child Mortality and Population Pressure in the D.I., Jogjakarta, Java, Indonesia," p. 354. Vrije Universiteit te Amsterdam, Amsterdam.

Tiwary, R. (1966). Intestinal infections and ocular lesions with particular reference to keratomalacia. *J. All-India Ophthal. Soc.* 14, 87–8.

Toskes, P., Currington, C. and Dawson, W. (1977). Visual dysfunction in patients with chronic pancreatitis. *Am. J. clin. Nutr.* 30, 623, (abstract).

Toureau, S., Sommer, A., McEvoy Doty, M. and Pettiss, S. T. (1976). "Assessment of the Prevalence of Xerophthalmia in Haiti." American Foundation for Overseas Blind, New York.

Trowell, H. C. (1937). Pellagra in African children. *Archs Dis. Child.* 12, 193–212.

Trowell, H. C., Moore, T. and Sharman, I. M. (1954). Vitamin E and carotenoids in the blood plasma in kwashiorkor. *Ann. N.Y. Acad. Sci.* 57, 734–6.

Turtz, C. A. and Turtz, A. I. (1960). Vitamin A intoxication. *Am. J. Ophthal.* 50, 165–166.

Ullerich, K. and Witte, A. (1961). Die zystriche Pankreasfibrose (Mucoviscidosis) als Ursache einer Keratomalazie. *Klin. Mbl. Augenheilk.* 139, 59–72.

Uyemura, M. (1928). Ueber eine Merkwürdige Augenhintergrundveränderung bei zwei Fallen von idiopathischer Hemeralopie. *Klin. Mbl. Augenheilk.* 81, 471–473.

Vahlquist, A., Sjölund, K., Nordén, Å., Peterson, P. A., Stigmar, G. and Johannson, B. (1978). Plasma vitamin A transport and visual dark adaptation in diseases of the intestine and liver. *Scand. J. clin. lab. Invest.* 38, 301–8.

Valenton, M. J. and Tan, R. V. (1975). Secondary ocular bacterial infection in hypovitaminosis A xerophthalmia. *Am. J. Ophthal.* 80, 673–677.

Van der Sar, A. (1951). Incidence and treatment of kwashiorkor in Curaçao. *Documenta Neerl. Indones. Morbis Trop.* 3, 25–44.

Van Eekelen, M. (1957). Diet in Thailand. *Voeding* 18, 336–341.

Van Stockum, M. J. (1938). De voeding van het inheemse kind en xeropthalmie. *Geneesk. Tijdschr. Ned.-Indië* 78, 856–880.

Vaughan, D. G. (1954). Xerophthalmia. *A.M.A. Archs Ophthal.* 51, 789–798.

Venkataswamy, G., Krishnamurthy, K. A., Chandra, P., Kalir, S. A. and Pirie, A. (1976). A nutrition rehabilitation centre for children with xerophthalmia. *Lancet* i, 1120–1122.

Vijayaraghavan, K., Naidu, A. N., Rao, N. P. and Srikantia, S. G. (1975). A simple method to evaluate the massive dose vitamin A prophylaxis programme in preschool children. *Am. J. clin. Nutr.* 28, 1189–1193.

Vidal, A. (1938). Avitaminosis compleja infantil en Honduras. *In* "Fifth Congreso Médico de Centro América y Panamá." (Summary in *Trop. Dis. Bull.* (1939) 36, 914.)

Von Ammon, F. A. (1830). Beobachtungen, Ansichten und Zweifel über die Entstehung der xerosis conjunctivae. *Ammon. Z. Ophthal.* 1, 65–79.

Von Graefe, A. (1866). Hornhautverschwärung bei infantiler Encephalitis. *Albrecht v. Graefes Arch. Ophthal.* 12, 250–256.

Von Szily, A. and Eckstein, A. (1923). Vitamin-mangel und Schichtstargenose. Katarakte als eine Erscheinungsform der Avitaminose mit Störung des Kalkstoffwechsels bei säugenden Ratten, herborgerufen durch qualitative Unterernährung der Muttertiere. *Klin. Mbl. Augenheilk.* 71, 545–583.

Voorhoeve, H. W. A. (1966). Xeropthalmia in the presence of kwashiorkor in Nigeria. *Trop. geogr. Med.* 18, 15–19.

Wald, G. (1935a). Vitamin A in eye tissues. *J. gen. Physiol.* **18**, 905–915.

Wald, G. (1935b). Pigments of the bull frog retina. *Nature, Lond.* **136**, 832–833.

Wald, G. (1943). Photoreceptor function of carotenoids and vitamins A. *Vitams Horm.* **1**, 195–227.

Wald, G. and Steven, D. (1939). Experiment in human vitamin A-deficiency. *Proc. natn. Acad. Sci. U.S.A.* **25**, 344–349.

Wald, G., Brouha, L. and Johnson, R. E. (1942). Experimental human vitamin A deficiency and the ability to perform muscular exercise. *Am. J. Physiol.* **137**, 551–556.

Wason, I. M. (1921). Ophthalmia associated with a dietary defiency in fat soluble vitamin (A). *J. Am. med. Ass.* **76**, 908–912.

Waters, J. W. (1950). Electroretinography of experimental animals. *Br. J. Ophthal.* **34**, 1–15.

Waters, J. W. (1952). Effect of vitamin A-deficiency on the dark adaptation of the pigeon. *Nature, Lond.* **169**, 413–414.

Weech, A. A. (1930). Association of keratomalacia with other deficiency diseases. *Am. J. Dis. Child.* **39**, 1153–1166.

Weekers, L. and Roussel, R. (1945). Utilisation de la campimétrie en lumière atténuée pour la misure de l'adaptation retinienne à l'obscurité. *Ophthalmologica* **110**, 242–258.

Welbourn, H. F. (1958). Bottle-feeding: a problem of modern civilization. *J. trop. Pediat.* **3**, 157–170.

Wickremesinghe, W. G. (1942). "Nutrition in Ceylon: Its Bearing on National Health and Well-being." Ceylon Daily News, Colombo.

Wiggert, B., Bergsma, D. R. and Helmsen, R. J. (1977). Retinol receptors in corneal epithelium, stroma and endothelium. *Biochem. biophys. Acta* **491**, 104–113.

Williams, C. D. (1933). A nutritional disease of childhood associated with a maize diet. *Archs Dis. Childh.* **8**, 423–433.

Williamson, A. D. (1948). Keratomalacia. *Med. J. Malaya* **3**, 68–9.

Williamson, A. D. and Leong, P. C. (1949). Keratomalacia in Singapore and its relation to vitamin A in milk. *Med. J. Malaya* **4**, 83–95.

Wilson, J. R. and Dubois, R. O. (1923). Report of a fatal case of keratomalacia in an infant, with postmorten examination. *Am. J. Dis. Child.* **26**, 431–446.

Witkovsky, P., Gallin, E., Hollyfield, J. G., Ripps, H. and Bridges, C. D. B. (1976). Vitamin A deprived *Xenopus* tadpoles. *J. Neurophysiol.* **39**, 1272–1287.

Wolbach, S. B. (1954). Effects of vitamin A deficiency and hypervitaminosis A in animals. *In* "The Vitamins" (Eds W. H. Sebrell, Jr and R. S. Harris), Vol. 1, 106–137. Academic Press, London, New York.

Wolbach, S. B. and Bessey, O. A. (1941). Vitamin A deficiency and the nervous system. *A.M.A. Archs Path.* **32**, 689–722.

Wolbach, S. B. and Howe, P. R. (1925). Tissue changes following deprivation of fat soluble A vitamin. *J. exp. Med.* **42**, 753–778.

Wolbach, S. B. and Howe, P. R. (1928). Vitamin A deficiency in the guinea-pig. *Archs Path. lab. Med.* **5**, 239–253.

Wolf, G. (1978). A historical note on the mode of administration of vitamin A for the cure of night blindness. *Am. J. clin. Nutr.* **31**, 290–292.

Wolf, I. J. (1958). Vitamin A deficiency in an infant. *J. Am. med. Ass.* **166**, 1859–1860.

Wong, V. G. and Collins, E. (1965). Optic atrophy in cystic fibrosis of the pancreas. *Am. J. Ophthal.* **59**, 763–769.

Woo, T. T. and Chu, F. T. (1940). The vitamin A content of the livers of Chinese infants, children and adults. *Chin. J. Physiol.* **15**, 83–99.

Wood, C. A. (1929). "Translation of *De oculis eorumque egritudinibus et curis* by Benevenutus Grassus of Jerusalem." Stanford University Press, Stanford.

W.H.O./F.A.O. Expert Committee (1967). Requirements of vitamin A, thiamine, riboflavin and niacin. *Tech. Rep. Ser. Wld Hlth Org.* No. 362.

World Health Organization (1976). Vitamin A deficiency and xerophthalmia. *Tech. Rep. Ser. Wld Hlth Org.* No. 590.

Wright, R. E. (1922). Keratomalacia in Southern India. *Br. J. Ophthal.* **6**, 164–175.

Yap Kie Tiong (1956). Protein deficiency in keratomalacia. *Br. J. Ophthal.* **40**, 502–503.

Yassur, Y. (1972). Keratomalacia. *Israel J. med. Sci.* **8**, 1192–4.

Yourish, N. B. (1953). Significance of Bitot's spots. *Am. J. Ophthal.* **36**, 109–110.

Yudkin, A. M. (1922). Ocular manifestations of the rat which result from a deficiency of vitamin A in the diet. *J. Am. med. Ass.* **79**, 2206–2208.

Yudkin, A. M. (1931). Presence of vitamin A in retina. *A.M.A. Archs Ophthal.* **6**, 510–517.

Yudkin, A. M. and Lambert, R. A. (1922a). Location of the earliest changes in experimental xerophthalmia of rats. *Proc. Soc. exp. Biol. Med.* **19**, 375.

Yudkin, A. M. and Lambert, R. A. (1922b). Lesions in the lacrimal glands of rats in experimental xerophthalmia. *Proc. Soc. exp. Biol. Med.* **19**, 376–7.

Yudkin, A. M. and Lambert, R. A. (1923). Pathogenesis of the ocular lesions produced by a deficiency of vitamine A. *J. exp. Med.* **38**, 17–24.

Zwart, P. (1966). Vitamine A gebrek bij moerasschildpadden. *Tijdschr. Diergeneesk.* **91**, 1657–1661.

Chapter 3

Adams, E. B. and Hift, W. (1961). Nutritional and other megaloblastic anaemias among Africans and Indians in Durban. *Trans. R. Soc. trop. Med. Hyg.* **55**, 374–382.

Agamanolis, D. P., Cherrer, E. M., Victor, M., Kark, J. A., Hines, J. D. and Harris, J. W. (1976). Neuropathology of experimental vitamin B_{12} deficiency in monkeys. *Neurology* **26**, 905–914.

Agarwal, L. P. and Datt, K. (1954). Role of nicotinic acid in healing of corneal ulcers. *Am. J. Ophthal.* **37**, 764–767.

Alexander, L. (1940). Wernicke's disease. *Am. J. Pathol.* **16**, 61–70.

Asahiuga, Y., and Goto, M. (1943). *Acta Soc. Ophthal. Japan* **47**, 938.

Aykroyd, W. R. and Verma, O. P. (1942). Superifical keratitis due to riboflavin deficiency. *Indian med. Gaz.* 77, 1–5.

Ayuyao, C. D. (1933). Corneal lesion in beriberi. *J. Philippine med. Ass.* 13, 158–161.

Baum, H. M., Michaelree, J. F. and Brown, E. B. (1942). Quantitative relationship of riboflavin to cataract formation in rats. *Science, N.Y.* 95, 24–25.

Beer (1817). *Lehre v.d. Augenkrankheiten, Wien* 2.

Bellows, J. G. and Chinn, H. (1943). Intraocular hemorrhages in choline deficiency. *A.M.A. Archs Ophthal.* 30, 105–109.

Bessey, O. A. and Wolbach, S. B. (1939). Vascularization of the cornea of the rat in riboflavin deficiency, with a note on corneal vascularization in vitamin A deficiency. *J. exp. Med.* 69, 1–12.

Birch-Hirschfeld, A. (1902). Zur Partogenase der chronischen Nicotinamblyopie. *Albrecht v. Graefes Arch. Ophthal.* 53, 79–112.

Bietti, A. (1901). *Klin. Mbl. Augenheilk.* 39, 337.

Bietti, G. (1940). "Le Vitamine in Oftalmologia," p. 225. Cappelli, Bologna.

Björkenheim, B. (1966). Optic neuropathy caused by vitamin B_{12} deficiency and carriers of the fish tapeworm. *Diphyllobothrium latum. Lancet* i, 688–690.

Boehrer, J. J., Stanford, C. E. and Ryan, E. (1943). Experimental riboflavin deficiency in man. *Am. J. med. Sci.* 205, 544–549.

Boerhaave, H. (1749). "Des maladies des yeux." Huart et Moreau Fils, Paris.

Bowles, L. L., Allen, L., Sydenstricker, V. P., Hock, C. W. and Hall, W. K. (1946). The development and demonstration of corneal vascularization in rats deficient in vitamin A and in riboflavin. *J. Nutr.* 32, 19–35.

Bowles, L. L., Hall, W. K., Sydenstricker, V. P. and Hock, C. W. (1949). Corneal changes in the rat with deficiencies of pantothenic acid and of pyridoxine. *J. Nutr.* 37, 9–20.

Boxer, G. E. and Rickards, J. C. (1952). Studies on the metabolism of the carbon of cyanide and thiocyanate. *Archs Biochem.* 39, 7–26.

Bradley, J. T. (1929). *Rep. Med. Hlth. Dept., Seychelles.*

Brown, K. H., Gaffar, A. and Alamgir, S. M. (1979). Xerophthalmia, protein-calorie malnutrition and infections in children. *J. Pediat.* 95, 651–656.

Browne, J. A. (1939). *Br. Guiana med. Ann.* 25.

Burgess, R. C. (1946). Deficiency diseases in prisoners-of-war at Changi, Singapore. *Lancet* ii, 411–418.

Burgess, R. C. (1958). Beriberi. I. Epidemiology. *Fedn Proc. Fedn Am. Socs exp. Biol.* 17, Suppl. 2, 3–8.

Burns, J. L. and Hartroft, W. S. (1949). Intraocular hemorrhages in young rats on choline-deficient diets. *Am. J. Ophthal.* 30, 735.

Calderini, L. (1847). "Votigia Med. Statistiche Sulla Pellagra," Milan.

Calhoun, F. P. (1918). *Am. J. Ophthal.* i, 834.

Carroll, F. D. (1944). Etiology and treatment of tobacco-alcohol amblyopia. *Am. J. Ophthal.* 27, 713.

Carroll, F. D. (1947). Nutritional retrobulbar neuritis. *Am. J. Ophthal.* 30, 172–176.

Carroll, F. D. (1966). Nutritional amblyopia. *Archs Ophthal.* 76, 406–411.

Carroll, F. D. (1971). Jamaican optic neuropathy in immigrants to the United States. *Am. J. Ophthal.* 71, 261–265.

Chen Tzu-Ta (1948). Angular blepharitis in ariboflavinosis—not well known clinical manifestation of riboflavin deficiency. *Chin. med. J.* 66, 1–4.

Chick, H. and Roscoe, M. H. (1927). On the composite nature of the water-soluble B vitamin. *Biochem. J.* 21, 698–711.

Chisholm, I. A., Bronte-Stewart, J. M. and Foulds, W. S. (1967). Hydroxocobalamin vs cyanocobalamin in the treatment of tobacco amblyopia. *Lancet* ii, 450–451.

Chisholm, I. A., Bronte-Stewart, J. M. and Awduche, E. O. (1970). Colour vision in tobacco amblyopia. *Acta ophthal.* 48, 1145–1156.

Clark, L. M. (1935–36). *Trans. Br. Med. Ass.* (Jamaica Branch), 201.

Clarke, C. A. and Sneddon, I. B. (1946). Nutritional neuropathy in prisoners-of-war and internees from Hong Kong. *Lancet* i, 734–738.

Clarke, C. A. and Sircus, W. (1952). Nutritional neuropathy in prisoners-of-war repatriated from Hong Kong. A follow-up. *Lancet* ii, 113–114.

Clarke, M. C. (1951). Some impressions of the Muruts of North Borneo. *Trans. R. Soc. trop. Med. Hyg.* 44, 453–464.

Cleckley, H. M., Sydenstricker, V. P. and Geeslin, L. E. (1939). Nicotinic acid in the treatment of atypical psychotic states associated with malnutrition. *J. Am. med. Ass.* 112, 2107–2110.

Cohen, H. (1936). Optic atrophy as the presenting sign in pernicious anaemia, *Lancet,* 11, 1202–1203.

Collins, R. A., Schreiber, M. and Elvehjem, C. A. (1953). The influence of relative humidity upon vitamin deficiencies in rats. *J. Nutr.* 49, 589–597.

Cosnett, J. E. and MacLeod, I. N. (1959). Retinal haemorrhages in severe anaemias. *Br. med. J.* 11, 1002–1004.

Cowan, M. J., Ward, D., Packman, S., Ammann, A. J., Yoshino, M., Sweetman, L. and Nyhan, W. (1979). Multiple biotin-dependent carboxylase deficiencies associated with defects in T-cell and B-cell immunity. *Lancet* ii, 115–118.

Crews, S. J. (1963). Bilateral amblyopia in West Indians. *Trans. ophthal. Soc. U.K.* 83, 653–667.

Cristini, G. (1950). Le alterazioni del cristallino provocate sperimentalmente con carenza di metili labili. *G. ital. oftal.* 3, 405–414.

Cruickshank, E. K. (1956). A neuropathic syndrome of uncertain origin. *West Indian med. J.* 5, 147–158.

Cruickshank, E. K. (1961). Neuromuscular disease in relation to nutrition. *Fedn Proc. Fedn Am. Socs exp. Biol.* 20, Suppl. 7, Part III, 345–352.

Dansey-Browning, G. C. and Rich, W. M. (1946). Ocular signs in the prisoner-of-war returned from the Far East. *Br. med. J.* 1, 20–21.

Dawson, J., Findlay, G. M. and Ward, R. D. (1948). Note on Vitamin B complex deficiency among Africans in Gold Coast. *Trans. R. Soc. trop. Med. Hyg.* 42, 277–282.

Day, P. L. (1934). Vitamin G deficiency. *Am. J. publ. Hlth* 24, 603–608.

Day, P. L. and Darby, W. J. (1936). The inverse relation between growth and incidence of cataract in rats given graded amounts of vitamin G-containing foods. *J. Nutr.* 12, 387–394.

Day, P. L., Langston, W. C. and O'Brien, C. S. (1931). Cataract and other ocular changes in vitamin G deficiency: experimental study on albino rats. *Am. J. Ophthal.* 14, 1005–1009.

Day, P. L., Langston, W. C. and Cosgrove, K. W. (1934). The appearance of cataract and dermatitis in experimental animals given vitamin G deficient diets containing casein and egg albumin. *J. Nutr.* 7, 12.

Degazon, D. W. (1956). Tropical amblyopia in Jamaica. *West Indian med. J.* 5, 223–230.

Denny-Brown, D. (1947). Neurological conditions resulting from prolonged and severe dietary restriction (case reports in prisoners-of-war, and general review). *Medicine* 26, 41–113.

Denny-Brown, D. (1958). Beriberi. VI. Special problems concerning beriberi. A. The neurological aspects of thiamine deficiency. *Fedn. Proc. Fedn Am. Socs exp. Biol.* 17, Suppl. 2, 35–39.

De Ocampo, G. (1941). Epithelial corneal dystrophy due to hypovitaminosis. *Acta med. Philippina* 3, 105–123.

De Ocampo, G., Yambao, C. V., Mañagas, P. J. and Sevilla, C. L. (1947). Epidemic retrobulbar neuritis in Philippines during Japanese occupation. *Am. J. Ophthal.* 30, 698–704.

Deschweinitz, G. E. (1896). "The Toxic Amblyopias." 51, 70, 85, Lea, Philadelphia.

De Wardener, H. E. and Lennox, B. (1947). Cerebral beriberi (Wernicke's encephalopathy). Review of 52 cases in a Singapore prisoner-of-war hospital. *Lancet* i, 11–17.

Dickenson, W. N. (1935–36). *Trans. Br. med. Ass. (Jamaica Branch)* 201.

Djacos, C. (1949). Les altérations oculaires dans la pellagre. *Annls Oculist. Paris,* 182, 279–294.

Dreyfus, P. M. (1976). Amblyopia and other neurological disorders associated with chronic alcoholism. *In.* "Handbook of Clinical Neurology" (Eds P. J. Vinken and G. W. Bruyn). Vol. 28, 331–347. North Holland, Amsterdam.

Duke-Elder, W. S. (1946). Nutritional aspects of ophthalmology. *IrishJ. med. Sci.* 6th Series, 177–189.

Durran, J. (1946). Ocular signs in the prisoner-of-war from the Far East. *Br. med. J.* 1, 626–7.

Edge, J. R. (1945). Partial starvation in prisoners-of-war. *Lancet* ii, 317–18.

Elliot, R. H. (1920). "Tropical Ophthalmology," 405. Oxford Med. Publs., London.

Ellis, P. P. and Hamilton, M. (1959). Retrobulbar neuritis in pernicious anaemia. *Am. J. Ophthal.* 48, 95–97.

Esser, A. M. (1928). Beiträge zur Geschichte der klassischantiken Augenheilkunde. 9. Die erste Erwähnung von Alkoholamblyopie in der Geschichte der Medizin. *Klin. Mbl. Augenheilk.* 80, 541.

Ferguson, W. J. W. (1944). Ocular signs of riboflavin deficiency. *Lancet* i, 431–433.

Figge, F. H. J. and Atkinson, W. B. (1941). Relation of water metabolism to porphyrin incrustations in pantothenic acid-deficient rats. *Proc. Soc. exp. Biol. Med.* 48, 112–124.

Fine, M. and Lachman, G. S. (1937). Retrobulbar neuritis in pellagra. *Am. J. Ophthal.* 20, 708–714.

Fisher, C. M. (1955). *Can. med. Serv. J.* 11, 157.

Förster, R. (1880). Beziehungen der Allgemeinleiden und Organ-Erkrankungen zu Veräuderungen und Krankheiten des Sehorgaus. *Handb. ges. Augenheilk.* 7.

Foulds, W. S. and Pettigrew, A. R. (1977). The biochemical basis of the toxic amblyopias. *In* "Scientific Foundations of Ophthalmology" (Ed. E. S. Perkins, and D. W. Hill), 50–54. Heinemann, London.

Foulds, W. S., Bronte-Stewart, J. M. and Chisholm, I. A. (1968a). Serum thiocyanate concentration in tobacco amblyopia. *Nature, Lond.* 218, 586.

Foulds, W. S., Cant, J. S., Chisholm, I. A., Bronte-Stewart, J. M. and Wilson, J. (1968b). Hydroxocobalamin in the treatment of Leber's hereditary optic atrophy. *Lancet* i, 896–897.

Foulds, W. S., Chisholm, I. A., Bronte-Stewart, J. M. and Wilson, T. M. (1969). Vitamin B_{12} absorption in tobacco amblyopia. *Br. J. Ophthal.* 53, 393–397.

Gershoff, S. N., Andrus, S. B. and Hegsted, D. M. (1959). The effect of the carbohydrate and fat content of the diet upon the riboflavin requirement of the cat. *J. Nutr.* 68, 75–88.

Gilbert, C. and Gillman, J. (1944). Diet and disease in the Bantu. *Science, N.Y.* 99, 398–399.

Gillman, J., Gilbert, C. and Gillman, T. (1947). The Bantu salivary glands in chronic malnutrition with a brief consideration of the parenchyma-interstitial tissue relationship. *S. Afr. J. med. Sci.* 12, 99–109.

Goldberger, J. and Lillie, D. R. (1926). A note on an experimental pellagralike condition in the albino rat. *Publ. Hlth Rep., Wash.* 41, 1025–1029.

Gordon, O. E. and Vail, D. (1950). *XVI Conc. Ophthal. Br. Acta* 2, 438.

Grande, F. and Peraita, M. (1941). "Avitaminosis y Sistema Nervioso," 1st edn. Servet, Madrid.

Gregory, M. K. (1943). The ocular criteria of deficiency of riboflavin. *Br. med. J.* ii, 134–135.

Griffith, W. H. and Wade, N. J. (1939). Choline metabolism I. The occurrence and prevention of hemorrhagic degeneration in young rats on a low choline diet. *J. biol. Chem.* 131, 567–577.

Guita, L. (1884). *Annali Ottal. Clin. ocul.* 13, 229.

György, P. and Eckardt, R. E. (1940). Further investigations on vitamin B_6 and related factors of the vitamin B_{12} complex in rats. Parts I and II. *Biochem. J.* 34, 1143–1153.

Halver, J. E. (1957). Nutrition of salmonoid fishes. III. Water-soluble vitamin requirements of Chinook salmon. *J. Nutr.* 62, 225–243.

Hamilton, H. E., Ellis, P. and Sheets, R. F. (1959). Visual impairment due to optic neuropathy in pernicious anaemia: report of a case and review of the literature. *Blood* 14, 378–385.

Harrington, D. O. (1962). Amblyopia due to tobacco alcohol and nutritional deficiency. Differential diagnosis with special reference to the character of the visual field defect. *Am. J. Ophthal.* 53, 967–972.

Hasegawa, Y. and Yagi, K. (1975). Electron microscopic study on the lens of riboflavin-deficient albino rat. *J. nutr. Sci. Vitamin* 21, 395–401.

Heaton, J. M. (1960). Vitamin B_{12} and the eye. *Proc. Nutr. Soc.* 19, 100–105.

Heaton, J. M., McCormick, A. J. A. and Freeman, A. G. (1958). Tobacco amblyopia: a clinical manifestation of vitamin B_{12} deficiency. *Lancet* ii, 286–290.

Helweg-Larsen, P., Hoffmeyer, H., Kieler, J., Thaysen, E. H., Thaysen, J. H., Thygeson, P. and Wulff, M. H. (1952). Famine disease in German concentration camps; complications and sequels, with special reference to tuberculosis, mental disorders and social consequences. *Acta med. scand.* 144, Suppl. 274.

Hills, O. W., Liebert, E., Steinberg, D. L. and Horwitt, M. K. (1951). Clinical aspects of dietary depletion of riboflavin. *A. M. A. Archs intern. Med.* 87, 682–693.

Hind, V. M. D. (1970). Degeneration in the peripheral visual pathway of vitamin B$_{12}$-deficient monkeys. *Trans. ophthal. Soc. U.K.* 90, 839–846.

Hinokuma, S. and Yamashita, K. (1950). *Ganka Rinsho Iho, Japan* 44, 58.

Hirschberg, J. (1879). Tobacco and alcohol amblyopia. *Br. med. J.* ii, 810–811.

Horner, F. (1878). Über die Intoxication—Amblyopia. *Corres. Bl. Schweiz. Ärtze* 8, 396.

Horwitt, M. K., Hills, O. W., Harvey, C. C., Liebert, E. and Steinberg, D. L. (1949). Effects of dietary depletion of riboflavin. *J. Nutr.* 39, 357–373.

Hoyt, C. S. III and Bilson, F. A. (1977). Low-carbohydrate diet optic neuropathy. *Med. J. Aust.* 1, 65–66.

Ichinohe, M. (1960). Experimental studies on ocular manifestations of biotin deficiency. *Acta Soc. Ophthal. Japan* 64, 1133–1149.

Irinoda, K. (1955). *XVII Conc. Ophthal. Acta (1954: Canda, U.S.)* 1, 661.

Irinoda, K. and Ichinohe, M. (1961). Experimental studies on ocular manifestation of biotin deficiency. *Jap. J. Ophthal.* 5, 32–42.

Irinoda, K. and Mikami, H. (1958). Angular blepharoconjunctivitis and pyridoxine (vitamin B$_6$) deficiency. *A.M.A. Archs Ophthal.* 60, 303–311.

Irinoda, K. and Sato, S. (1954). Contribution to the ocular manifestations of riboflavin deficiency. *Tohoku J. exp. Med.* 61, 93–104.

Irinoda, K. and Yamada, S. (1956). Ocular manifestations in niacin deficiency and its reciprocity to riboflavin deficiency. *J. Vitaminol., Osaka* 2, 83–94.

Ironside, R. (1938–39). Neuritis complicating pregnancy. *Proc. R. Soc. Med.* 32, 588–595.

Ishida. (1918). Cited by A. S. Fernando (1923). *Am. J. Ophthal.* 6, 385.

Jaensch, P. A. (1930). Augenerkrankungen und Pellagra. *Mschr. Psychiat. Neurol.* 76, 355–363.

Jiménez Garcia, F. (1940). Estudio clinico de los trastornas carenciales observados en la poblacion civil de Madrid divante la guerra (1936–39); glositis surple. *Rev. clin. españ.* 1, 231–237.

Johnson, L. V. and Eckardt, R. E. (1940). Rosacea keratitis and conditions with vascularization of cornea treated with riboflavin. *A.M.A. Archs Ophthal.* 23, 899–907.

Jolliffe, N. (1939). Effects of vitamin deficiency on mental and emotional processes. *Ass. Res. nerv. ment. Dis. (Res. Publ.)* 19, 144–153.

Jolliffe, N., Bowman, K. M., Rosenblum, L. A. and Fein, H. D. (1940). Nicotinic acid deficiency encephalopathy. *J. Am. med. Ass.* 114, 307–312.

Kagawa, S. (1938). Studies on the relation of neuritis axialis to beriberi in Japan. *Jap. J. med. Sci.* 5, 1–16, 17–41, 43–60.

Kagoshima, S. (1918). Uber die Veränderung des N. opticus bei beriberi. *Verh. path. Ges., Tokyo* 8, 190.

Kimble, M. S. and Gordon, E. S. (1939). The importance of riboflavin and ascorbic acid in the utilization of vitamin A. *J. biol. Chem.* **128**, lii–liii.

King, J. H. and Passmore, J. W. (1955). Nutritional amblyopia; study of American prisoners-of-war in Korea. *Am. J. Ophthal.* **39**, 173–186.

Knuettgen, H. (1955). Über ein Ataxiesyndrom bei liberianischen Eingeborenen (Strachan-Svelt-Syndrom). *Z. Tropenmed. Parasit.* **6**, 472–491.

Konta, S. (1960). Experimental studies on ocular manifestations of choline deficiency. *Acta Soc. Ophthal. Japan* **64**, 1118–1132.

Koyanagi, T., Sone, K. and Sugihara, S. (1966). Effect of riboflavin deficiency on rat electroretinogram. *J. Vitaminol., Osaka* **12**, 281–285.

Krause, A. C. and Weekers, R. (1938). Inositol in ocular tissues. *A.M.A. Archs Ophthal.* **20**, 299–303.

Krehl, W. A. (1949). Niacin in amino acid metabolism. *Vitams Horm.* **7**, 111–146.

Kruse, H. D., Sydenstricker, V. P., Sebrell, W. H. Jr and Cleckley, H. M. (1940). Ocular manifestations of ariboflavinosis. *Pub. Hlth Rep. Wash.* **55**, 157–169.

Krylov, T. (1932). Eye disturbances in pellagra. *Sov. Vest. Oftal.* **1**, 388–390.

Kunze, K. and Leitenmaier, K. (1976). Vitamin B_{12} deficiency and subacute combined degeneration of the spinal cord (funicular spinal disease). *Handb. clin. Neurol.* **28**, 173–198.

Landor, J. V. and Pallister, R. A. (1935). Avitaminosis B_2. *Trans. R. Soc. trop. Med. Hyg.* **29**, 121–134.

Langston, W. C., and Day, P. L. (1933). Nutritional cataract in Norway rat (*Mus norvegicus*). *Sth. med. J.* **26**, 128–129.

Langston, W. C., Day, P. L. and Cosgrove, K. W. (1933). Cataract in albino mouse resulting from deficiency of vitamin G (B_2). *A.M.A. Archs Ophthal.* **10**, 508–514.

Lee, O. S. Jr and Hart, W. M. (1944). Metabolism of cornea, studies of oxygen consumption of corneas of riboflavin- and vitamin A-deficient rats. *Am. J. Ophthal.* **27**, 488–500.

Lee, P. N. (1975). Tobacco consumption in various countries. *Tobacco Res. Coun. Paper* No. 6, 4th edn.

Leigh, A. G. (1948). Review: nutritional amblyopia. *Ophthal. Lit. Lond.* **2**, 53, 163–173.

Leishman, R. (1952). Gastric function in tobacco amblyopia. *Trans. ophthal. Soc. U.K.* **71**, 319–327.

Lele, R. D., Solank, B. R. and Bhagwatt, R. S. (1964). Retinal haemorrhages in anaemia. *J. Ass. Physns, India* **12**, 599–602.

Lessell, S. (1971). Experimental cyanide optic neuropathy. *Archs Ophthal.* **86**, 194–204.

Levine, J. (1934). Pellagra as cause of optic neuritis, report of a case. *A.M.A. Archs Ophthal.* **12**, 902–909.

Leyton, G. B. (1946). Effects of slow starvation. *Lancet* ii, 73–79.

Lippincott, S. W. and Morris, H. P. (1942). Pathologic changes associated with riboflavin deficiency in mouse. *J. natn. Cancer Inst.* **2**, 601–610.

Lombroso, C. (1892). "Trattato Profilattico e Clinico Della Pellagra." Turin.

Lowry, O. H. and Bessey, O. A. (1945). The effects of light, trauma, riboflavin, and ariboflavinosis on the production of corneal vascularity and on healing of corneal lesions. *J. Nutr.* **30**, 285–292.

McDonald, R. A., Robbins, S. L. and Mallory, G. K. (1958). Morphologic effects of serotonin (5-hydroxytryptamine). *A.M.A. Archs Path.* **65**, 369–377.

McElroy, L. W., Salomon, K., Figge, F. M. J. and Cowgill, G. R. (1941). On porphyrin nature of fluorescent "blood-caked" whiskers of pantothenic acid deficient rats. *Science, N.Y.* **94**, 467.

McLaren, D. S. (1959). The eye and related glands of the rat and pig in protein deficiency. *Br. J. Ophthal.* **43**, 78–87.

McLaren, D. S. (1960a). Ocular manifestations of vitamin B complex deficiency. *5th Int. Congr. Nutr.* Abstr. No. 41.

McLaren, D. S. (1960b). Malnutrition and eye disease in Tanganyika. *Proc. Nutr. Soc.* **19**, 89–91.

Mann, I. (1945). Ariboflavinosis. *Am. J. Ophthal.* **28**, 243–7.

Markar, M. A. H., Peiris, J. B., de Silva, G. V. and Prematilleka, N. (1969). Retinopathy in megaloblastic anaemias. *Trans. R. Soc. trop. Med. Hyg.* **63**, 398–406.

Martini, V. (1955). Ricerche sulla rigenerazione della fibre nervose corneali: azione della vitamina B_{12}. *Boll. Soc. ital. Biol. sper.* **31**, 745–6.

Mason, M. (1953). The metabolism of tryptophan in riboflavin-deficient rats. *J. biol. Chem.* **201**, 513–8.

Masuda, K. and Aoyama, J. (1951). Endemic occurrence of ariboflavinosis and pellagra; clinical observations of so-called "shibi" or "gatchaki" in Tsugaru district. *Tohoku J. exp. Med.* **55**, 1–5.

Mathur, S. P. (1969). Maculopathy in pellagra. *Br. J. Ophthal.* **53**, 350–1.

Mathur, S. P., Shah, D. R. and Makhija, J. M. (1968). Ocular manifestations of pellagra. *Proc. All-India Ophthal. Soc.* **23**, 195–197.

Medical Research Council (Brit.) (1951). Studies of undernutrition, Wuppertal 1946–49. *Spec. Rep. Ser. med. Res. Counc.* No. 275.

Mendoza González, E. (1941). La neuritis optica en la pellagra. *Annls Soc. oftal. Mexico* **16**, 189–193.

Menna, F. and Rosati, P. (1953). Azione della vitamina B_{12} e della leropterina sui tagli corneali. Ricerche sperimentali in Lepus cuniculus. *Boll. Soc. ital. Biol. sper.* **29**, 1191–1193.

Métivier, V. M. (1941). Eye disease due to vitamin deficiency in Trinidad; tropical nutrition amblyopia; essential corneal epithelial dystrophy; conjunctival bleeding in newborn. *Am. J. Ophthal.* **24**, 1265–1280.

Mikami, H. (1956). Experimental studies on ocular manifestations of vitamin B_6 deficiency. *Acta Soc. Ophthal. Japan* **60**, 1236–1255.

Miller, P. J., Johnston, R. L., Hoefer, J. A. and Luecke, R. W. (1954). The riboflavin requirement of the baby pig. *J. Nutr.* **52**, 405–413.

Mitsui, Y., and Hinokuma, S. (1950). *Ganka Rinsho Iho, Japan* **44**, 157.

Miyashita, S. (1923). Zur klinik der keratitis superficialis diffusa. *Klin. Mbl. Augenheilk.* **70**, 88–90.

Monekosso, G. L. and Ashby, P. H. (1963). The natural history of an amblyopia syndrome in Western Nigeria. *W. Afr. med. J.* **12**, 226–233.

Money, G. L. (1958). Endemic neuropathies in the Epe district of Southern Nigeria. *W. Afr. med. J.* 7, 58–62.

Money, G. L. (1959). Clinical aspects of tropical ataxic neuropathies related to malnutrition. *W. Afr. med. J.* 8, 3–17.

Money, G. L. (1961). Obscure funnicular myelopathies in Uganda. *Cent. Afr. J. Med.* 7, 121–4.

Moore, D. G. F. (1930). Partial loss of central acuity of vision for reading and far distance in schoolchildren and its possible association with food deficiency. *W. Afr. med. J.* 4, 46–48.

Moore, D. G. F. (1934). Retrobulbar neuritis cum avitaminosis. *W. Afr. med. J.* 7, 119–120.

Moore, D. F. (1937). Nutritional retrobulbar neuritis, followed by partial optic atrophy. *Lancet* i, 1225–7.

Moore, D. F. (1939). Retrobulbar neuritis cum pellagra in Nigeria. *J. trop. Med. Hyg.* 42, 109–114.

Moore, D. F. (1940). Pellagra or pellagra-like conditions in association with deficiency of vitamin A. *J. trop. Med. Hyg.* 43, 190–194.

Moore, D. F. (1958). Amblyopia. *Lancet* ii, 527.

Mueller, J. F. and Vilter, R. W. (1950). Pyridoxine deficiency in human beings induced with desoxypyridoxine. *J. clin. Invest.* 29, 193–201.

Musini, A. (1954). Lesioni oculari indotte in ratti a diete carenzate di vitamina A a B₆ con riguardo al metabolismo del triptofano. *Atti 40 Congr. Soc. oftalmol. ital.* 14, 220.

Murray, W. C. G. and Asregadoo, E. R. (1959). Some common eye diseases in British Guiana. *W. Indian med. J.* 8, 225–228.

Musselman, M. M. (1945). Nutritional disease in Cabanatuan. *War Med.* 8, 325–332.

Musselman, M. M. (1946). Pellagra in Americans in Japanese prisons. *Bull. U.S. Army Med. Dept.* 5, 403–411.

Naessens, W. M. (1930). Beriberi in infants. *Geneesk. Tijdschr. Ned.-Indië.* 74, 211–218.

Nañagas, P. J. (1953). Nutritional dystrophy of corneal epithelium. *A.M.A. Archs Ophthal.* 49, 536–552.

Nicholls, L. (1933). Phrynoderma: condition due to vitamin deficiency. *Indian med. Gaz.* 68, 681–6.

Nicholls, L. (1934). Study of vitamin A deficiency in Ceylon with special reference to statistical incidence of phrynoderma and "sore mouth". *Indian med. Gaz.* 69, 241–251.

Nikoskelainen, E., Sogg, R. L., Rosenthal, R., Friberg, T. R. and Dorfman, L. J. (1977). The early phase in Leber hereditary optic atrophy. *Am. J. Ophthal.* 95, 969–983.

North, J. D. K. and Sinclair, H. M. (1956). Nutritional neuropathy. *A.M.A. Archs Pathol.* 62, 341–353.

North, J. D. K. and Sinclair, H. M. (1957). The effect of a combined deficiency of thiamine and of pantothenic acid on the nervous system of the rat. *J. Nutr.* 61, 219–234.

374   NUTRITIONAL OPHTHALMOLOGY

Ohta, K. (1930). Zur Klinik der Säuglings-Beriberi. *Jb. Kinderheilk.* **128**, 1–9.

Oleson, J. J., Bird, H. R., Elvehjem, C. A. and Hart, E. B. (1939). Additional nutritional factors required by the rat. *J. biol. Chem.* **127**, 23–42.

Osuntokun, B. O., Durowoju, J. E., McFarlane, H. and Wilson, J. (1968). Plasma amino acids in the Nigerian nutritional ataxic neuropathy. *Br. med. J.* **3**, 647–649.

Osuntokun, B. O. and Osuntokun, O. (1971). Tropical amblyopia in Nigerians. *Am. J. Ophthal.* **72**, 708–716.

Ottolenghi, S. (1890). Cited by J. D. Spillane (1947).

Owen, R. A. (1966). Defective vision in West Indian immigrants. *Br. J. Ophthal.* **50**, 561–569.

Patek, A. J., Post, J. and Victor, J. (1941). Riboflavin deficiency in the pig. *Am. J. Physiol.* **133**, 47–55.

Pettigrew, A. R. and Fell, G. S. (1972). The simplified colorimetric determination of thiocyanate in biological fluids, and its application to investigation of the toxic amblyopias. *Clin. Chem.* **18**, 996–998.

Pettigrew, A. R., Fell, G. S. and Chisholm, I. A. (1972). Red cell glutathione in tobacco amblyopia. *Expl. Eye Res.* **14**, 87–90.

Philipsen, W. M. J. G. and Hommes, O. R. (1970). Atrophy of the optic nerve in vitamin B_6 deficiency. *Ophthalmologica* **160**, 103–104.

Phillips, C. I., Wang, M. K. and van Peborgh, (1970). Some observations on the mechanism of tobacco amblyopia and its treatment with sodium thiosulphate. *Trans. ophthal. Soc. U.K.* **90**, 809–826.

Philpot, F. J. and Pirie, A. (1943). Riboflavin and riboflavin adenine dinucleotide in ox ocular tissues. *Biochemistry, N.Y.* **37**, 250–254.

Pirie, A. (1943). The relation of riboflavin to the eye. *Br. J. Opthal.* **27**, 291–301.

Pirie, A. (1959). Crystals of riboflavin making up the tapetum lucidum in the eye of a lemur. *Nature, Lond.* **183**, 985–986.

Pock-Steen, P. H. (1939). Eye symptoms in patients with leiodystonia and sprue: aknephascopia. *Geneesk. Tijdschr. Ned.-Indië* **79**, 1986–2006.

Pock-Steen, P. H. (1947). Adaptation tests by vitamin B_2 deficiency. *Acta med. scand.* **126**, 554–564.

Pohlman, M. E. and Ritter, E. F. (1952). Observations on vitamin deficiency in eye, ear, nose and throat clinics of Japanese prison hospital. *Am. J. Ophthal.* **35**, 228–230.

Potter, R. L., Axelrod, A. E. and Elvehjem, C. A. (1942). The riboflavin requirement of the dog. *J. Nutr.* **24**, 449–460.

Potts, A. M. (1973). Tobacco amblyopia. *Surv. Ophthal.* **17**, 313–339.

Prickett, C. O. (1934). The effect of a deficiency of Vitamin B_1 upon the central and peripheral nervous systems of the rat. *Am. J. Physiol.* **107**, 459–470.

Prickett, C. O., Salmon, W. D. and Schrader, G. A. (1939). Histopathology of the peripheral nerves in acute and chronic vitamin B_1 deficiency in the rat. *Am. J. Path.* **15**, 251–260.

Quéré, M. A., Diallo, J., Graveline, J., Cros, J. and Giordano, G. (1967). Tropical nutritional optical neuritis in West Africa. *Annls Oculist Paris* **200**, 745–763.

Raman, T. K. and Abbu, C. (1941). Lesions of optic nerve in vitamin B_1 deficiency. *J. Indian med. Ass.* **10**, 417–422.

Rampoldi, R. (1885). La pellagra e il mal d'oochi. *Annali Ottal. Clin. ocul.* **14**, 99–112.

Riad, M. (1929). *XIII Conc. Ophthal. Acta* 2, 477.

Ridley, H. (1945). Ocular manifestations of malnutrition in released prisoners-of-war from Thailand. *Br. J. Ophthal.* 29, 613–618.

Rinehart, J. F., Friedman, M. and Greenberg, L. D. (1949). Effect of experimental thiamine deficiency on the nervous system of the rhesus monkey. *A.M.A. Archs Path.* 48, 129–139.

Rodger, F. C. (1953). Experimental thiamin deficiency as a cause of degeneration in the visual pathway of the rat. *Br. J. Ophthal.* 37, 11–29.

Rodger, F. C. (1954). Degenerative changes in the rat visual pathway when thiamin and riboflavin deficiencies are combined. *Br. J. Ophthal.* 38, 144–155.

Rodger, F. C. (1959). "Blindness in West Africa," 128. Lewis, London.

Rönne, H. (1910). Pathologische-anatomische Untersuchungen über alkoholische Intoxicatious-Amblyopie. *Albrecht v. Graefes Arch. Ophthal.* 17, 1–95.

Ross, J. F., Beddington, H. and Paegel, B. L. (1948). The development and progression of subacute combined degeneration of the spinal cord in patients with pernicious anaemia treated with synthetic folic acid. *Blood* 3, 68–90.

Sachs, T. (1889). Anatomical and clinical contributions to the knowledge of central scotoma in affections of the optic nerve. *Archs Ophthal.* 18, 133.

Salmon, W. D. and Engel, R. W. (1940). Pantothenic acid and hemorrhagic adrenal necrosis in rats. *Proc. Soc. exp. Biol. Med.* 45, 621–623.

Salmon, W. D., Hays, I. M. and Guerrant, N. B. (1928). Etiology of dermatitis of experimental pellagra in rats. *J. infect. Dis.* 43. 426–441.

Samelsohn, J. (1882). Zue Anatomie und Nosologie der retrobulbaren Neuritis (Amblyopia Neuritis). *Albrecht v. Graefes Arch. Ophthal.* 28, 1–110.

Schreiber, M. and Elvehjem, C. A. (1954). The influence of flavonoid compounds on the nasal excretion of a red pigment by rats subjected to stress conditions. *J. Nutr.* 54, 257–270.

Scott, H. H. (1918). An investigation into an acute outbreak of central neuritis. *Ann. trop. Med. Parasit.* 12, 109–196.

Scott, J. G. (1944). Corneal vascularity as sign of ariboflavinosis. *Jl. R. Army Med. Corps* 82, 133–135.

Sebrell, W. H. Jr, and Butler, R. E. (1938). Riboflavin deficiency in man. *Publ. Hlth Rep. Wash.* 53, 2282–2284.

Sekino, I. (1960). Experimental studies on the ocular manifestations in folic acid deficiency. *Acta Soc. Ophthal. Japan* 64, 2218–2233.

Shapland, C. D. (1946). Ocular disturbances associated with malnutrition. *Jl R. Army Med. Corps* 87, 253–265.

Sharples, L. R. (1929). Condition of "burning feet" or "foot burning" in labourers on sugar plantations in Corentyne district of British Guiana. *J. trop. Med. Hyg.* 32, 358–360.

Sherman, H. C. and Sandels, M. R. (1931). Further experimental differentiation of vitamins B and G. *J. Nutr.* 3, 395–409.

Shih, V. E., Abroms, I. F., Johnson, J. L., Carney, M., Mandell, R., Robb, R. M., Cloherty, J. P. and Rajagopalan, K. V. (1977). Sulfite oxidase deficiency: biochemical and clinical investigations of a hereditary metabolic disorder in sulfur metabolism. *New Eng. J. Med.* 297, 1022–1028.

Shinozuka, S. (1959). Studies on the riboflavin metabolism in epidemic keratoconjunctivitis. *Acta Soc. Ophthal. Japan* 63, 682–696.

Sichel, J. (1837). "Traite de l'ophtalmologie, cataract et de l'amaurose." Manson, Paris.

Sichel, J. (1865). Nouvells recherches pratiques sur l'amblyopie et l'amaurose causées par l'abus du tabac à fumer, avec des remarques sur l'amblyopie et l'amaurose des buvents. *Annls Oculist. Paris* 54, 122.

Sie Boen Lian. (1947). Camp amblyopia. *Ophthalmoligica* 113, 38–44.

Silvette, H., Haag, H. B. and Larson, P. S. (1960). Tobacco amblyopia. *Am. J. Ophthal.* 50, 71–100.

Smith, A. D. M. (1961). Retrobulbar neuritis in Addisonian pernicious anaemia. *Lancet* i, 1001–1002.

Smith, A. D. M. and Duckett, S. (1965). Cyanide, vitamin B_{12}, experimental demyelination and tobacco amblyopia. *Br. J. exp. Path.* 46, 615–622.

Smith, D. A. and Woodruff, M. F. A. (1951). Deficiency diseases in Japanese prison camps. *Spec. Rep. Ser. med. Res. Coun.* No. 274.

Spies, T. D., Vilter, R. W. and Ashe, W. F. (1939). Pellagra, beriberi and riboflavin deficiency in human beings. *J. Am. med. Ass.* 113, 931–7.

Spies, T. D., Perry, D. J., Cogswell, R. C. and Frommeyer, W. B. (1945). Ocular disturbances in riboflavin deficiency. *J. Lab. clin. Med.* 30, 751–765.

Spillane, J. D. (1947). "Nutritional Disorders of the Nervous System." Livingstone, Edinburgh.

Srivastava, S. K. and Beutler, E. (1972). Galactose cataract in riboflavin deficient rats. *Biochem. Med.* 6, 372–379.

Stambolian, D. and Behrens, M. (1977). Optic neuropathy associated with vitamin B_{12} deficiency. *Am. J. Ophthal.* 83, 465–8.

Stannus, H. S. (1912). Pellagra in Nyasaland. *Trans. R. Soc. trop. Med. Hyg.* 5, 112–9.

Stannus, H. S. (1913). Pellagra in Nyasaland. *Trans. R. Soc. trop. Med. Hyg.* 7, 32–56.

Stannus, H. S. (1936). Pellagra and pellagra-like conditions in warm climates. *Trop. Dis. Bull.* 33, Section I 729–741, Section II 815–825, Section III 885–901.

St John, C. H. (1936). "Malnutrition in Patients Attending the Eye Department of Barbados General Hispital." Cited by D. F. Moore (1937).

Strachan, H. (1888). "Annual of the Universal Medical Sciences," 139. Philadelphia.

Strachan, H. (1897). On a form of multiple neuritis prevalent in the West Indies. *Practitioner* 59, 477–484.

Strambio, C. (1789). "De Pellagra." Milan.

Street, H. R., Cowgill, G. R. and Zimmerman, H. M. (1941). Further observations of riboflavin deficiency in the dog. *J. Nutr.* 22, 7–24.

Swank, R. L. and Prados, M. (1942). Avian thiamine deficiency. II. Pathologic changes in the brain and cranial nerves (especially the vestibular) and their relation to the clinical behavior. *A.M.A. Archs Neurol. Psychiat.* 47, 97–131.

Sydenstricker, V. P., Sebrell, W. H. Jr, Cleckley, H. M. and Kruse, H. D. (1940). The ocular manifestations of ariboflavinosis. *J. Am. med. Ass.* 114, 2437–2445.

Sysi, R. (1946). Investigations on the effect of vitamin B_1 on the accommodation of man. *Acta Ophthal.* Suppl. No. 25.

Takada (1934). Cited by W. S. Duke-Elder (1946).

Takahashi, H. (1958). Ocular manifestation of vitamin B_{12} deficiency. *Acta Soc. Ophthal. Japan* 62, 1683–1697.

Takahashi, K. (1959). *Acta Soc. Ophthal. Japan* 63, 1787.

Thygeson, P. (1957). Aetiology and differential diagnosis of non-trachomatous follicular conjunctivitis. *Bull. Wld Hlth Org.* 16, 995–1011.

Tomizawa, A. (1959). Ocular manifestation of deficiency of pantothenic acid. *Acta Soc. Ophthal. Japan* 63, 3314–3339.

Uthoff, W. (1886). Untersuchungen über den Einfluß des chronischen Alkoholismus auf das manschliche Schorgan. *Albrecht v. Graefes Arch. Ophthal.* 32, 95–167.

Van Bijsterveld, O. P. (1976). Pyridoxine deficiency and the conjunctiva. *Ophthalmologica* 173, 324–9.

Van Bogaert, L. (1927). La polyneurite anemique. *Annls Méd.* 22, 321.

Van Heyningen, R. (1957). Meso inositol in the lens of mammalian eyes. *Biochem. J.* 65, 24–28.

Venkataswamy, G. (1967). Ocular manifestations of vitamin B-complex deficiency. *Br. J. Ophthal.* 51, 749–754.

Verma, O. P. (1942). Partial degeneration of optic nerve associated with vitamin deficiency. *Indian med. Gaz.* 77, 646–650.

Verma, O. P. (1944). Note on treatment of angular conjunctivitis with riboflavin. *Indian med. Gaz.* 79, 258–259.

Victor, M., Adams, R. D. and Collins, G. H. (1971). The Wernicke-Korsakoff syndrome. A clinical and pathological study of 245 patients, 82 with postmortem examinations. *Contemp. neurol. Ser.* 7, 1–206.

Victor, M. and Dreyfus, P. M. (1965). Tobacco–alcohol amblyopia. Further comments on its pathology. *Archs Ophthal.* 74, 649–657.

Victor, M., Mancall, E. L. and Dreyfus, P. M. (1960). Deficiency amblyopia in the alcoholic patient. *Archs Ophthal.* 64, 1–33.

Vilter, R. W., Mueller, J. F. and Glazer, H. S. (1953). The effect of vitamin B_6 deficiency induced by desoxypyridoxine in human beings. *J. Lab. clin. Med.* 42, 335–357.

Wadia, N. H., Desai, M. M., Quadros, E. J. and Dastur, D. K. (1972). Role of vegetarianism, smoking and hydroxocobalamin in optic neuritis. *Br. med. J.* 3, 264–267.

Waisman, H. A. (1944). Production of riboflavin deficiency in the monkey. *Proc. Soc. exp. Biol. Med.* 55, 69–71.

Walker, R. (1958). Age changes in the rat's exorbital lacrimal gland. *Anat. Rec.* 132, 49–70.

Walsh, F. B. (1957). "Clinical Neuro-Ophthalmology," 920–921. Williams and Wilkins, Baltimore.

Watson-Williams, E. J., Bottomley, A. C., Ainley, R. G. and Phillips, C. J. (1969). Absorption of vitamin B_{12} in tobacco amblyopia. *Br. J. Ophthal.* 53, 549–552.

Whaley, E. M. (1909). *Trans. Nat. Conf. Pellagra* Columbia, South Carolina 1, 279.

Whitbourne, D. (1947). Nutritional retrobulbar neuritis in children in Jamaica. *Am. J. Ophthal.* 30, 169–171.

Wilkinson, P. B. and King, A. (1944). Amblyopia due to a vitamin deficiency. *Lancet* i, 528–531.

Wilson, J. and Langman, M. J. S. (1966). Relation of subacute combined degeneration of the cord to vitamin B_{12} deficiency. 212, 787–789.

Wintrobe, M. M., Buschke, W., Follis, R. H. Jr and Humphreys, S. (1944). Riboflavin deficiency in swine. *Johns Hopkins Hosp. Bull.* 75, 102–114.

Wokes, F. (1958). Tobacco amblyopia. *Lancet* ii, 526–527.

Wolbach, S. B. and Howe, P. R. (1925). Tissue changes following deprivation of fat-soluble A vitamin. *J. exp. Med.* 42, 753–777.

Wright, E. J. (1928). Disease due to A and B avitaminosis in Sierra Leone. *W. Afr. med. J.* 2, 127–130.

Wright, E. J. (1930). "A and B Avitaminosis Diseases of Sierra Leone."

Yasuda, S. and Goto, E. (1940). *Ganka Rinsho Iho, Japan* 21, 993.

Chapter 4

American Pediatric Society (1898). *Archs Pediat.* 15, 481.

Barber, A. and Nothaker, W. G. (1952). Effects of cortisone on non-perforating wounds of cornea in normal and scorbutic guinea pigs. *A.M.A. Archs Path.* 54, 334–342.

Bellows, J. (1936). Biochemistry of lens; influence of vitamin C and sulfydryls on production of galactose cataract. *A.M.A. Archs Ophthal.* 16, 762–769.

Bessesen, B. S. (1923). Changes in organ weights of the guinea pig during experimental study. *Am. J. Physiol.* 63, 245–256.

Biernacka-Biesiekierska, J. and Szczygowa, M. (1954). The significance of ascorbic acid in the physiology of colour perception. *Klin. Oczna* 24, 1–6.

Boyd, T. A. S. (1955). Influence of local ascorbic acid concentration on collagenous tissue healing in the cornea. *Br. J. Ophthal.* 39, 204–214.

Bunce, G. E. and Hess, J. L. (1976). Lenticular opacities in young rats as a consequence of maternal diets low in tryptophan and/or vitamin E. *J. Nutr.* 106, 222–9.

Campbell, F. W. and Ferguson, I. D. (1950). The role of ascorbic acid in corneal vascularization. *Br. J. Ophthal.* 34, 329–334.

Campbell, F. W., Ferguson, I. D. and Garry, R. C. (1950). Ascorbic acid and healing of heat injuries in the guinea pig cornea. *Br. J. Nutr.* 4, 32–42.

Cohen, C. (1906). Uber den Einfluss des Lebensalters auf die Adaptation. *Klin. Mbl. Augenheilk.* 45, 120–134.

Cristiansson, J. (1957). Changes in the vitreous body in scurvy. Studies on guinea pigs *in vivo.* I. The biopolymers of the vitreous body. II. Studies on the aqueous content. III. Studies on electrolytes. *Acta Ophthal.* 35, 336–360, 420–8, 429–440.

Demole, V. and Knapp, P. (1941). Augenerkrankungen bei einigen Vitamin-E-frei ernährten Ratten. *Ophthalmologica* 101, 65–73.

Demole, V. and Pfaltz, H. (1940). Syndromes neuromusculaires précoces et tardifs des rats atteints d'avitaminose E. Caractères différentiels. *Revue méd. Suisse romande* 60, 464–476.

D'Esposito, M. (1957). Ricerche istochimiche sui rapporte fra vitamina "E" e mucopolisaccaride corneale. *Annali Ottal. Clin. Ocul.* 83, 323–328.

Devi, A., Raina, P. L. and Singh, A. (1965). Abnormal protein and nucleic acid metabolism as a cause of cataract formation induced by nutritional deficiency in rabbit. *Br. J. Ophthal.* 49, 271–275.

Duke-Elder, W. S. (1946). The nutritional aspects of ophthalmology. *Ir. J. med. Sci.* 6th Series, 177–189.

Falls, H. F. and Jurrow, H. N. (1946). Effect of antepartum with vitamin K on retinal hemorrhage. *J. Am. med. Ass.* 131, 203–205.

Geever, E. F. and Levenson, S. M. (1960). Pathogenesis of the collagen defect in experimental scurvy. *Archs Ophthal.* 63, 812–820.

Giles, C. L. (1960). Retinal hemorrhages in the newborn. *Am. J. Ophthal.* 49, 1005–1011.

Hayes, K. C. (1974). Retinal degeneration in monkeys induced by deficiencies of vitamin E or A. *Invest. Ophthal.* 13, 499–510.

Hood, J. and Hodges, R. E. (1969). Ocular lesions in scurvy. *Am. J. clin. Nutr.* 22, 559–567.

Jacobsthal, H. (1900). *Beitr. path. Anat.* 27, 173.

Jaeger, E. (1861). "Ueber die Einstellungindes dioptrischen Apparates in menschlichen Auge." Seidel, Vienna.

Johnson, L., Schaffer, D. and Boggs, T. R. Jr (1974). The premature infant, vitamin E deficiency and retrolental fibroplasia. *Am. J. clin. Nutr.* 27, 1158–1173.

Kitamura, S. (1910). Ein Beitrag zur Kerntrus der Netzhautveränderungen beim Skorbut. *Dt. med. Wschr.* 36, 403.

Knapp, A. A. (1939). Vitmain-D complex in progressive myopia; etiology, pathology, and treatment; preliminary study. *Am. J. Ophthal.* 22, 1329–1337.

Knapp, A. A. (1943). Night blindness, improvement with vitamin D, including experimental production of retinitis pigmentosa and its treatment in humans with vitamin D. *U.S. Naval med. Bull.* 41, 373–377.

Lecoq, R., and Isidor, P. (1949). Studies on histopathology of vitamin E deficiency. *Ann. N.Y. Acad. Sci.* 52, 139–141.

Linnér, E. (1964). Intraocular pressure regulation and ascorbic acid. *Acta Soc. Med. upsal.* 69, 225–232.

Löwenstein, A. (1917). *Klin. Mbl. Augenheilk.* 59, 583.

Malatesta, C. (1951). *Boll. oculist* 30, 541.

Maumenee, A. E., Hellmann, L. M. and Shettles, L. B. (1941). Factors influencing plasma prothrombin in the newborn infant. IV. The effect of antenatal administration of vitamin K on the incidence of retinal hemorrhage in the newborn. *Johns Hopkins Hosp. Bull.* 68, 158–168.

Maxwell, J. P. and Pi, H. T. (1940). Cataract in adult rickets (osteomalacia). *Proc. R. Soc. Med.* 33, 777–782.

Meinert (1887). Tetanie in der Schwangerschaft. *Arch. Gynäkol.* 30, 444–455.

Mellanby, E. (1919). An experimental investigation on rickets. *Lancet* i, 407–412.

Müller, W. and Nover, A. (1955). Kernveranderungen in den Ganglienzellen der Nethaut bei experimentellen Vitamin-C-Mangel. *Z. Vitam.- Horm.- u. Fermentforsch.* 7, 277–280.

Owens, W. C. and Owens, E. U. (1949). Retrolental fibroplasia in premature infants. II. Studies on the prophylaxis of the disease: The use of alpha-tocopherol acetate. *Am. J. Ophthal.* 32, 1631–1637.

Phelps, D. L. and Rosenbaum, A. L. (1977). The role of tocopherol in oxygen-induced retinopathy: kitten model. *Pediatrics* 59, Suppl. No. 6, 998–1005.

Pi, H. T. (1934). Subcapsular cataract in osteomalacia. *Chin. med. J.* 48, 948–964.

Pray, L. G., McKeown, H. S. and Pollard, W. E. (1941). Hemorrhagic diathesis of the newborn: effect of vitamin K prophylaxis and therapy. *Am. J. Obstet. Gynec.* 42, 836–845.

Purcell, E. F., Lerner, L. H. and Kinsey, V. E. (1954). Ascorbic acid in aqueous humor and serum of patients with and without cataract. Physiological significance of relative concentrations. *A.M.A. Archs Ophthal.* 51, 1–6.

Rainess, L. (1930). Eye symptom in rachitis. *Archs Pediat.* 47, 55–57.

Sabatine, P. L., Rosen, H., Geever, E. F. and Levenson, S. M. (1961). Scurvy, ascorbic acid concentration and collagen formation in the guinea pig eye. *A.M.A. Archs Ophthal.* 65, 32–37.

Simonelli, M. (1950). Intossicazione sperimentale de vitamina K e manifestazioni oculari. *G. ital. oftal.* 3, 183–187.

Stewart, C. P. (1941). Nutritional factors in dark adaptation. *Edinb. med. J.* 48, 217–237.

Sulkin, D. F., Sulkin, N. M. and Nushan, H. (1972). Corneal fine structure in experimental scorbutus. *Invest. Ophthal.* 11, 633–643.

Terroine, T. (1953). Protection par l'acide ascorbique contre carence en biotine chez le rat. *C. r. hebd. Séanc. Acad. Sic.* 237, 1030–1032.

Wille, H. (1944). Investigations in influence of K avitaminosis on occurrence of retinal haemorrhages in newborn. *Acta Ophthal.* 22, 261–269.

Yudkin, A. M., Farquhar, L. R. and Wakeman, A. J. (1934). Some abnormalities in rats subsisting on diets poor in mineral nutrients. *A.M.A. Archs Path.* 17, 40–45.

Zilva, S. S. and Still, G. F. (1920). Orbital haemorrhage with proptosis in experimental scurvy. *Lancet* i, 1008.

Chapter 5

Belkin, M., Zeimer, R., Chajek, T., Friedman, G. and Melamed, E. (1976). Non-invasive quantitation of corneal copper in hepatolenticular degeneration (Wilson's disease). *Lancet* i, 391–392.

Bellows, J. G. (1944). "Cataract and Anomalies of the Lens," 296. Kimpton, London.

Berlyne, G. M. (1968). Microcrystalline conjunctival calcification in renal failure. A useful clinical sign. *Lancet* ii, 366–370.

Berlyne, G. M., Benari, J., Danovitch, G. M. and Blumenthal, M. (1972). Cataracts of chronic renal failure. *Lancet* i, 509–511.

Beutler, E., Fairbanks, V. F. and Fahey, J. L. (1963). "Clinical Disorders of Iron Metabolism," 131–132, Grune and Stratton, New York.

Bietti, G. (1940). Ueber einen rein tetanischen Ernährungskatarakt. *Klin. Mbl. Augenheilk.* 105, 299–312.

Bowness, J. M., Morton, R. A., Shakir, M. H. and Stubbs, A. L. (1952). Distribution of copper and zinc in mammalian eyes. Occurrence of metals in melanin fractions from eye tissues. *Biochem. J.* 51, 521–430.

Brenner, R. L., Smith, J. L., Cleveland, W. W., Bejar, R. L. and Lockhart, W. S. Jr (1969). Eye signs of hypophosphatasia. *Archs Ophthal.* 81, 614–7.

Budinger, J. M. (1961). Diphenylthiocarbazone blindness in dogs. *A.M.A. Archs Pathol.* 71, 304–310.

Cogan, D. G., Albright, F. and Bartter, F. C. (1948). Hypercalcemia and band keratopathy. *A.M.A. Archs Ophthal.* 40, 624–638.

Davies, G., Dymock, I., Harry, J. and Williams, R. (1972). Deposition of melanin and iron in ocular structures in haemochromatosis. *Br. J. Ophthal.* 56, 338–342.

Demco, T. A., McCormick, A. Q. and Richards, J. S. F. (1974). Conjunctival and corneal changes in chronic renal failure. *Can. J. Ophthal.* 9, 208–213.

Duke-Elder, W. S. (1940). "Textbook of Ophthalmology," Vol. 3, p. 3156. Mosby, St Louis, Missouri.

Ehlers, N. and Bülow, N. (1977). Clinical copper metabolism parameters in patients with retinitis pigmentosa and other tapetoretinal degenerations. *Br. J. Ophthal.* 61, 595–596.

Ehlers, N., Kruse Hansen, F., Hansen, H. E. and Jensen, O. A. (1972). Corneo-conjunctival changes in uraemia. Influence of renal allotransplantation. *Acta Ophthal.* 50, 83–94.

Ellis, P. P. (1969). Ocular deposition of copper in hypercupremia. *Am. J. Ophthal.* 68, 423–7.

Erdheim, J. (1906). Letania parathyreopriva. *Mitt. Grenzgeb. Med. Chir.* 16, 632–744.

Fanconi, G., Girardet, P., Schlesinger, B., Butler, N. and Black, J. (1952). Chronische Hypercalcamie, kombirnest mit Osteosklerose, Hyperazotämie, Minderwirchs und kungentalen Missbildungen. *Helv. paediat. acta* 7, 314–349.

Follis, R. H. Jr, Day, H. G. and McCollum, E. V. (1941). Histological studies of the tissues of rats fed a diet extremely low in zinc. *J. Nutr.* 22, 223–237.

Follis, R. H. Jr. Orent-Keiles, E. and McCollum, E. V. (1942). Histological studies of the tissues of rats fed a diet extremely low in sodium. *A.M.A. Archs Pathol.* 33, 504–512.

François, J. (1972). Ocular manifestations in aminoacidopathies. *Adv. Ophthal.* 25, 28–103.

Frommer, D., Morris, J., Sherlock, S., Abrams, J. and Newman, S. (1977). Kayser–Fleischer-like rings in patients without Wilson's disease. *Gastroenterology* 72, 1331–1335.

Gahlot, D. K., Khosla, P. K., Makashir, P. D., Vasuki, K. and Basu, N. (1976). Copper metabolism in retinitis pigmentosa. *Br. J. Ophthal.* 60, 770–774.

Galton, D. J. (1965). Diabetic retinopathy and haemochromatosis. *Br. med. J.* i, 1169.

Gartner, S. and Rubner, K. (1955). Calcified scleral nodules in hypervitaminosis D. *Am. J. Ophthal.* 39, 658–663.

Gerard-Lefebvre (1959). Concerning hypervitaminosis D₂ and idiopathic hypercalcemia: a closely related syndrome. *Pédiatrie* 14, 576–580.

Gillman, T. (1957). Nutrition, liver disease and some aspects of ageing in Africans. *Ciba Fdn. Colloq. Ageing* 3, 104–111.

Goldberg, M. F. and von Noorden, G. K. (1966). Ophthalmologic findings in Wilson's hepatolenticular degeneration with emphasis on ocular motility. *Archs Ophthal.* 75, 162–170.

Goldmann, H. (1929). Experimentelle Letaniekatarakt. *Albrecht v. Graefes Arch. Ophthal.* 122, 146–197.

Hanselmayer, H., Pogglitsch, H. and Schmidberger, H. (1974). Calcification in the conjunctiva and cornea in chronic renal failure treated with haemodialysis. *Klin. Mbl. Augenheilk.* 164, 98–105.

Harris, L. S., Cohn, K., Toyofuku, H., Lonergan, E. and Galin, M. A. (1971). Conjunctival and corneal calcific deposits in uremic patients. *Am. J. Ophthal.* 72, 130–133.

Hubbard, G. B., Herron, B. E., Andrews, J. S. and Elliott, J. H. (1969). Influence of topical and oral zinc upon corneal wound healing. *Br. J. Ophthal.* 53, 407–411.

Ireland, A. W., Hornbrook, J. W., Neale, F. C. and Posen, S. (1968). The crystalline lens in chronic surgical hypoparathyroidism. *Archs invest. Med.* 122, 408–411.

Knopik, A. and Stankiewicz, A. (1972). Pathomorphology of cataract caused by experimental potassium and magnesium deficiency. *Klin. Oczna* 42, 549–552.

Knopik, A., Stankiwicz, A., Kulig, A. and Krawczyk, Z. (1973). Studies on the pathomorphology of cataract induced by experimental potassium and magnesium deficiency. *Acta med. pol.* 14, 177–184.

Kobayashi, F. and Mimuran, N. (1974). Uraemic retinopathy after long-term dialysis. *Acta Soc. Ophthal. Japan* 78, 1473–1483.

Kolker, A. E. (1966). Ocular manifestations of hematologic disease. In "Progress in Hematology" (Eds E. B. Brown and C. V. Moore), Vol. 5, 354–389. Heinemann, London.

Lemp, M. A. and Ralph, R. A. (1977). Rapid development of band keratopathy in dog eyes. *Am. J. Ophthal.* 83, 657–659.

Lessell, S. and Norton, E. W. D. (1964). Band keratopathy and conjunctival calcification in hypophosphatasia. *Archs Ophthal.* 71, 497–499.

Levi, A. J., Sherlock, S., Scheuer, P. J. and Cumings, J. N. (1967). Presymptomatic Wilson's disease. *Lancet* ii, 575–579.

Levy, N. S., Dawson, W. W., Rhodes, B. J. and Garnica, A. (1974). Ocular abnormality in Menkes's kinky-hair syndrome. *Am. J. Ophthal.* 77, 319–325.

Lubeck, M. J. (1959). Papilledema caused by iron-deficiency anemia. *Trans. Am. Acad. Ophthal. Oto-lar.* 63, 306–310.

Lyle, D. J. (1948). Ocular syndrome of cataract and papilledema in manifest form of parathyroid deficiency. *Am. J. Ophthal.* 31, 580–584.

Martin, G. D., Stanley, J. A. and Davidson, I. W. F. (1972). Corneal lesions in squirrel monkeys maintained on a low-chromium diet. *Invest. Ophthal.* 11, 153–158.

Matta, C. S., Felker, G. V. and Ide, C. H. (1975). Eye manifestations in acrodermatitis enteropathica. *Archs Ophthal.* 93, 140–142.

Meesmann, A. (1938). *Klin. Mbl. Augenheilk.* 100, Suppl. 1.

Morrison, S. A., Russell, R. M., Carney, E. A. and Oaks, E. V. (1978). Zinc deficiency: a cause of abnormal dark adaptation in cirrhotics. *Am. J. clin. Nutr.* 31, 276–281.

Nishimura, H. (1953). Zinc deficiency in suckling mice deprived of colostrum. *J. Nutr.* 49, 79–97.

Orent-Keiles, E., Robinson, A. and McCollum, E. V. (1937). The effects of sodium deprivation on the animal organism. *Am. J. Physiol.* 119, 651–661.

Pirie, A. and van Heyningen, R. (1956). "Biochemistry of the Eye." Blackwell, Oxford.

Roginski, E. E. and Mertz, W. (1967). An eye lesion in rats fed low chromium diets. *J. Nutr.* 93, 249–251.

Roth, A. M. and Foos, R. Y. (1972). Ocular pathological changes in primary hemochromatosis. *Archs Ophthal.* 87, 507–514.

Schwarz, K. and Milne, D. B. (1972). Growth-promoting effects of silicon in rats. *Nature, Lond.* 239, 333–334.

Sprinkler, L. H., Harr, J. R., Newberne, P. M., Whanger, P. M. and Weswig, P. H. (1971). Selenium deficiency lesions in rats fed vitamin E supplemented rations. *Nutr. Rep. Int.* 4, 335–340.

Stankiewicz, A., Krawczykowa, Z. and Bocian, J. (1972). Lenticular metabolism in experimental cataract in rabbits caused by deficiency of potassium and magnesium. *Klin. Oczna* 42, 553–557.

Swan, K. C. and Salit, P. W. (1941). Lens opacities associated with experimental calcium deficiency: preliminary report. *Am. J. Ophthal.* 24, 611–614.

Toskes, P., Currington, C. and Dawson, W. (1977). Visual dysfunction in patients with chronic pancreatitis. *Am. J. clin. Nutr.* 30, 623.

Turpeinen, O. (1938). Studies on sodium deficiency: the effects of sodium deprivation on young puppies. *Am. J. Hyg.* 28, 104–110.

Vallee, B. L., Wacker, W. E. C., Bartholomay, A. F. and Hoch, F. L. (1959). Zinc metabolism in hepatic dysfunction. *Ann. intern. Med.* 50, 1077–1091.

von Bahr, G. (1936). Studies on aetiology and pathogenesis of cataracta zonularis. *Acta Ophthal.* Suppl. 11, 1–236.

von Bahr, G. (1940). Influence of calcium deficiency on surviving rabbit's lens. Experimental study on pathogenesis of cataracta tetanica. *Acta Ophthal.* 18, 170–189.

Wamoto, T. and DeVoe, A. G. (1976). Electron microscopical study of the Fleischer ring. *Archs Ophthal.* 94, 1579–1584.

Warshawsky, R. S., Hill, C. W., Doughman, D. J. and Harris, J. E. (1975). Acrodermatitis enteropathica. Corneal involvement with histochemical and electron micrograph studies. *Archs Ophthal.* 93, 194–197.

Weitzel, G., Strecker, F. J., Roester, U., Buddecke, E. and Fretzdorff, A. M. (1954). Zink im Tapetum lucidum. *Hoppe-Seyler's Z. physiol. Chem.* 296, 19–30.

Wirsching, L. Jr (1962). Eye symptoms in acrodermatitis enteropathica. *Acta Ophthal.* 40, 567–574.

Wray, S. H., Kuwabara, T. and Sanderson, P. (1976). Menke's kinky hair disease: a light and electron microscopic study of the eye. *Invest. Ophthal.* 15, 128–138.

Yu, J. S., Oates, R. K., Walsh, K. H. and Stuckey, S. J. (1971). Osteopetrosis. *Archs Dis. Child.* 46, 257–263.

Yudkin, A. M. (1924). An experimental study of ophthalmia in rats on rations deficient in vitamin A. *A.M.A. Archs Ophthal.* 53, 416–425.

Chapter 6

Alam, S. Q., Becker, R. V., Stucki, W. P., Rogers, Q. R. and Harper, A. E. (1966). Effect of threonine on the toxicity of excess tyrosine and cataract formation in the rat. *J. Nutr.* 89, 91–96.

Aurbach, E., Guggenheim, K., Kaplansky, J. and Rowe, H. (1964). Effect of protein depletion on the electric response of the retina in albino rats. *J. Physiol., Lond.* 172, 417–424.

Bagchi, K. (1959a). The effects of dietary protein on the sulphydryl content of crystalline lens. *Indian J. med. Res.* 47, 184–199.

Bagchi, K. (1959b). The effects of methionine-sulphoximine-induced methionine deficiency on the crystalline lens of albino rats. *Indian J. med. Res.* 47, 437–447.

Balcet, C. (1948). Manifestazioni oculari da insufficiente alimentazione. *Rass. ital. ottal.* 17, 271–275.

Bardiger, M., Miller, D. S. and Nicholson, A. L. (1968). The effect of diet on ocular refraction in the rat. *Proc. Nutr. Soc.* 27, 22–23a.

Berg, J. L., Pund, E. R., Sydenstricker, V. P., Hall, W. K., Bowles, L. L. and Hock, C. W. (1947). The formation of capillaries and other tissue changes in the cornea of the methionine-deficient rat. *J. Nutr.* 33, 271–281.

Berson, E. L., Hayes, K. C., Rabin, A. R., Schmidt, S. Y. and Watson, G. (1976a). Retinal degeneration in cats fed casein. II. Supplementation with methionine, cystine or taurine. *Invest. Ophthal.* 15, 52–58.

Berson, E. L., Schmidt, S. Y. and Rabin, A. R. (1976b). Plasma amino acids in hereditary retinal disease: ornithine, lysine and taurine. *Br. J. Ophthal.* 60, 142–147.

Bietti, G. B. (1950). Ophthalmic aspects of protein deficiency and disordered protein metabolism. *Documenta Ophthal.* 4, 200–226.

Bourne, M. C. and Pyke, M. A. (1935). The occurrence of cataract in rats fed on diets deficient in vitamin B. *Biochem. J.* 29, 1865–1871.

Bowles, L. L., Hall, W. K. and Sydenstricker, V. P. (1950). Ocular changes in the rat resulting from high levels of tyrosine and phenylalanine in the diet. *Anat. Rec.* 106, 265–266.

Brown, E. F. and Morgan, A. F. (1948). The effect of vitamin A deficiency upon the nitrogen metabolism of the rat. *J. Nutr.* 35, 425–438.

Buist, N. R., Kennaway, N. G. and Burns, R. P. (1973). Eye and skin lesions in tyrosinaemia. *Lancet* i, 620–621.

Bürger, M. (1920). Die Oedemkrankheit. *Ergebn. inn. Med. Kinderheilk.* 23, 189–238.

Burns, R. P. (1972). Soluble tyrosine aminotransferase deficiency: an unusual cause of corneal ulcers. *Am. J. Ophthal.* 73, 400–402.

Buschke, W. (1943). Classification of experimental cataracts in the rat. Recent observations on cataract associated with tryptophan deficiency and with some other experimental conditions. *A.M.A. Archs Ophthal.* 30, 735–750.

Cartwright, G. W., Wintrobe, M. M., Buschke, W. H., Follis, R. H. Jr, Suksta, A. and Humphreys, S. (1945). Anemia, hypoproteinemia, and cataracts in swine fed casein hydrolysate or zein. Comparison with pyridoxine-deficiency anemia. *J. clin. Invest.* 24, 268–277.

Cogan, D. G. and Kuwabara, T. (1960). Ocular pathology of cystinosis, with particular reference to the elusiveness of the corneal crystals. *Archs Ophthal.* 63, 51–57.

Cole, A. S. and Scott, P. P. (1954). Tissue changes in the adult tryptophan-deficient rat. *Br. J. Nutr.* 8, 125–138.

Curtis, P. B., Hauge, S. M. and Kraybill, H. R. (1932). The nutritive value of certain animal protein concentrates. *J. Nutr.* 5, 503–517.

David, J. C. (1976). Evidence for the possible formation of a toxic tyrosine metabolite by the liver microsomal drug metabolizing system. *Naunyn-Schmeidebergs Arch. exp. Path. Pharmak.* 292, 79–86.

Day, P. L., Langston, W. C. and Cosgrove, K. W. (1934). The appearance of cataract and dermatitis in experimental animals given vitamin G deficient diets containing casein and egg albumin. *J. Nutr.* 7, 12.

Donaldson, H. H. and King, H. D. (1936). On the growth of the eye in three strains of the Norway rat. *Am. J. Anat.* 60, 203–229.

Emiru, V. P. (1971). The cornea in kwashiorkor. *J. trop. Pediat.* 17, 117–134.

Ferraro, A. and Roizin, L. (1947). Ocular changes in rats on amino-acid (valine) deficient diet. *Am. J. Ophthal.* 30, 330–331.

Ferraro, A., Roizin, L. and Givner, I. (1947). Ocular changes in rats on diets deficient in amino acids: corneal dystrophy due to valine deficiency. *A.M.A. Archs Ophthal.* 38, 342–352.

François, J. (1972). Ocular manifestations in aminoacidopathies. *Adv. Ophthal.* 25, 28–103.

François, J. and Rabaey, M. (1959). Agar microelectrophoresis at high tension of soluble lens proteins in cataract. *A.M.A. Archs Ophthal.* 62, 991–1000.

Fromm, H. J. and Nordlie, R. C. (1959). Redistribution of methionine and cystine during experimental wound healing. *Biochim. biophys. Acta* 31, 357–364.

Gardiner, P. A. and Macdonald, I. (1957). Relationship between refraction of the eye and nutrition. *Clin. Sci.* 16, 435–442.

Gardiner, P. A. and Macdonald, I. (1958). Dietary intake and refractive errors: an experimental correlation. *Proc. Nutr. Soc.* 17, xx.

Giles, C. L. and Wong, V. G. (1969). Occurrence of adult cystinosis in childhood. Report of two cases. *J. Pediat. Ophthal.* 6, 195–197.

Groschke, A. C., Anderson, J. O. and Briggs, G. M. (1948). Peculiar enlargement of eyeballs in chicks caused by feeding a high level of glycine. *Proc. Soc. exp. Biol. Med.* **69**, 488–491.

Gunter, R., Brown, W. J. and Schalock, R. (1972). Cataractogenesis in infant rats with model phenylketonuria. *Percept. Mot. Skills Res. Exch.* **35**, 47–9.

Halasa, A. H. (1969). Tonography in normal and malnourished children. *Archs Ophthal.* **81**, 328–330.

Halasa, A. H. and McLaren, D. S. (1964). The refractive state of malnourished children. *Archs Ophthal.* **71**, 827–831.

Hall, W. K., Sydenstricker, V. P., Hock, C. W. and Bowles, L. L. (1946). Protein deprivation as a cause of vascularization of the cornea in the rat. *J. Nutr.* **32**, 509–523.

Hall, W. K., Bowles, L. L., Sydenstricker, V. P. and Schmidt, H. L. (1948). Cataracts due to deficiencies of phenylalanine and of histidine in the rat. A comparison with other types of cataracts. *J. Nutr.* **36**, 277–295.

Hayes, K. C., Rabin, A. R. and Berson, E. L. (1975a). An ultrastructural study of nutritionally induced and reversed retinal degeneration in cats. *Am. J. Path.* **78**, 504–524.

Hayes, K. C., Carey, R. E. and Schmidt, S. Y. (1975b). Retinal degeneration associated with taurine deficiency in the cat. *Science, N.Y.* **188**, 949–951.

Helmsen, R. J., Gaasterland, D. E. and Rubin, M. (1973). Induction of buphthalmos in chicks fed an excess of glycine. *Invest. Ophthal.* **12**, 348–353.

Hess, W. N. (1937–38). Production of nutritional cataract in trout. *Proc. Soc. exp. Biol. Med.* **37**, 306–309.

Hueper, W. C. and Martin, G. J. (1943). Tyrosine poisoning in rats. *A.M.A. Archs Pathol.* **35**, 685–694.

Irreverre, F., Mudd, S. H., Heizer, W. D. and Lester, L. (1967). Sulfite oxidase deficiency: Studies of a patient with mental retardation, dislocated ocular lenses, and abnormal urinary excretion of S-sulfo-L-cysteine, sulfite and thiosulfite. *Biochem. Med.* **1**, 187–217.

Jackson, C. M. (1936). Recovery in rats upon refeeding after prolonged suppression of growth by dietary deficiency of protein. *Am. J. Anat.* **58**, 179–193.

Johnson, R. M. and Baumann, C. A. (1948). Relative significance of growth and metabolic rate upon the utilization of vitamin A by the rat. *J. Nutr.* **35**, 703–715.

Kauffman, R. G. and Norton, H. W. (1966). Growth of the procine eye lens during insufficiencies of dietary protein. *Growth* **30**, 463–470.

Kaunitiz, H., Wiesinger, H., Blodi, F. C., Johnson, R. E. and Slanetz, C. A. (1954). Relation of protein and fat intake to growth and corneal vascularization in galactoflavin-produced ariboflavinosis. *J. Nutr.* **52**, 467–482.

Kenyon, K. R. and Sensenbrenner, J. A. (1974). Electron microscopy of cornea and conjunctiva in childhood cystinosis. *Am. J. Ophthal.* **78**, 68–76.

Khetarpal, S. K. (1964). Electroretinographic changes in undernourished children. *Br. J. Ophthal.* **48**, 154–7.

Klemens, F. (1948). *Klin. Mbl. Augenheilk,* **113**, 183.

Kobak, M. W., Benditt, E. P., Wissler, R. W. and Steffee, C. H. (1947). The relation of protein deficiency to experimental wound healing. *Surgery Gynec. Obstet.* **85**, 751–756.

Kubíček, R. and Dolének, A. (1958). Taurine et acides aminés dans la rétine des animaux. *J. Chromat.* **1**, 266–8.

La Du, B. N. and Gjessing, L. R. (1972). Tyrosinosis and tyrosinaemia. *In "The Metabolic Basis of Inherited Disease,"* 3rd edn (Eds J. B. Stanbury, J. B. Wyngaarden and D. S. Fredrickson) 296–307. McGraw-Hill, New York.

Lafon, M. (1939). Recherches sur quelques aspects du bessoin qualitatif d'azote; esquisse d'une analyse biométrique et physiologique et de la carence en lysine et en cystine; étude sur le rat et sur la souris. *Ann. Physiol. physiochem. Biol.* 15, 1–94.

Lieberman, T. W., Podos, S. M. and Harstein, J. (1966). Acute glaucoma, ectopia lentis and homocystinuria. *Archs Ophthal.* 75, 252–255.

Limson, M. and Jackson, C. M. (1932). Changes in the weights of various organs and systems of young rats maintained on a low-protein diet. *J. Nutr.* 5, 163–174.

Localis, S. A., Morgan, M. E. and Hinton, J. W. (1948). The biological chemistry of wound healing. I. The effect of DL-methionine on the healing of wounds in protein-depleted animals. *Surgery Gynec. Obstet.* 86, 582–590.

McDonald, J. E. (1954). Cysteine protection of the cornea against beta radiation. *A.M.A. Archs Ophthal.* 51, 301–310.

McLaren, D. S. (1958a). Growth and water content of the eyeball of the albino rat in protein deficiency. *Br. J. Nutr.* 12, 254–259.

McLaren, D. S. (1958b). Involvement of the eye in protein malnutrition. *Bull. Wld Hlth Org.* 19, 303–314.

McLaren, D. S. (1959a). The eye and related glands of the rat and pig in protein deficiency. *Br. J. Ophthal.* 43, 78–87.

McLaren, D. S. (1959b). Influence of protein deficiency and sex on the development of ocular lesions and survival time of the vitamin A-deficient rat. *Br. J. Ophthal.* 43, 234–241.

McLaren, D. S. (1960). The effects of malnutrition on the eye, with special reference to work with experimental animals. *Wld Rev. Nutr. Dietet.* 2, 29–51.

Maun, M. E., Cahill, W. M. and Davis, R. M. (1945a). Morphologic studies of rats deprived of essential amino acids. II. Leucine. *A.M.A. Archs Path.* 40, 173–178.

Maun, M. E., Cahill, W. M. and Davis, R. M. (1945b). Morphologic studies of rats deprived of essential amino acids. I. Phenylalanine. *A.M.A. Archs Path.* 39, 294–300.

Maun, M. E., Cahill, W. M. and Davis, R. M. (1946). Morphologic studies of rats deprived of essential amino acids. III. Histidine. *A.M.A. Archs Path.* 41, 25–31.

Mitchell, H. S., Cook, G. M. and Henderson, M. D. (1940). Anticataractogenic action of certain nitrogenous factors. *A.M.A. Archs Ophthal.* 24, 990–998.

Morris, M. L. Jr (1965). Feline degenerative retinopathy. *Cornell Vet.* 55, 295–308.

Niedermeier, S. (1950). Zur Nachtblindheit bei Russlandheimkehrern. *Klin. Mbl. Augenheilk.* 116, 416–417.

Niven, C. F., Washburn, M. R. and Spreling, G. A. (1946). Growth retardation and corneal vascularization with tyrosine and phenylalanine in a purified diet. *Proc. Soc. exp. Biol. Med.* 63, 106–108.

Ogino, S. and Tojo, H. (1956). Biochemical studies on cataract. VII. Relation of tyrosine metabolism to production of galactose cataract. *Med. J. Osaka Univ.* 7, 445–457.

Park, M. M. and Schwilk, N. Jr (1963). Bilateral lamellar type cataracts in a case of phenylketonuria. *Am. J. Ophthal.* 56, 140–2.

Patch, E. M. (1934). Cataract as a result of dietary deficiency in larval amblystoma tigrinum. *Science, N.Y.* 79, 57–58.

Patch, E. M. (1941). Dietary production of cataracts in larval amblystoma tigrinum. *J. Nutr.* 22, 365–381.

Patch, E. M. (1943). Relation of diet to lenticular changes in larvae of amblystoma tigrinum. *Archs Ophthal.* 29, 69–84.

Pirie, A. (1948). Comparison of eye changes in riboflavin deficiency and in tryptophan deficiency in the rat. *Br. J. Nutr.* 2, 14–20.

Poston, H. A., Riis, R. C., Rumsey, G. L. and Ketola, H. G. (1977). Supplementary dietary methionine prevents cataracts in lake trout fed isolated soybean protein. *Fedn Proc. Fedn Am. Soc. exp. Biol.* 36, Abstract 4369, 1098.

Presley, G. D., Stinton, I. N. and Sidbury, J. B. (1969). Ocular defects associated with homocystinuria, *Sth. med. J.* 62, 944–946.

Rabin, A. R., Hayes, K. C. and Berson, E. L. (1973). Cone and rod responses in nutritionally induced retinal degeneration in the cat. *Invest. Ophthal.* 12, 694–704.

Ramsey, M. S., Daitz, L. D. and Beaton, J. W. (1975). Lens fringe in homocystinuria. *Archs Ophthal.* 93, 318.

Rezende, C. and De Moura Campos, F. A. (1942). Cataract in rats fed low-protein diet. *A.M.A. Archs Ophthal.* 28, 1038–1041.

Rich, L. F., Beard, M. E. and Burns, R. P. (1973). Excess dietary tyrosine and corneal lesions. *Expl. Eye Res.* 17, 87–97.

Roy, F. H. and Kelly, M. L. (1973). Maple syrup urine disease. *J. pediat. Ophthal.* 10, 70–3.

Schaeffer, A. J. (1946). Effect of certain amino acids on healing of experimental wounds of the cornea. *Proc. Soc. exp. Biol. Med.* 61, 165–6.

Schaeffer, A. J. (1950). Attempt to influence corneal wound healing by local application of certain amino acids. *Am. J. Ophthal.* 33, 741–750.

Schaeffer, A. J. and Murray, J. D. (1950). Tryptophan determination in cataracts due to deficiency or delayed supplementation of tryptophan. *A.M.A. Archs Ophthal.* 43, 202–216.

Schaeffer, A. J. and Shankman, S. (1950). Amino-acid composition of proteins of ocular tissues. *Am. J. Ophthal.* 33, 1049–1054.

Schmidt, S. Y., Berson, E. L. and Hayes, K. C. (1976). Retinal degeneration in cats fed casein. I. Taurine deficiency. *Invest. Ophthal.* 15, 47–52.

Schweizer, W. (1947). Studies on the effect of L-tyrosine on the white rat. *J. Physiol., Lond.* 106, 167–176.

Scott, P. P., Greaves, J. P. and Scott, M. G. (1964). Nutritional blindness in the cat. *Expl. Eye Res.* 3, 357–364.

Shih, V. E., Berson, E. L., Mandell, R. and Schmidt, S. Y. (1978). Ornithine ketoacid transaminase deficiency in gyrate atrophy of the choroid and retina. *Am. J. hum. Genet.* 30, 174–179.

Simell, O., and Takki, K. (1973). Raised plasma-ornithine and gyrate atrophy of the choroid and retina. *Lancet* i, 1031–1033.

Smith, T. H., Holland, M. G. and Woody, W. C. (1971). Ocular manifestations of familiar hyperlysinemia. *Trans. Am. Acad. Ophthal. Oto-lar.* 75, 355–360.

Sood, N. N. and Gupta, S. (1966). Refractive changes in malnourished children. *Orient. Archs Ophthal.* 4, 264–269.

Sydenstricker, V. P., Hall, W. K., Hock, C. W. and Pund, E. R. (1946). Amino acid and protein deficiencies as causes of corneal vascularization: A preliminary report. *Science, N.Y.* 103, 194–6.

Sydenstricker, V. P., Bowles, L. L., Hall, W. K. and Schmidt, H. L. (1947). The corneal vascularization resulting from deficiencies of amino acids in the rat. *J. Nutr.* 34, 481–490.

Totter, J. R. and Day, P. L. (1942). Cataract and other ocular changes resulting from tryptophan deficiency. *J. Nutr.* 24, 159–166.

Trowell, H. C., Davies, J. N. P. and Dean, R. F. A. (1954). "Kwashiorkor," 249. Arnold, London.

Udupa, K. N., Woessner, J. F. and Dunphy, J. E. (1956). The effect of methionine on the production of mucopolysaccharides and collagen in healing wounds of protein depleted animals. *Surgery Gynec. Obstet.* 102, 639–645.

Uyama, Y., Ogino, S. and Odahara, H. (1956). Biochemical studies on cataract. 4. Relationship between tyrosine metabolism and development of diabetic cataracts. *Med. J. Osaka Univ.* 7, 329–341.

Uyama, Y., Ogino, S. and Yamada, Y. (1955). Biochemical studies on cataract. 2. Relationship between abnormal metabolism of tyrosine and cataract formation. *Med. J. Osaka Univ.* 6, 519–528.

von Sallmann, L., Reid, M. E., Grimes, P. A. and Collins, E. M. (1959). Tryptophan-deficiency cataract in guinea pigs. *A.M.A. Archs Ophthal.* 62, 662–672.

Vozza, R. (1957). Cataract in rats fed on human milk. *Am. J. Ophthal.* 44, 387–393.

Ward, P. J. (1965). Refractive error in the rat. *Proc. Nutr. Soc.* 24, xxxv-vi.

Weekers, R. (1942). Symptômes oculaires de l'oedème de carence. Protéines plasmatiques et ophtalmotonus. *Ophthalmologica* 103, 81–87.

Williamson, M. B. and Fromm, H. J. (1952). Effect of cystine and methionine on healing of experimental wounds. *Proc. Soc. exp. Biol. Med.* 80, 623–626.

Williamson, M. B. and Fromm, H. J. (1955). The incorporation of sulfur amino acids into the proteins of regenerating wound tissue. *J. biol. Chem.* 212, 705–712.

Wilson, R. S. and Ruiz, R. S. (1969). Bilateral central retinal artery occlusion in homocystinuria. *Archs Ophthal.* 82, 267–268.

Wong, V. G., Leitman, P. S. and Seegmiller, J. E. (1967). Alterations of pigmentary epithelium in cystinosis. *Archs Ophthal.* 77, 361–369.

Zaleski, W. A., Hill, A. and Murray, R. G. (1973). Corneal erosions in tyrosinosis. *Can. J. Ophthal.* 8, 556–559.

Zee, D. S., Freeman, J. M. and Holtzman, N. A. (1974). Ophthalmoplegia in maple syrup urine disease. *J. Pediat.* 84, 113–115.

Zivkov, E. and Teoharov, B. (1958). Clinical and pathological aspects of retinal oedema in alimentary dystrophy. *Arkh. Patol.* No. 2, 71–76.

Zuidema, P. J. (1955). Calcification and cirrhosis of pancreas in patients with deficient nutrition. *Documenta Med. geogr. trop.* 7, 229–251.

Chapter 7

Armaly, M. F. (1967). Diabetes mellitus and the eye. II. Intraocular pressure and aqueous outflow facility. *Archs Ophthal.* 77, 493–502.

Armaly, M. F. and Baloglou, P. J. (1967). Diabetes mellitus and the eye. I. Changes in the anterior segment. *Archs Ophthal.* 77, 485–492.

Bailey, C. C., Bailey, O. T. and Leech, R. S. (1944). Alloxan diabetes with diabetic complications. *New Engl. J. Med.* 230, 533–536.

Bankes, J. L. K. (1971). The sparkling vitreous—a sign of diabetes? *Trans. ophthal. Soc. U.K.* 91, 167–172.

Bellows, J. G. (1944). "Cataract and Anomalies of the Lens," 508. Kimpton, London.

Bellows, J. G. and Chinn, H. (1941). Biochemistry of lens: production of lens opacities by injection of hypertonic solutions. *A.M.A. Archs Ophthal.* 25, 796–810.

Beutler, E., Matsumoto, F., Kuhl, W., Krill, A., Levy, N., Sparkes, R. and Degnan, M. (1973). Galactokinase deficiency as a cause of cataract. *New Engl. J. Med.* 288, 1203–6.

Butturini, U., Grignolo, A. and Baronchelli, A. (1953). "Diabete" da ditizone: aspetti metabolici oculair ed istologici. *G. Clin. med.* 34, 1253–1347.

Caird, F. I., Pirie, A. and Ramsell, T. G. (1969). "Diabetes and the Eye." Oxford, Blackwell.

Chacko, C. M., Christian, J. C. and Nadler, H. L. (1971). Unstable galactose-1-phosphate uridyl transferase: A new variant of galactosemia. *J. Pediat.* 78, 454–460.

Chaikoff, I. L. and Lachman, G. S. (1933). Occurrence of cataract in experimental pancreatic diabetes. *Proc. Soc. exp. Biol. Med.* 31, 237–241.

Charalampous, F. C. and Hegsted, D. M. (1950). Effects of age and diet on development of cataracts in the diabetic rat. *Am. J. Physiol.* 161, 540–544.

Cohen, A. M., Michaelson, I. C. and Yanko, L. (1972). Retinopathy in rats with disturbed carbohydrate metabolism following a high sucrose diet. I. Vascular changes. *Am. J. Ophthal.* 73, 863–869.

Craig, J. M. and Maddock, C. E. (1953). Observations on nature of galactose toxicity in rats. *A.M.A. Archs Pathol.* 55, 118–130.

Darby, W. J. and Day, P. L. (1939). Xylose as a cataractogenic agent. *Proc. Soc. exp. Biol. Med.* 41, 507–8.

Darby, W. J. and Day. P. L. (1940). Blood sugar levels in rats receiving the cataractogenic sugars galactose and xylose. *J. biol. Chem.* 133, 503–509.

Dohan, F. C., Fish, C. A. and Lukens, F. D. W. (1941). Induction and course of permanent diabetes produced by anterior pituitary extract. *J. Endocr.* 28, 341–357.

Dvornik, D., Simard-Duquesne, N., Krami, M., Sestanj, K., Gabtay, K. H., Kinoshita, J. H., Varma, S. D. and Merda, L. O. (1973). Polyol accumulation in galactosemic and diabetic rats: Control by an aldose reductase inhibitor. *Science, N.Y.* 182, 1146–1148.

Engerman, R. L. and Bloodworth, J. M. B. Jr (1965). Experimental diabetic retinopathy in dogs. *Archs Ophthal.* 73, 205–210.

Foglia, V. G. and Cramer, F. K. (1944). Experimental production of diabetic cataract in the rat. *Proc. Soc. exp. Biol. Med.* **55**, 218–219.

François, J., Rabaey, M., Wieme, R. J. and Neetens, A. (1954). Étude des protéins cristalliniennes hydrosolubles par l'ectrophorèse dans la cataracte expérimentale. *Annls Oculist. Paris* **187**, 593–610.

Gifford, S. R. and Bellows, J. G. (1939). Histologic changes in lens produced by galactose. *A.M.A. Archs Ophthal.* **21**, 346–358.

Gitzelmann, R., Curtius, H.-C. and Schneller, I. (1967). Galactitol and galactose-1-phosphate in the lens of a galactosaemic infant. *Expl Eye Res.* **6**, 1–3.

Greiner, J. V. and Chylack, L. J. Jr (1976). Anatomy of the experimental "hypoglycemic" cataract in the rat lens. *Ophthal. Res.* **8**, 133–145.

Harley, J. D., Irvine, S., Mutton, P. and Gupta, J. D. (1974). Maternal enzymes of galactose metabolism and the inexplicable infantile cataract. *Lancet* ii, 259–261.

Harris, J. E., Hauschildt, J. D. and Nordquist, L. T. (1954). Lens metabolism as studied with reversible cation shift; role of glucose. *Am. J. Ophthal.* **38**, 141–147.

Hatcher, H. and Andrews, J. S. (1970). Changes in lens fatty acid composition during galactose cataract formation. *Invest. Ophthal.* **9**, 801–806.

Heggeness, F. W. (1960). Calorigenic response to high carbohydrate intake in weanling rats. *Fedn Proc. Fedn Am. Socs exp. Biol.* **19**, 324.

Heggeness, F. W. and Lerman, S. (1960). Relationship between metabolism of xylose and cataractogenesis in the weanling rat. *J. Nutr.* **72**, 309–313.

Hörmann, E. (1954). Uber die Pathogenese des Milchzuckerstats der weissen Ratte. *Albrecht v. Graefes Arch. Ophthal.* **154**, 561–573.

Huggert, A. (1954). The appearance of the crystalline lens during different stages of transitory changes of refraction. Part II. *Acta ophthal.* **32**, 37–47.

Hutton, J. C., Schofield, P. J., Williams, J. F., Regtop, H. L. and Hollows, F. C. (1976). The effect of an unsaturated-fat diet on cataract formation in streptozotocin-induced diabetic rats. *Br. J. Nutr.* **36**, 161–177.

Janes, R. G. and Ellis, P. P. (1957). Vascular changes in eyes of diabetic rats: alterations in the anterior segment. *A.M.A. Archs Ophthal.* **57**, 218–223.

Keen, H. and Smith, R. (1959). Vitamin B_{12} and the course of diabetic retinopathy. *Lancet* i, 849–852.

King, R. C., Dobree, J. H., Kok, D. A., Foulds, W. S. and Dangerfield, W. G. (1963). Exudative diabetic retinopathy: spontaneous changes and effects of a corn oil diet. *Br. J. Ophthal.* **47**, 666–672.

Kinoshita, J. H. (1955). Carbohydrate metabolism of lens. *A.M.A. Archs Ophthal.* **54**, 360–8.

Kinoshita, J. H. (1965). Cataracts in galactosemia. *Invest. Ophthal.* **4**, 786–799.

Kinoshita, J. H., Dvornik, D., Kraml, M. and Gabbay, K. H. (1968). The effect of an aldose inhibitor on the galactose-exposed rabbit lens. *Biochim. Biophys. Acta.* **158**, 472–475.

Kinoshita, J. H., Merola, L. O. and Dikmak, E. (1962). Osmotic changes in experimental galactose cataracts. *Expl. Eye Res.* **1**, 405–410.

Lerman, S. (1959). Enzymatic factors in experimental galactose cataract. *Science, N.Y.* **130**, 1473–4.

Lerman, S. and Heggeness, F. M. (1961). The metabolism of xylose by the ocular lens of the rat. *Biochem. J.* **79**, 224–229.

Levy, N. S., Krill, A. E. and Beutler, E. (1972). Galactokinase deficiency and cataracts. *Am. J. Ophthal.* 74, 41–48.

Lou, M. F. and Kinoshita, J. H. (1967). Cataract of lens glycolysis. *Biochem. biophys. Acta* 141, 547–549.

Lundbaek, K., Christensen, N. J., Jensen, V. A., Johansen, K., Olsen, T. S., Hansen, A. P., Ørskov, H. and Østerby, R. (1970). Diabetes, diabetic angiopathy and growth hormone. *Lancet* ii, 131–133.

McDaniel, E. G., Hundley, J. M. and Sebrell, W. H. Jr (1956). Tryptophan-niacin metabolism in alloxan diabetic rats. *J. Nutr.* 59, 407–423.

McKinna, A. J. (1966). Neonatal hypoglycaemia—some ophthalmic observations. *Can. J. Ophthal.* i, 56–59.

McLaren, D. S. (1963). "Malnutrition and the Eye." 272–3, Academic Press, London, New York.

Merril, C. R., Geier, M. R. and Petricciani, J. C. (1971). Bacterial virus gene expression in human cells. *Nature, Lond.* 233, 398.

Mesropian, E. I. (1970). Anterior segment lesions in diabetes mellitus. *Oftal. Zh.* 24, 598–601.

Mitchell, H. S. (1935). Cataract in rats fed on galactose. *Proc. Soc. exp. Biol. Med.* 32, 971–973.

Mitchell, H. S. and Cook, G. M. (1937). Influence of protein or cystine intake on cataract-producing action of galactose. *Proc. Soc. exp. Biol. Med.* 36, 806–808.

Mitchell, H. S. and Dodge, W. M. (1935). Cataract in rats fed on high lactose rations. *J. Nutr.* 9, 37–49.

Mitchell, S. W. (1860). On the production of cataract in pigs by the administration of sugar. *Am. J. med. Sci. N. S.* 39, 67.

Obazawa, H., Merola, L. O. and Kinoshita, J. H. (1974). The effects of xylose on the isolated lens. *Invest. Ophthal.* 13, 204–9.

O'Brien, C. S., Molsberry, J. M. and Allen, J. H. (1934). Diabetic cataract; incidence and morphology in 126 young diabetic patients. *J. Am. med. Ass.* 103, 892–897.

Patterson, J. W. (1952). Development of diabetic cataracts. *Am. J. Ophthal.* 35, 68–72.

Patterson, J. W. (1953). Cataracts caused by carbohydrates. *Am. J. Ophthal.* 36, 143–9.

Patterson, J. W. (1955). Cataractogenic sugars. *Archs Biochem. Biophys.* 58, 24–30.

Patterson, J. W. and Bunting, K. W. (1965). Changes associated with the appearance of mature sugar cataracts. *Invest. Ophthal.* 4, 167–173.

Patterson, J. W. and Patterson, M. E. (1965). Point of irreversibility of galactose cataracts in the rat. *Proc. Soc. exp. Biol. Med.* 118, 324–6.

Patz, A. (1953). Cataracts in galactosemia: observations in three cases. *Am. J. Ophthal.* 36, 453–462.

Pirie, A. and Van Heyningen, R. (1956). "Biochemistry of the Eye," 103. Blackwell, Oxford.

Roderiguez, R. R. and Krehl, W. A. (1951). The influence of diet and insulin on the incidence of cataracts in diabetic rats. *Yale J. Biol. Med.* 24, 103–108.

Safir, A. and Rogers, S. H. (1970). Ocular effects of juvenile-onset diabetes. *Am. J. Ophthal.* 69, 387–392.

Schwartz, D. E. (1974). Corneal sensitivity in diabetics. *Archs Ophthal.* 91, 174–8.

Schwarz, V. and Golberg, L. (1955). Galactose-1-phosphate in galactose cataract. *Biochim. biophys. Acta* 18, 310–1.

Sibay, T. M. and Hausler, H. R. (1967). Eye findings in two spontaneously diabetic related dogs. *Am. J. Ophthal.* 63, 289–294.

Smith, M. E. and Glickman, P. (1975). Diabetic vacuolation of the iris pigment epithelium. *Am. J. Ophthal.* 79, 875–877.

Stephens, T., Irvine, S., Mutton, P., Gupta, J. D. and Harley, J. D. (1974). The case of the cataractous kangaroo. *Med. J. Aust.* ii, 910–911.

Sterling, R. E. and Day. P. L. (1951). Blood sugar levels and cataract in alloxan-treated, galactose-fed and xylose-fed weanling rats. *Proc. Soc. exp. Biol. Med.* 78, 431–433.

Van Heyningen, R. (1958). Metabolism of xylose by the lens: calf lens *in vitro*. *Biochem. J.* 69, 481–491.

Van Heyningen, R. (1959a). Metabolism of xylose by the lens. 2. Rat lens *in vivo* and *in vitro*. *Biochem. J.* 73, 197–207.

Van Heyningen, R. (1959b). Formation of polyols by the lens of the rat with "sugar" cataract. *Nature, Lond.* 184, 194–195.

Van Heyningen, R. (1962). The sorbitol pathway in the lens. *Expl Eye Res.* 1, 396–404.

Van Heyningen, R. (1969). Xylose cataract: a comparison between the weanling and the older rat. *Expl Eye Res.* 8, 379–385.

Vannas, A., Hogan, M. J., Golbus, M. S. and Wood, I. (1975). Lens changes in a galactosemic fetus. *Am. J. Ophthal.* 80, 726–733.

Vere, D. W. and Verel, D. (1955). Relation between blood sugar level and the optical properties of the lens of the human eye. *Clin. Sci.* 14, 183–196.

Von Sallmann, L., Caravaggio, L., Grimes, P. añd Collins, E. M. (1958). Morphological study on alloxan-induced cataract. *A.M.A. Archs Ophthal.* 59, 55–67.

Wilson, W. A. (1970). Ocular findings in ketotic hypoglycaemia. *Trans. Am. Ophthal. Soc.* 67, 355–368.

Yanko, L., Michaelson, I. C. and Cohen, A. M. (1972a). Retinopathy in rats with disturbed carbohydrate metabolism following a high sucrose diet. 2. Neural changes. *Am. J. Ophthal.* 73, 870–875.

Yanko, L., Michaelson, I. C. and Cohen, A. M. (1972b). The retinopathy of sucrose-fed rats. *Israel J. med. Sci.* 8, 1632–6.

Chapter 8

Anderson, R. E. and Maude, M. B. (1972). Lipids of ocular tissues. VIII. The effects of essential fatty acid deficiency on the phospholipids of the photoreceptor membrane of the rat retina. *Archs Biochem.* 151, 270–277.

Anderson, R. E., Landis, D. J. and Dudley, P. A. (1976). Essential fatty acid deficiency and renewal of rod outer segments in the albino rat. *Invest. Ophthal.* 15, 232–236.

Baum, J. L., Tannenbaum, M. and Kolodny, E. H. (1965). Refsum's syndrome with corneal involvement. *Am. J. Ophthal.* 60, 699–708.

Berman, E. R. (1974). Biochemical diagnostic tests in genetic and metabolic eye diseases. *In* "Genetic and Metabolic Eye Diseases" (Ed. B. Goldberg). Little Brown, Boston.

Bolmers, D. J. M. (1975). Ocular anomalies in the types of Fredrickson. *Ophthalmologica* 171, 86–90.

Bron, A. J. and Williams, H. P. (1972). Lipaemia of the limbal vessels. *Br. J. Ophthal.* 56, 543–546.

Charalampous, F. C. and Hegsted, D. M. (1950). Effects of age and diet on development of cataracts in the diabetic rat. *Am. J. Physiol.* 161, 540–544.

Cogan, D. G. and Kuwabara, T. (1955). *XVII Conc. Ophthal. (1954; Canada, U.S.) Acta* 1, 523.

Cogan, D. G. and Kuwabara, T. (1959a). Ocular changes in experimental hypercholesterolemia. *A.M.A. Archs Ophthal.* 61, 219–225.

Cogan, D. G. and Kuwabara, T. (1959b). Arcus senilis. *A.M.A. Archs Ophthal.* 61, 553–560.

Connor, W. E. and Connor, S. L. (1972). The key role of nutritional factors in the prevention of coronary heart disease. *Prev. Med.* i, 49–83.

Dudley, P. A., Landis, D. J. and Anderson, R. E. (1975). Further studies on the chemistry of photoreceptor membranes of rats fed an essential fatty acid deficient diet. *Expl Eye Res.* 21, 523–530.

Finley, J. K., Berkowitz, D. and Croll, M. N. (1961). The physiological significance of gerontoxon. *Archs Ophthal.* 66, 211–23.

Forrest, G. L. and Futterman, S. (1972). Age-related changes in the retinal capillaries and the fatty-acid composition of retinal tissue of normal and essential fatty-acid-deficient rats. *Invest. Ophthal.* 11, 760–764.

Forsius, H. (1954). Arcus senilis cornae; its clinical development and relationship to serus lipids, proteins and lipoproteins. *Acta Ophthal.* Suppl. No. 42, 1–78.

Fredrickson, D. S., Goldstein, J. L. and Brown, M. S. (1978). The familial hyperlipoproteinaemias. *In* "The Metabolic Basis of Inherited Disease," 4th edn (Eds J. S. Stanbury, J. B. Wyngaarden and D. S. Fredrickson), 604–655. McGraw-Hill, New York.

Friedman, M. and Rosenman, R. H. (1959). Association of specific overt behavior pattern with blood and cardiovascular findings: blood cholesterol level, blood clotting time, incidence of arcus senilis and clinical coronary artery disease. *J. Am. med. Ass.* 169, 1286–1296.

Futterman, S., Rollins, M. H. and Vacano, E. (1968). The effect of alloxan diabetes on polyenoic fatty acid synthesis by retinal tissue. *Biochem. biophys. Acta* 164, 433–434.

Gouras, P., Carr, R. E. and Gunkel, R. D. (1971). Retinitis pigmentosa in abetalipoproteinemia: effects of vitamin A. *Invest. Ophthal.* 10, 784–793.

Hands, A. R., Sutherland, N. S. and Bartley, W. (1965). Visual acuity of essential fatty acid-deficient rats. *Biochem. J.* 94, 279–283.

Hollenhorst, R. W. (1961). Significance of bright plaques in the retinal arterioles. *J. Am. med. Ass.* 178, 23–29.

Hollenhorst, R. W. (1966). Vascular status of patients who have cholesterol emboli in the retina. *Am. J. Ophthal.* 61, 1159–1165.

Jampel, R. S. and Falls, H. F. (1958). Atypical retinitis pigmentosa, acanthocytosis and heredodegenerative neuromuscular disease. *Archs. Ophthal.* 59, 818–820.

Janes, R. G. (1964). Changes in the rabbit's eye caused by cholesterol feeding. *Am. J. Ophthal.* 58, 819–828.

Kaunitz, H., Wiesinger, H., Blodi, F. C., Johnson, R. E. and Slanetz, C. A. (1954). Relation of protein and fat intake to growth and corneal vascularization in galactoflavin-produced ariboflavinosis. *J. Nutr.* 52, 467–482.

Khachadurian, A. K., Freyha, R., Shamma'a, M M. and Baghdassarian, S. A. (1971). Abetalipoproteinaemia and colour-blindness. *Archs Dis. Childh.* 46, 871–873.

Kurz, G. H., Shakib, M., Sohmer, K. K. and Friedman, A. H. (1976). The retina in type 5 hyperlipoproteinaemia. *Am. J. Ophthal.* 82, 32–43.

Laughlin, R. C. (1962). Cataracts in patients treated with triparanol. *J. Am. med. Ass.* 181, 339–340.

Light, A. E., Solomon, C. and De Beer, E. J. (1956). Effects of dietary supplements in preventing or augmenting the production of cataracts in rats by 1,4-dimethane-sulphonoxybutane. *J. Nutr.* 60, 157–172.

Lijo Pavia, J. (1954). Fondo de ojo en la hipercolesterolemia experimental. *Revta ass. méd. argent.* 68, 9–13.

Macaraeg, P. V. J. Jr, Lasagna, L. and Snyder, B. (1968). Arcus not so senilis. *Int. Med.* 68, 345–354.

Muller, D. P. R., Lloyd, J. K., and Bird, A. C. (1977). Long term management of abetalipoproteinaemia. *Archs Dis. Childh.* 52, 209–214.

Nieman, C. (1955). Influence of dietary fat on incidence of alloxan diabetes in growing rats. *Am. J. Physiol.* 181, 183–186.

Pirie, A., and van Heyningen, R. (1956). "Biochemistry of the Eye," 26, 151, 226. Blackwell, Oxford.

Rifkind, B. M. (1972). Corneal arcus and hyperlipoproteinemia. *Surv. Ophthal.* 16, 295–304.

Roderiguez, R. R. and Krehl, W. A. (1951). The influence of diet and insulin on the incidence of cataracts in diabetic rats. *Yale J. Biol. Med.* 24, 103–108.

Rubenstein, R. A., Whereat, A. F. and Nazarian, I. (1967). Effect of hypercholesterolemia on the eye and on aortic transplants in the anterior chamber. *Am. J. Ophthal.* 63, 972–978.

Russell-Ross, R. W. (1963). Atheromatous retinal embolism. *Lancet* ii, 1354–1356.

Samochowiec, L. (1976). On the action of essential phospholipids in experimental atherosclerosis. *In* "Phosphatidyl-choline" (Ed. H. Peeters), 211–216. Springer, Berlin.

Sperling, M. A., Hiles, D. A. and Kennerdell, J. S. (1972). Electroretinographic responses following vitamin A therapy in abetalipoproteinemia. *Am. J. Ophthal.* **73**, 342–351.

Steinberg, D. (1978). Phytanic acid storage disease: Refsum's syndrome. *In* "The Metabolic Basis of Inherited Disease, 4th edn (Eds J. B. Stanbury, J. B. Wyngaarden and D. S. Fredrickson). McGraw-Hill, New York.

Suga, J. (1960). Experimental cholesterol arteriosclerosis in rabbits. *Acta Soc. ophthal. Japan* **64**, 1980–1989.

Toussaint, D. and Danis, P. (1971). An ocular pathologic study of Refsum's syndrome. *Am. J. Ophthal.* **72**, 342–347.

Vinger, P. F. and Sachs, B. A. (1970). Ocular manifestations of hyperlipoproteinaemia. *Am. J. Ophthal.* **70**, 563–573.

von Sallmann, L., Gelderman, A. H. and Laster, L. (1969). Ocular histopathologic changes in a case of abetalipoproteinemia. *Doc. Ophthal.* **26**, 451–460.

Wheeler, T. G., Benolken, R. N. and Anderson, R. E. (1975). Visual membranes: specificity of fatty acid precursors for the electrical response to illumination. *Science, N.Y.* **188**, 1312–1314.

Wyman, M. and McKissick, G. E. (1973). Lipemia retinalis in a dog and cat: case repots. *J. Am. anim. Hosp. Ass.* **9**, 288–291.

Yee, R. D., Cogan, D. G. and Zee, D. S. (1976a). Ophthalmoplegia and dissociated nystagmus in abetalipoproteinaemia. *Archs Ophthal.* **94**, 571–5.

Yee, R. D., Herbert, P. N., Bergsma, D. R. and Biemer, J. J. (1976b). Atypical retinitis pigmentosa in familial hypobetalipoproteinemia. *Am. J. Ophthal.* **82**, 64–71.

Chapter 9

Alden, E. R., Kalina, R. E. and Hodson, W. A. (1973). Transient cataracts in low-birth-weight infants. *J. Pediat.* **82**, 314–318.

Aterman, K. (1952). Some local factors in the restoration of the rat's liver after partial hepatectomy. *A.M.A. Archs Pathol.* **53**, 197–208.

Bannon, S. L., Higginbottom, R. M., McConnell, J. M. and Kaan, H. W. (1945). Development of galactose cataract in the albino rat embryo. *A.M.A. Archs Ophthal.* **33**, 224–228.

Blamberg, D. L., Blackwood, U. B., Supplee, W. C. and Combs, G. F. (1960). Effect of zinc deficiency in hens on hatchability and embryonic development. *Proc. Soc. exp. Biol. Med.* **104**, 217–220.

Brinsmade, A. B. (1957). Developmental disorders in rabbit embryo after glucose deficiency in mother during pregnancy. *Beitr. path. Anat.* **117**, 140–153.

Callison, E. C. and Orent-Keiles, E. (1951). Abnormalities of the eye occurring in young vitamin E-deficient rats. *Proc. Soc. exp. Biol. Med.* **76**, 295–297.

Chamberlain, J. G. and Nelson, M. M. (1962). Effects of the niacin antimetabolite, 6-amino-nicotinamide, during pregnancy in the Long-Evans rat. (Demonstration). *Anat. Rec.* **142**, 337.

Cheng, D. W., Chang, L. F. and Bairnson, T. A. (1957). Gross observations on developing abnormal embryos induced by maternal vitamin E deficiency. *Anat. Rec.* 129, 167–185.

Chernoff, G. F. (1975). A mouse model of the fetal alcohol syndrome. *Teratology* 2, 14A.

Cohlan, S. Q. (1953). Excessive intake of vitamin A as a cause of congenital anomalies in the rat. *Science, N.Y.* 117, 535–536.

Curtiss, C. (1953). Effects of a low protein intake on the pregnant rat. *Metabolism* 2, 344–353.

Dann, M., Levine, S. L. and New, E. V. (1964). A long-term follow-up study of small premature infants. *Pediatrics* 33, 945–955.

de Meyer, R. (1959). Action tératogène du galactose administré à la rate gravide. *Annls Endocr.* 20, 203–211.

Duncan, J. P. and Hurley, L. S. (1978). An interaction between zinc and vitamin A in pregnant and fetal rats. *J. Nutr.* 108, 1431–1438.

Eames, T. H. (1964). Comparison of the eye conditions of hypermature, premature and full-term schoolchildren. *Eye Ear Nose Throat Mon.* 43, 36–41.

Elchlepp, J. G. (1956). Development of the chick eye: relation of ground substance change to organ growth. *Anat. Rec.* 126, 425–432.

Ferguson, T. M. and Couch, J. R. (1954). Further gross observations on the B_{12}-deficient chick embryo. *J. Nutr.* 54, 361–370.

Ferguson, T. M., Rigdon, R. H. and Couch, J. R. (1956). Cataracts in vitamin E deficiency: an experimental study in the turkey embryo. *A.M.A. Archs Ophthal.* 55, 346–355.

Fledelius, H. (1976). Prematurity and the eye. Ophthalmic 10-year follow-up of children of low and normal birth weight. *Acta Ophthal.* Suppl. 128, 245.

Fletcher, M. C. and Brandon, S. (1955). Myopia of prematurity. *Am. J. Ophthal.* 40, 474–481.

Fujino, J., Tsuruhara, T., Akena, G., Fukui, T., Isono, H. and Kono, J. (1959). Experimental studies on the malformations in newborn rats due to strontium salt. *J. Osaka Cy med. Cent.* 8, 1729–1733.

Gerhard, J. P. (1974). The lens of the premature infant. *J. Med. Strasbourg* 5, 147–9

Gersh, I. and Catchpole, H. R. (1949). The organization of ground substance and basement membrane and its significance in tissue injury, disease and growth. *Am. J. Anat.* 85, 457–521.

Giroud, A. (1959). The nutritional requirements of embryos and the repercussions of deficiencies. *Wld Rev. Nutr. Dietet.* 1, 229–263.

Giroud, A. and Boisselot, J. (1947). Répercussions de l'avitaminose B_2 sur l'embryon du rat. *Archs fr. Pédiat.* 4, 317–327.

Giroud, A. and Martinet, M. (1955). Hypervitaminose "A" et anomalies chez le foetus de rat. *Int. Z. Vitaminforsch.* 26, 10–18.

Giroud, A. and Martinet, M. (1959). Ocular malformations with fibrosis of the vitreous body in rabbit embryos subjected to hypervitaminosis A. *Bull. Soc. ophthal.* 72, 191–201.

Goldberg, I. D., Goldstein, H., Quade, D. and Rogot, E. (1967). Association of perinatal factors with blindness in children. *Publ. Hlth Rep.* 82, 519–531.

Graham, M. V. and Gray, O. P. (1963). Refraction of premature babies' eyes. *Br. med. J.* i, 1452–1454.

Grainger, R. B., O'Dell, B. L. and Hogan, A. G. (1954). Congenital malformations as related to deficiencies of riboflavin and vitamin B_{12}, source of protein, calcium to phosphorus ratio and skeletal phosphorus metabolism. *J. Nutr.* 54, 33–48.

Grau, C. R., Austic, R. E. and Matteson, G. C. (1965). Degeneration of the eyes of tyrosine-deficient chick embryos. *Science, N.Y.* 148, 1743–1765.

Grignolo, A. and Rivara, A. (1968). Observations biométriques sur l'oeil des enfants nés à terme et des prématures au cours de la première année. *Annls Oculist. Paris* 201, 817–826.

Gruenwald, P. (1958). Malformations caused by necrosis in the embryo: illustrated by the effect of selenium compounds on chick embryos. *Am. J. Path.* 34, 77–103.

Grunëberg, H. (1943). "The Genetics of the Mouse." Cambridge University Press.

Guilbert, H. R., and Goss, H. (1932). Some effects of restricted protein intake on the estrous cycle and gestation in the rat. *J. Nutr.* 5, 251–265.

Hale, F. J. (1935). Relation of vitamin A to anophthalmos in pigs. *Am. J. Ophthal.* 18, 1087–1093.

Härtel, A. and Härtel, G. (1960). Experimental study of teratogenic effect of emotional stress in rats. *Science, N.Y.* 132, 1483–1484.

Hosaka, A. (1963). The ocular findings in premature infants, especially on the premature signs. *Jap. J. Ophthal.* 7, 77–81.

Hurley, L. S. and Swenerton, H. (1966). Congenital malformations resulting from zinc deficiency in rats. *Proc. Soc. exp. Biol. Med.* 123, 692–696.

Jones, K. L., Smith, D. W., Ulleland, C. N. and Streissguth, P. (1973). Pattern of malformation in offspring of chronic alcoholic mothers. *Lancet* i, 1267–1271.

Kalter, H. (1964). Teratogenetically induced congenital aphakia. *Expl Eye Res.* 3, 228–9.

Kochhar, D. M. (1967). Teratogenic activity of retinoic acid. *Acta path. microbiol. scand.* 70, 398–454.

Kuck, J. Jr. (1961). The formation of fructose in the ocular lens. *A.M.A. Archs Ophthal.* 65, 840–846.

Lamba, P. A. and Sood, N. N. (1968). Congenital primary aphakia with retinal dysplasia and heart defect. *J. All-India Ophthal. Soc.* 16, 29–31.

Lamming, G. E., Salisbury, G. W., Hays, R. L. and Kendall, K. A. (1954). The effect of incipient vitamin A deficiency on reproduction in the rabbit. II. Embryonic and fetal development. *J. Nutr.* 52, 227–239.

Langman, J. and van Faassen, F. (1955). Congenital defects in rat embryo after partial-thyroidectomy of mother animal: preliminary report on eye defects. *Am. J. Ophthal.* 40, 65–76.

Lefebvres-Boisselot, J. (1951). Role tératogène de la déficience en acide pantothénique chez le rat. *Annls méd.* 52, 225–298.

Lefebvres-Boisselot, J. (1965). Teratogenic character of pantothenic acid deficiency and conditions in which an antivitamin, sodium DL-ω-methylpantothenate, is effective. *Archs Sci. Physiol.* 19, 223–230.

Lepkovsky, S. and Borson, H. J. (1955). Nutrition and nutritional disease. *Ann. Rev. Med.* 6, 93–124.

Lepkovsky, S., Borson, H. J., Bouthilet, R., Pencharz, R., Singman, D., Dimick,

M. K. and Robbins, R. (1951). Reproduction in vitamin B_{12}-deficient rats with emphasis upon intrauterine injury. *Am. J. Physiol.* 165, 79–86.

Luckhaus, G. and Machemer, L. (1978). Histological examinations of perinatal eye development in the rat after injection of sodium cyclamate and sodium saccharin during pregnancy. *Fd Cosmet. Toxicol.* 16, 7–8.

McCormick, A. Q. (1968). Transient cataract in premature infants. A new clinical entity. *Can. J. Ophthal.* 3, 202–6.

McDonald, A. D. (1962). Neurological and ophthalmic disorders in children of very low birth weight. *Br. med. J.* i, 895–900.

McDonald, A. D. (1964). Cataract in children of very low birth weight. *Guy's Hosp. Rep.* 113, 296–304.

McLaren, D. S. (1960). The effects of malnutrition on the eye: with special reference to work with experimental animals. *Wld Rev. Nutr. Dietet.* 2, 25–51.

Millen, J. W. and Woollam, D. H. M. (1957). Influence of cortisone on teratogenic effects of hypervitaminosis-A. *Br. med. J.* ii, 196–7.

Millen, J. W. and Woollam, D. H. M. (1958). Effect of vitamin B complex on the teratogenic activity of hypervitaminosis A. *Nature, Lond.* 182, 940.

Millen, J. W., Woollam, D. H. M., and Lamming, G. E. (1953). Hydrocephalus associated with deficiency of vitamin A. *Lancet* ii, 1234–1236.

Moore, L. A., Billinger, I., Miller, M. N. and Hellman, L. M. (1942). Abortion in rabbits fed vitamin K deficient diet. *Am. J. Obstet. Gynec.* 43, 1007–1012.

Nelson, M. M. and Evans, H. M. (1953). Relation of dietary protein levels to reproduction in the rat. *J. Nutr.* 51, 71–84.

Nelson, M. M., Wright, H. V., Asling, C. W. and Evans, H. M. (1955). Multiple congenital abnormalities resulting from transitory deficiency of pteroylglutamic acid during gestation in the rat. *J. Nutr.* 56, 349–369.

Nelson, M. M., Baird, C. D. C., Wright, H. V. and Evans, H. M. (1956). Multiple congenital abnormalities in the rat resulting from riboflavin deficiency induced by the antimetabolite galactoflavin. *J. Nutr.* 58, 125–134.

O'Dell, B. L., Hardwick, B. C. and Reynolds, G. (1961). Mineral deficiencies of milk and congenital malformations in the rat. *J. Nutr.* 73, 151–7.

O'Toole, B. A., Fradkin, R., Warkany, J., Wilson, J. G. and Gann, G. V. (1974). Vitamin A deficiency and reproduction in rhesus monkeys. *J. Nutr.* 104, 1513–1524.

Palludan, B. (1966). "A-avitaminosis in swine. A Treatise on the Importance of Vitamin A for Reproduction." Munksgaard, Copenhagen.

Pearson, P. B., Hart, E. B. and Bohstedt, G. (1937). The effect of the quality of protein on the oestrous cycle. *J. Nutr.* 14, 329–339.

Pelagalli, G. V. (1963). Cristalino ed ipervitaminosi A. Ricerche in embrioni di pollo. *Boll. Soc. ital. Biol. sper.* 39, 1626–1628.

Permutt, S. and Johnson, F. B. (1953). Histochemical studies on the lens following radiation injury. *A.M.A. Archs Pathol.* 55, 20–30.

Pike, R. L. (1951). Congenital cataract in albino rat fed different amounts of tryptophan and niacin. *J. Nutr.* 44, 191–204.

Pilman, N. I. and Weinbaum, D. S. (1974). Congenital ocular defects in premature infants. *Oftal. Zh.* 29, 346–348.

Potier de Courcy, G. (1966). Caractères globaux des metabolismes nucleique et proteique chez le foetus de rat carancé en acide pantothénique. *Archs Sci. Physiol.* 20, 43–63.

Ransdell, J. F. (1956). Eye abnormalities in vitamin B_{12}-deficient rats. *Int. Z. Vitaminforsch.* 26, 412–413.

Reif-Lehrer, L., Bergenthal, J. and Hanninen, L. (1975). Effects of monosodium glutamate on chick embryo retina in culture. *Invest. Ophthal.* 14, 114–124.

Richter, C. P. and Duke, J. R. (1970). Cataracts produced in rats by yogurt. *Science, N.Y.* 168, 1372–1374.

Rivara, A. and Gemme, G. (1965). Misurazione dell'asse oculare autero-postenore e del potere diottrico oculare vei prematuri. *Annali Ottal. Clin. Ocul.* 91, 1328–1334.

Rivara, A. and Gemme, G. (1966). Miopia degli immaturi. Valutazione della refrazione oculare in rapporto alla prematurita all'eta al peso e all'ossigenoteropsia. *AHi XLIX Cay. Soc. Oftal. Iral. Mrg.* 23, 395–404.

Sarma, V. (1959). Maternal vitamin A deficiency and fetal microcephaly and anophthalmia. *Obstet. Gynec.* 13, 299–301.

Šeba, J. (1974). Ophthalmological findings in newborn children. Part 3. Premature births. *Čslká Oftal.* 30, 55–58.

Smithells, R. W. (1976). Environmental teratogens of man. *Br. med. Bull.* 32, 27–33.

Tabuchi, A., and Yamamoto, M. (1974). Clinical follow-up of refractive errors in premature infants. *Folia Ophthal. Jap.* 25, 256–263.

Waddington, C. H. and Perry, M. (1958). Effects of some amino-acid and purine antagonists on chick embryos. *J. Embryol. exp. Morph.* 6, 365–372.

Warkany, J. (1945). Manifestations of prenatal nutritional deficiency. *Vitams Horm.* 3, 73–103.

Warkany, J. (1954). Disturbance of embryonic development by maternal vitamin deficiencies. *J. cell. comp. Physiol.* 43, Suppl. 1, 207–236.

Warkany, J. and Schraffenberger, E. (1946). Congential malformations induced in rats by maternal vitamin A deficiency. I. Defects of the eye. *A.M.A. Archs Ophthal.* 35, 150–169.

Warkany, J., Beaudry, P. H. and Hornstein, S. (1959). Attempted abortion with aminopterin (4-amino-pteroylglutamic-acid); malformations of the child. *Am. J. Dis. Child.* 97, 274–281.

Chapter 10

Anderson, D. E., Pope, L. S. and Stephens, D. (1970). Nutrition and eye cancer in cattle. *J. natn. Cancer Inst.* 45, 697–707.

Anon (1969). Thiamine deficiency in ruminants? *Nutr. Abstr. Rev.* 27, 176–178.

Barger, G. (1931). "Ergot and Ergotism." Oxford Med. Publs, London.

Barnett, K. C. and Watson, W. A. (1970). Bright blindness in sheep. A primary retinopathy due to feeding bracken (*Pteris aquilina*). *Res. vet. Sci.* 11, 289–291.

Baron, J. B. (1972). Effects of alcoholic intoxication on the eye. *Semaine Hôp.* 48, 705–708.

Bellows, J. G. (1944). "Cataract and Anomalies of the Lens," 362. Kimpton, London.

Berggren, L. (1957). Lack of effect of citral on ocular tension. *Acta Ophthal.* 35, 451–453.

Čavka, V. (1963). New ophthalmological symptoms in cirrhosis of the liver (in Serbo-Croat). *Jugoslav. Oftal. Arh.* 1, 5–44.

Chopra, R. N., Pasricha, C. L., Goyal, R. K., Lal, S. and Sen, A. K. (1939). Experimental production of syndrome of epidemic dropsy in man. *Indian med. Gaz.* 74, 193–195.

Choremis, C., Joannides, T. and Kyriakides, B. (1960). Severe ophthalmic complications following favism. *Br. J. Ophthal.* 44, 353–356.

Cruz-Coke, R. (1965). Colour-blindness and cirrhosis. *Lancet* i, 1131–1133.

Dobbie, G. C. and Langham, M. E. (1961). Reaction of animal eyes to sanguinarine and argemone oil. *Br. J. Ophthal.* 45, 81–95.

Duke-Elder, W. S. (1954). "Textbook of Ophthalmology," Vol. 6, p. 6186, 6856 Mosby, St Louis, Missouri.

Dutt, S. C. (1950). *XVI Conc. Ophthal. Br. Acta* 2, 872.

Fialkow, P. J., Thuline, H. C. and Fenster, F. (1966). Lack of association between cirrhosis and the common types of colour blindness. *New Engl. J. Med.* 275, 584–587.

Flecker, (1944). Sudden blindness after eating "finger cherries" (*Rhodomyrtus macrocarpa*). *Med. J. Aust.* 2, 183–185.

Garner, A. (1974). Retinal oxalosis. *Br. J. Ophthal.* 58, 613–619.

Hakim, S. A. E. (1954). Argemone oil, sanguinarine and epidemic-dropsy glaucoma. *Br. J. Ophthal.* 38, 193–216.

Hakim, S. A. E. (1957). Poppy alkaloids and glaucoma. *J. Physiol., Lond.* 138, 40–41P.

Hart, L. (1941). The toxicity of seeds of argemone mexicana for fowls. *Aust. vet. J.* 17, 69–71.

Kaunitz, J. (1932). Chronic endemic ergotism; its relation to thrombo-angiitis obliterans. *A.M.A. Archs Surg.* 25, 1135–1151.

Kirwan, E. W. O'G. (1934). Primary glaucoma; symptom complex of epidemic dropsy. *A.M.A. Archs Ophthal.* 12, 1–20.

Kirwan, E. W. O'G. (1935). Ocular complications of epidemic dropsy. *Indian med. Gaz.* 70, 485–9.

Kirwan, E. W. O'G. (1936). Aetiology of chronic primary glaucoma. *Br. J. Ophthal.* 20, 321–331.

Lal, R. B. and Roy, S. C. (1937). Investigations into epidemiology of epidemic dropsy; experiments to test validity of infection theory in semi-isolated community. *Indian J. med. Res.* 25, 233–238.

Lal, R. B., Das Gupta, A. C., Mukherji, S. P. and Adak, B. (1941). Investigations into epidemiology of epidemic dropsy; feeding experiments on human subjects to test toxicity of some of the derivatives and modifications of argemone oil. *Indian J. med. Res.* 29, 839–849.

Lal, R. B., Mukherji, S. P., Das Gupta, A. C., and Chatterji, S. R. (1940). Investigations into epidemiology of epidemic dropsy; quantitative aspects of problem of toxicity of mustard oil. *Indian J. med. Res.* 28, 163–196.

Leach, E. H. (1955). Ocular changes in monkeys fed with sanguinarine and other substances. *Trans. ophthal. Soc. U.K.* 75, 425–430.

Leach, E. H. and Lloyd, J. P. (1956). Experimental ocular hypertension in animals. *Trans. ophthal. Soc. U.K.* 76, 453–460.

Levett, J. and Karras, L. (1977). Effects of alcohol on human accommodation. *Aviation space environ. Med.* 48, 434–437.

Lieb, W. A. and Scherf, H.-J. (1956). Papaversieae-Alkaloide und Augendruck. *Klin. Mbl. Augenheilk.* 128, 686–705.

Maynard, F. P. (1909). Preliminary note on increased intraocular tension met with in cases of epidemic dropsy. *Indian med. Gaz.* 44, 373.

Meier, I. (1862). *Albrecht v. Graefes Arch. Ophthal.* 8, Pt. 2, 120.

Newman, H. and Fletcher, E. (1941). The effect of alcohol on vision. *Am. J. med. Sci.* 202, 723–731.

Peters, A. (1902). Uber Veränderungen an den Ciliarepithelien bei Naphthalin- und Ergotininvergiftung. *Ber. d. Versamm. ophthal. Gés.* 30, 20–25.

Rapidis, P., Andreanos, D. and Krystallis, A. (1975). Uveal manifestations of chronic alcoholism. (In Greek). *Archs Soc. Ophthal. Grèce Nord* 22, 398–406.

Rodger, F. C., Grover, A. D. and Saiduzzafar, H. (1960a). The effect of citral on intra-ocular dynamics in monkeys. *A.M.A. Archs Ophthal.* 63, 77–83.

Rodger, F. C., Saiduzzafar, H. and Grover, A. D. (1960b). The effect of citral and vitamin A on the intra-ocular dynamics of rabbits. *Am. J. Ophthal.* 50, 309–313.

Rosen, E. S., Edgar, J. T. and Smith, J. L. S. (1969). Male fern retrobulbar neuropathy in cattle. *Trans. ophthal. Soc. U.K.* 89, 285–299.

Ross, M. and Bras, G. (1965). Tumour incidence patterns and nutrition in the rat. *J. Nutr.* 87, 245–260.

Rothstein, T. B., Shapiro, M. W. Sacks, J. G. and Weis, M. J. (1973). Dyschromatopsia with hepatic cirrhosis: relation to serum B_{12} and folic acid. *Am. J. Ophthal.* 75, 889–895.

Scott, J. G. (1962). Does ergot cause cataract? *Med. Proc.* 8, 4–8.

Summerskill, W. H. J. and Molnar, G. D. (1962). Eye signs in hepatic cirrhosis. *New Engl. J. Med.* 226, 1244–1248.

Timm, G. (1963). Oxalose und Auge. *Ophthalmologica* 146, 1–8.

Travinskaya, M. A. and Shtilman, E. A. (1973). Visual field and colour perception changes in patients with chronic alcoholism. *Oftal. Zh.* 28, 83–6.

Van Kampen, K. R. and James, L. F. (1971). Ophthalmic lesions in locoweed poisoning of cattle, sheep and horses. *Am. J. vet. Res.* 32, 1293–1295.

Watson, W. A., Terlecki, S., Patterson, D. S. P., Sweasey, D., Herbert, C. N. and Done, J. T. (1972). Experimentally produced progressive retinal degeneration (bright blindness) in sheep. *Br. vet. J.* 128, 457–469.

Yamashita, S. (1972). Studies on the ocular changes of experimental lathyrism. Report 1. Changes of rat cornea treated by 1-iminodipropionitrile (IDPN). *Acta Soc. Ophthal. Japan* 76, 587–594.

Yamashita, S. (1973). Studies on the ocular changes of experimental lathyrism. 2. Electron-microscopic observations on epithelial, stromal and endothelial cells of β1-Iminodipropionitrile (1DPN)-treated rat cornea. *Acta Soc. Ophthal. Japan* 77, 834–846.

Chapter 11

Airaksinen, E. M., Sihvola, P., Airaksinen, M. M., Sivhola, M. and Tuovinen, E. (1979). Uptake of taurine by platelets in retinitis pigmentosa. *Lancet* i, 474–475.

Anon (1959). Diet and myopia in children. *Nutr. Rev.* 17, 36–38.

Anon (1976). Riboflavin deficiency, galactose metabolism and cataract. *Nutr. Rev.* 34, 77–79.

Armengaud, M. V., Frament, V., Diop, B. and Diop, J. M. (1961). Les kératites de la rougeole en milieu africain à Dakar. *Bull. Soc. méd. d'Afrique noire de langue française* 6, 36–44.

Azizi, A. and Krakovsky, D. (1965). Keratoconjunctivitis as a constant sign of measles. *Ann. Paediat.* 204, 397–405.

Balcet, C. (1948). Manifestazioni oculari da insufficiente alimentazione. *Rass. ital. ottal.* 17, 271–5.

Bellows, J. G. (1944). "Cataract and Anomalies of the Lens," 522. Kimpton, London.

Bergsma, D. R., Wiggert, B. N., Funahashi, M., Kuwabara, T. and Chader, G. J. (1977). Vitamin A receptors in normal and dystrophic retina. *Nature, Lond.* 265, 66–67.

Bhat, K. S. and Gopalan, C. (1974a). Human cataract and galactose metabolism. *Nutr. Metab.* 17, 1–8.

Bhat, K. S. and Gopalan, C. (1974b). Human cataract and galactose metabolism. *Nutr. Metab.* 16, 111–118.

Bietti, G. B. (1955). Some contributions to problems of trachoma. *Am. J. Ophthal.* 39, 112–130.

Bietti, G. (1956). Some contributions to the problems of trachoma. *Rev. int. Trachome* 33, 201–228.

Bird, A. C., Anderson, J. and Fuglsang, H. (1976). Morphology of posterior segment lesions of the eye in patients with onchocerciasis. *Br. J. Ophthal.* 60, 2–20.

Blumenthal, C. J. (1950). Malnutritional keratoconjunctivitis disease of South African Bantu. *S. Afr. med. J.* 24, 191–8.

Blumenthal, C. J. (1954). Blindness and malnutrition in eastern Cape Province. *S. Afr. med. J.* 28, 967–971.

Blumenthal, C. J. (1961). Kwashiorkor. *Br. med. J.* i, 822.

Budden, F. H. (1956). Proc. Conf. African Onchocerciasis, 1954 (Bamako, Afrique Occidentale Francaise) *W.H.O. Document* WHO/Onchocerciasis/23.

Campbell, D. A. and Tonks, E. L. (1962). Biochemical findings in human retinitis pigmentosa with particular reference to vitamin A deficiency. *Br. J. Ophthal.* **46**, 151–164.

Chatterjee, A. (1973). Cataract in Punjab. *Ciba Fdn Symp.* No. 19, 265–279.

Chatzinoff, A., Nelson, F., Stahl, N. and Clahane, A. (1968). 11-*cis*-Vitamin A in the treatment of retinitis pigmentosa. A negative study. *Archs Ophthal.* **80**, 417–419.

Cooper, S. N. (1960). Cited by A. Fuchs (1960).

Cotlier, E. and Sharma, Y. R. (1980). Plasma tryptophan in senile cataract. *Lancet* i, 607.

D'Haussy, R., Rit, J. M. and Legraulet, J. (1958). Lesions of eye fundus in onchocerciasis. *Med. trop.* **18**, 340–367.

Duke-Elder, W. S. (1954). Pathological myopia. *"Textbook of Ophthalmology,"* Vol. 4, 4313–4359. Mosby, St Louis, Missouri.

Duke-Elder, W. S. (1959). "Parson's Diseases of the Eye," 13th edn, 276. Churchill, London.

Duke-Elder, W. S. (1965). "System of Ophthalmology," Vol. 8, Part I, p. 338. London, Kimpton.

Expert Committee on Trachoma (1956). *Second Report. Tech. Rep. Ser. W.H.O.* No. 16.

Falcone, G. (1952). Ariboflavinosi oculare a tropici. *Arch. ital. Sci. med. trop. parasit.* **33**, 619–632.

Foster, J. and Benson, J. (1935). Percentage incidence and sugical significance of different forms of senile cataract. *Trans. ophthal. Soc. U.K.* **54**, 127–145.

Franken, S. (1974). Measles and keratomalacia in East Africa. *Trop. geogr. Med.* **26**, 39–44.

Frederique, G., Howard, R. O. and Boniuk, V. (1969). Corneal ulcers in rubeola *Am. J. Ophthal.* **68**, 996–1003.

Fuchs, A. (1960). Geographic distribution of senile cataract. *Am. J. Ophthal.* **49**, 1039–1043.

Futterman, S., Swanson, D. and Kalina, R. E. (1974). Retinol in retinitis pigmentosa: evidence that retinol is in normal concentration in serum and the retinol-binding protein complex displays unaltered fluorescence properties. *Invest. Ophthal.* **13**, 798.

Gardiner, P. A. (1956). Observations on the food habits of myopic children. *Br. med. J.* ii, 699–700.

Gardiner, P. A. (1958). Dietary treatment of myopia in children. *Lancet* i, 1152–5.

Goldschmidt, E. (1966). Myopia and height. *Acta Ophthal.* **44**, 751–761.

Goldschmidt, E. (1968). On the aetiology of myopia. An epidemiological study. *Acta Ophthal.* Suppl. 98, 171.

Heinz, K., Schabel, F. and Günther, R. (1971). Augenbefunder bei Gicht und Hyperurikämie. *Wien. Klin. Wschr.* **83**, 42–4.

Holm, S. (1937). Les états de la réfraction oculaire che les palénégrides au Gabon, Afrique Equatoriale française; étude de race pour éclairer la gèrise de la réfraction. *Acta Ophthal.* Suppl. No. 13, 1–299.

Hyams, S. W., Pokotilo, E. and Shkurko, G. (1977). Prevalence of refractive errors in adults over 40: a survey of 8102 eyes. *Br. J. Ophthal.* **61**, 428–432.

Johnstone, W. W. and McLaren, D. S. (1963). Refraction anomalies in Tanganyikan children. *Br. J. Ophthal.* 47, 95–108.

Kirkby, D. B., (1936). *In* "The Eye and its Diseases" (Ed. C. Berens), 462 Saunders, Philadelphia.

Lagraulet, J. and Bard, J. (1967). Lésions oculaire de la rougeole dans les milieux nefaux en Afrique noire. *Bull. Soc. Path. exot.* 60, 203–205.

Liu, H. Y., Giday, Z. and Moore, B. F. (1973). Certain bovine milk protein inducible eye signs in patients with allergic malabsorption. *J. pediat. Ophthal.* 10, 7–11.

Livingston, P. C. and Ridley, H. (1946). Discussion: Ocular disturbances associated with malnutrition. *Trans. ophthal. Soc. U.K.* 66, 19–131.

McLaren, D. S. (1960a). Nutrition and eye disease in East Africa: experience in Lake and Central Provinces in Tanganyika. *J. trop. Med. Hyg.* 63, 101–122.

McLaren, D. S. (1960b). Malnutrition and eye disease in Tanganyika. *Proc. Nutr. Soc.* 19, 89–91.

McLaren, D. S. (1960c). The effects of malnutrition on the eye: with special reference to work with experimental animals. *Wld Rev. Nutr. Dietet.* 2, 25–51.

McLaren, D. S. (1961). The refraction of Indian schoolchildren: a comparison of data from East Africa and India. *Br. J. Ophthal.* 45, 604–613.

McLaren, D. S. (1970). Corneal ulcers in rubeola. *Am. J. Ophthal.* 70, 442–443.

Majima, A., Nakajima, A., Ichikawa, H. and Watanabe, M. (1960). Prevalence of ocular anomalies among schoolchildren. *Am. J. Ophthal.* 50, 139–146.

Mann, I. (1959). Researches into the regional distribution of eye disease. *Am. J. Ophthal.* 47, 134–144.

Maraini, G. (1974). The vitamin A transporting protein complex in human hereditary pigmentous retinal dystrophy. *Invest. Ophthal.* 13, 288–290.

Maraini, G., Fadda, G. and Gozzoli, F. (1975). Serum levels of retinol-binding protein in different genetic types of retinitis pigmentosa. *Invest. Ophthal.* 14, 236.

Massoud, W. H., Bird, A. C. and Perkins, E. S. (1975). Plasma vitamin A and beta-carotene in retinitis pigmentosa. *Br. J. Ophthal.* 59, 200–204.

Mingelen, R. (1933). "Cataracta Seniles," N.I. Thesis, Djakarta.

Morales, M., Taricgo, S. and Phillipi, O. (1965). Complicaciones oculares del sarampión. *Res. Child. Pediat.* 36, 717–723.

Murray, W. C. G. and Asregadoo, E. R. (1959). Some common eye diseases in British Guiana. *West Indian med. J.* 8, 225–8.

Oomen, J. M. V. (1971). Xerophthalmia in Northern Nigeria. *Trop. geogr. Med.* 23, 246–250.

Peckham, C. S., Gardiner, P. A., and Goldstein, H. (1977). Acquired myopia in 11-year-old children. *Br. med. J.* i, 542–545.

Pendse, G. S. (1954). Refraction and body growth. *Indian med. Res. Mem.* No. 38, 1–94.

Pfeiffer, C. E. (1921). Untersuchungen über die Häufigkeit und Lokalisation von Wasser-spaltenbildungen souler Lensen, nach Spaltampermikroskopie von 219 Augen gesunder Personen. *Albrecht v. Graefes Arch. Ophthal.* 106, 71–91.

Pi, H. T. (1934). Cataract among Chinese. *Chin. med. J.* 48, 928–947.

Potter, D. F. and Duncan, R. B. (1976). The role of food in extraocular allergy. *Tr. Ophthal. Soc. NZ.* 28, 103–106.

Pratt-Johnson, J. A. (1959). Studies on the anatomy and pathology of the peripheral cornea. *Am. J. Ophthal.* 47, 478–487, disc. 487–8.

Prchal, J. T., Conrad, M. E. and Skalka, H. W. (1978). Association of presenile cataracts with heterozygosity for galactosaemic states and with riboflavin deficiency. *Lancet* i, 12–13.

Quéré, M. A. (1964). Les complications oculaire de la rougéole, cause majeure de cécité chez l'enfant en pays tropical. *Ophthalmologica* 148, 107–120.

Rahi, A. H. S. (1972). Retinol-binding protein (RBP) and pigmentary dystrophy of the retina. *Br. J. Ophthal.* 56, 647–651.

Reed, J. G. (1947). Ocular symptoms in prisoners-of-war in Sumatra. *Trans. R. Soc. trop. Med. Hyg.* 40, 411–420.

Rich, W. M. (1946). Ocular signs in prisoners -of-war from the Far East. *Br. med. J.* i, 330–331.

Ridley, H. (1945). Ocular manifestations of malnutrition in released prisoners-of-war from Thailand. *Br. J. Ophthal.* 29, 613–618.

Rodger, F. C. (1957). The pathogenesis of ocular onchocerciasis. *Trans. ophthal. Soc. U.K.* 77, 267–289.

Rodger, F. C. (1960). The pathogenesis and pathology of ocular onchocerciasis. *Am. J. Ophthal.* 49, 327–337.

Sato, T. (1965). Discussion on myopia in Japan. *Trans. Ophthal. Soc. N.Z.* 17, 109–115.

Sauter, J. J. M. (1976). "Xerophthalmia and Measles in Kenya." Drukkerij van Denderen B. V., Groningen.

Scheifele, D. and Forbes, C. (1973). The biology of measles in African children. *E. Afr. med. J.* 50, 168–173.

Skeller, E. (1954). "Anthropological and Ophthalmological Studies on the Angmagssalik Eskimos." Lunos, Copenhagen.

Smith, D. A. and Woodruff, M. F. A. (1951). Deficiency diseases in Japanese prison camps. *Spec. Rep. Ser. med. Res. Coun.* No. 274.

Sorsby, A. (1950). The incidence and causes of blindness: an international survey. *Br. J. Ophthal.* Monograph Suppl. 14.

Sorsby, A., Benjamin, B., Sheridan, M. and Tanner, J. M. (1957). Emmetropia and its aberrations: a study in the correlation of the optical components of the eye. *Spec. Rep. Ser. med. Res. Coun.* No. 293.

Sorsby, A., Leary, G. A. and Richards, M. J. (1962a). The optical components in anisometropia. *Vision Res.* 2, 43–51.

Sorsby, A., Leary, G. A. and Richards, M. J. (1962b). Correlation ametropia and component ametropia. *Vision Res.* 2, 309–313.

Spillane, J. D. (1947). "Nutritional Disorders of the Nervous System," 38. Livingstone, Edinburgh.

Suringa, D. W. R., Bank, L. J. and Ackerman, B. (1970). Role of measles virus in skin lesions and Koplik's spots. *New Engl. J. Med.* 283, 1139–1142.

Thygeson, P. (1959). Ocular viral diseases. *Med. Clin. Nth. Amer.* 43, 1419–1440.

Torokhova, L. F. (1947). Role of vitamin insufficiency in pathogenesis of cataract. *Sov. Vest. Oftal.* 26, 33–35.

Vanneste, L. (1956). Ophthalmological observations in patients from the East Province of the Belgian Congo. *Annls Soc. belge med. trop.* 36, 271–297.

Wangspa, S. and Limpaphayom, P. (1965). Vision of schoolchildren in Thailand. *Trans. Ophthal. Soc. N.Z.* 17, 106–109.

Whittle, H., Duggan, M., Kogbe, O. and Smith, J. S. (1978). Herpes simplex corneal ulcers in malnourished African children with measles. Paper read at *1st General Assembly of the International Agency for the Prevention of Blindness* Oxford, July, 1978.

Wright, R. E. (1936). Incidence of cataract at certain age periods in South Indian districts. *Br. J. Ophthal.* 20, 545.

Young, F. A., Leary, G. A., Baldwin, W. R., West, D. C., Box, R. A., Harris, E. and Johnson, C. (1969). The transmission of refractive errors with Eskimo families. *Am. J. Optom.* 46, 676–685.

Zuidema, P. J. (1955). Calcifications and cirrhosis of the pancreas in patients with deficient nutrition. *Documenta Med. geogr. trop.* 7, 229–251.

Zuidema, P. J. (1959). Cirrhosis and disseminated calcifications of the pancreas in patients with malnutrition. *Trop. geogr. Med.* 11, 70–4.

Author Index

Harris, J. W., 137, *365*
Harris, L. S., 208, *382*
Harris, W. A., 44, *350*
Harry, J., 211, *381*
Harstein, J., 248, *387*
Hart, E. B., 22, 124, 295, *362, 374, 399*
Hart, L., 309, *401*
Hart, W. M., 25, 128, *353, 371*
Härtel, A., 285, *398*
Härtel, G., 285, *398*
Hartmann, E., 45, *350*
Hartroft, W. S., 139, *366*
Harvey, C. C., 143, 187, *370*
Hasegawa, Y., 130, *369*
Hatcher, H., 259, *391*
Hauge, S. M., 234, *385*
Hausler, H. R., 265, *393*
Hauschildt, J. D., 264, *391*
Havener, W. H., 120, *356, 357*
Hayes, K. C., 32, 33, 194, 195, 240, 241, *350, 379, 384, 386, 388*
Hays, I. M., 130, *375*
Hays, R. L., 288, *398*
Hays, V. W., 40, *349*
Hazzard, D. G., 42, *347*
Heaton, J. M., 160, 178, *369*
Hecht, S., 74, *350*
Heggeness, F. M., 258, *391*
Heggeness, F. W., 260, *391*
Hegsted, D. M., 23, 112, 128, 132, 264, 271, *349, 351, 369, 390, 394*
Heinsius, E., 11, *342*
Heinz, K., 340, *404*
Heizer, W. D., 251, *386*
Helgebostad, A., 45, *350*
Helig, P., 78, *362*
Heller, J., 14, *350*
Helleströem, B. E., 6, *342*
Hellmann, L. M., 200, 288, *379, 399*
Helmboldt, D. F., 42, *347*
Helmsen, R. J., 14, 223, *364, 386*
Helweg-Larsen, P., 174, *370*
Henderson, M. D., 239, *387*
Hendley, C. D., 74, *350*
Henschel, A., 9, *342*
Herbert, C. N., 311, *402*
Herbert, H., 51, *350*
Herbert, P. N., 279, 280, *396*
Herlinger, H., 112, *350*
Herron, B. E., 205, *382*

Herron, W. L., 39, *350*
Hess, C., 29, 79, *350*
Hess, J. L., 195, *378*
Hess, W. N., 239, *386*
Hetler, R. A., 20, *350*
Hicks, R. J., 52, 96, *350*
Hift, W., 178, 187, *365*
Higginbottom, R. M., 303, *396*
Hiles, D. A., 279, 280, *395*
Hill, A., 252, *389*
Hill, C. W., 213, *383*
Hills, O. W., 143, 187, *370*
Hime, J. M., 23, *350*
Hind, V. M. D., 137, *370*
Hines, J. D., 137, *365*
Hinokuma, S., 149, *370, 372*
Hinton, J. W., 233, *387*
Hirschberg, J., 152, *370*
Hoch, F. L., 212, *383*
Hock, C. W., 20, 127, 129, 228, 229, 246, *346, 366, 384, 386, 389*
Hodges, R. E., 37, 54, 74, 103, 198, *350, 360, 379*
Hodson, W. A., 304, 305, *396*
Hoefer, J. A., 128, 131, *372*
Hoffmeyer, H., 174, *370*
Hogan, A. G., 292, 293, *398*
Hogan, M. J., 266, *393*
Höglund, G., 44, *346*
Holland, M. G., 249, *388*
Hollenhorst, R. W., 277, 278, *395*
Hollows, F. C., 265, *391*
Holly, F. J., 63, *353*
Hollyfield, J. G., 37, *364*
Holm, E., 30, *349, 350*
Holm, K., 117, *350*
Holm, S., 320, 321, *404*
Holtzman, N. A., 251, *389*
Hommes, O. R., 162, *374*
Hong, K., 37, *351*
Hood, D. C., 37, *360*
Hood, J., 37, 54, 74, 103, 198, *360, 379*
Hoogenkamp, P. A., 108, *351*
Hörmann, E., 257, *391*
Hornbrook, J. W., 208, *382*
Horner, F., 152, *370*
Hornstein, S., 307, *400*
Horwitt, M. K., 143, 187, *370*
Hosaka, A., 305, 306, *398*
Houet, R., 87, *351*

420   AUTHOR INDEX

Lal, S., 315, *401*
Lamb, A. R., 22, *356*
Lamba, P. A., 306, *398*
Lambert, R. A., 17, *352, 365*
Lamming, G. E., 42, 43, 288, *355, 398, 399*
Lamotte, M., 11, *342*
Lamotte-Barillon, S., 11, *342*
Lamy, M., 11, *342*
Landis, D. J., 274, *393, 394*
Landor, J. V., 168, *371*
Langham, M. E., 309, 315, *401*
Langman, J., 285, *398*
Langman, M. J. S., 137, *378*
Langston, W. C., 126, 130, 238, *367, 371, 385*
Larson, P. S., 160, *376*
Lasagna, L., 277, *395*
Laster, L., 279, *396*
Latham, M. C., 109, 116, *361*
Laughlin, R. C., 276, *395*
Lawas, I., 109, *362*
Leach, E. H., 20, 26, 32, 309, 310, *359, 402*
Leary, G. A., 319, 322, *406, 407*
Lebas, P., 56, *344*
Leber, T., 14, 51, *353*
Lechat, M. F., 111, *353*
Lecomte-Ramioul, S., 87, *351*
Lecoq, R., 195, *379*
Lee, O. S. Jr., 25, 128, *353, 371*
Lee, P. N., 160, *371*
Lee, Y., 6, *342*
Leech, R. S., 262, *390*
Lefebvres-Boisselot, J., 290, 292, *398*
Legraulet, J., 324, *404*
Leigh, A. G., 174, *371*
Leishman, R., 178, *371*
Leitenmaier, K., 151, *371*
Leitman, P. S., 246, *389*
Leitner, Z. A., 100, *353*
Leitzmann, C., 109, *361*
Lele, R. D., 187, *371*
Lemp, M. A., 55, 63, 209, *353, 382*
Lennox, B., 180, 181, *368*
Lentini, E. A., 23, *349*
Leong, P. C., 89, *364*
Lepkovsky, S., 292, 295, *398, 399*
Lerman, S., 258, 260, *391*
Lerner, L. H., 196, *380*

Lessell, S., 137, 138, 210, *371, 382*
Lester, L., 251, *386*
Levenson, S. M., 192, *379, 380*
Levett, J., 313, *402*
Levi, A. J., 215, *382*
Levine, J., 172, 177, *371*
Levine, R. A., 56, *353*
Levine, S. L., 305, 306, *397*
Levy, N. S., 81, 214, 267, *353, 382, 390, 392*
Lew, W., 5, *341*
Leyton, G. B., 11, 174, *342, 371*
Lieb, W. A., 309, *402*
Lieberman, T. W., 248, *387*
Liebert, E., 143, 187, *370*
Lienhardt, H. F., 39, 40, *351*
Lietman, P. S., 118, *353*
Light, A. E., 272, *395*
Lijo Pavia, J., 273, *395*
Lillie, D. R., 123, *369*
Lim, K. H., 109, *353*
Limpaphayom, P., 321, *407*
Limson, M., 219, *387*
Linnér, E., 197, *379*
Lippincott, S. W., 128, 131, *371*
Lipson, E. D., 44, *350*
Liu, H. Y., 339, *405*
Livingston, P. C., 76, 322, *353, 405*
Livrea, M. A., 39, *357*
Lloyd, J. K., 280, *395*
Lloyd, J. P., 309, 310, *402*
Localis, S. A., 233, *387*
Lockhart, W. S. Jr., 210, *381*
Lodato, G., 4, 7, *342, 343*
Loewenthal, L. J. A., 102, *353*
Loh, R. C. K., 109, *353*
Lombroso, C., 152, *371*
Lonergan, E., 208, *382*
Lou, M. F., 254, *392*
Löwenstein, A., 196, *379*
Lowrey, L. G., 2, *343*
Lowry, L., 100, *359*
Lowry, L. K., 37, 54, 74, 103, *360*
Lowry, O. H., 128, *371*
Lubeck, M. J., 210, *382*
Lucas, D. R., 6, *343*
Luckhaus, G., 303, *399*
Luecke, R. W., 128, 131, *372*
Lukens, F. D. W., 262, *390*
Lund, C. J., 100, *353*

Nguyen Dinh Cat, 109, *356*
Nicholls, L., 58, 102, 168, *357, 373*
Nicholson, A. L., 223, *384*
Nicotra, C., 39, *357*
Niedermeier, S., 245, *387*
Nieman, C., 272, *395*
Niemeyer, H., 112, *355*
Nikoskelainen, E., 179, *373*
Nimalasuriya, A., 58, *357*
Nishimura, H., 205, *383*
Niven, C. F., 232, *387*
Noeggerath, C. T., 14, *348*
Noell, W. K., 34, 37, 39, *347, 357*
Noorden, G. K. von, 216, *382*
Nordén, A., 75, 117, 118, *357, 363*
Nordlie, R. C., 233, *385*
Nordquist, L. T., 264, *391*
Norn, M. S., 55, *357*
North, J. D. K., 134, 135, *373*
Norton, E. W. D., 210, *382*
Norton, H. W., 3, 237, *342, 386*
Nothaker, W. G., 192, *378*
Nover, A., 193, *380*
Nushan, H., 192, *380*
Nyhan, W., 189, *367*

O

Oaks, E. V., 118, 212, *359, 383*
Oates, R. K., 209, *384*
Obal, A., 11, *343*
Obazawa, H., 258, *392*
O'Brien, C. S., 126, 130, 268, *367, 392*
Odahara, H., 239, *389*
O'Dell, B. L., 292, 293, 294, *398, 399*
Ogino, S., 239, *387, 389*
Ohta, K., 185, *374*
Okumoto, M., 29, *361*
Oleson, J. J., 124, *374*
Oliver, T. K., 120, *357*
Olsen, T. S., 269, *392*
Olson, J. A., 87, 109, *362*
Olson, R. E., 109, *361*
Ong, D. E., 14, *357*
Oomen, H. A. P. C., 46, 51, 55, 69, 92, 93, 97, 99, 100, 101, 104, 108, 109, 110, 115, *354, 357*
Oomen, J. M. V., 111, 328, *357, 405*
Ören, C., 60, *349*
Orent-Keiles, E., 204, 293, *381, 383, 396*

Organisciak, D. T., 39, *347*
Oropeza, P., 112, *357*
Østerby, R., 269, *392*
Ørskov, H., 269, *392*
Osuntokun, B. O., 167, *374*
Osuntokun, O., 167, *374*
O'Toole, B. A., 288, *399*
Ottolenghi, S., 152, *374*
Ottoway, C. W., 42, *345*
Ourgaud, A. G., 70, 72, 74, 87, *351*
Ouwehand, C. D., 51, *357*
Overall, M., 23, 24, *358*
Owen, R. A., 164, *374*
Owens, E. U., 199, *380*
Owens, W. C., 199, *380*

P

Packman, S., 189, *367*
Paegel, B. L., 178, *375*
Pagola, J. G., 112, *358*
Palich-Szántó, O., 8, *343*
Pallister, R. A., 168, *371*
Palludan, B., 287, *399*
Parinaud, 51, *358*
Park, M. M., 251, *387*
Parlindungan Dinaga, H. S. R., 55, *352*
Pasricha, C. L., 315, *401*
Passmore, J. W., 170, 172, *371*
Patch, E. M., 238, *387, 388*
Patek, A. J., 118, 128, *358, 374*
Paton, D., 56, 59, 60, 99, *347, 358*
Patterson, D. S. P., 311, *402*
Patterson, J. W., 6, 257, 258, 262, 264, 265, 268, *343, 392*
Patterson, M. E., 258, *392*
Patwardhan, V. N., 97, 110, *358, 361*
Patz, A., 256, *392*
Pearson, P. B., 295, *399*
Peckham, C. S., 322, *405*
Peiris, J. B., 187, *372*
Pelagalli, G. V., 289, *399*
Pencharz, R., 292, *399*
Pendse, G. S., 320, *405*
Peraita, M., 174, *369*
Perera, A., 107, *346*
Perkins, E. S., 339, *405*
Permutt, S., 301, *399*
Pernetta, C., 112, *358*
Perry, D. J., 141, *376*

Subject Index